D0122916

Health Informatics

(formerly Computers in Health Care)

Kathryn J. Hannah   Marion J. Ball
Series Editors

Health Informatics Series
(formerly Computers in Health Care)

Series Editors
Kathryn J. Hannah   Marion J. Ball

Dental Informatics
Integrating Technology into the Dental Environment
L.M. Abbey and J. Zimmerman

Health Informatics Series
Evaluating the Organizational Impact of Healthcare Information Systems, Second Edition
J.G. Anderson and C.E. Aydin

Ethics and Information Technology
A Case-Based Approach to a Health Care System in Transition
J.G. Anderson and K.W. Goodman

Aspects of the Computer-Based Patient Record
M.J. Ball and M.F. Collen

Performance Improvement Through Information Management
Health Care's Bridge to Success
M.J. Ball and J.V. Douglas

Strategies and Technologies for Healthcare Information
Theory into Practice
M.J. Ball, J.V. Douglas, and D.E. Garets

Nursing Informatics
Where Caring and Technology Meet, Third Edition
M.J. Ball, K.J. Hannah, S.K. Newbold, and J.V. Douglas

Healthcare Information Management Systems
A Practical Guide, Second Edition
M.J. Ball, D.W. Simborg, J.W. Albright, and J.V. Douglas

Healthcare Information Management Systems
Cases, Strategies, and Solutions, Third Edition
M.J. Ball, C.A. Weaver, and J.M. Kiel

Clinical Decision Support Systems
Theory and Practice
E.S. Berner

Strategy and Architecture of Health Care Information Systems
M.K. Bourke

Information Networks for Community Health
P.F. Brennan, S.J. Schneider, and E. Tornquist

Informatics for the Clinical Laboratory
A Practical Guide for the Pathologist
D.F. Cowan

Charles P. Friedman   Jeremy C. Wyatt

Evaluation Methods in Biomedical Informatics

Second Edition

Foreword by Edward H. Shortliffe
With contributions by Joan S. Ash, Allen C. Smith III,
P. Zoë Stavri, and Mark S. Roberts

With 49 Illustrations

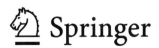 Springer

Charles P. Friedman, PhD
Professor, Center for Biomedical Informatics
University of Pittsburgh
Pitttsburgh, PA 15260
and
Senior Scholar and Program Officer
National Library of Medicine
Division of Extramural Programs
Bethesda, MD 20894
USA

Jeremy C. Wyatt, MD
Professor of Health Informatics
University of Dundee
Dundee, Scotland DD1 4NH
and
Director, Health Informatics Centre
Ninewells Hospital
Dundee
Scotland DD1 9SY
UK

Series Editors:
Kathryn J. Hannah, PhD, RN
Adjunct Professor, Department of
  Community Health Sciences
Faculty of Medicine
University of Calgary
Calgary, Alberta T2N 4N1
Canada

Marion J. Ball, EdD
Vice President, Clinical Informatics
  Strategies Healthlink, Inc.
Baltimore, MD 21210
and
Adjunct Professor
The Johns Hopkins University School of
  Nursing
Baltimore, MD 21205
USA

Library of Congress Control Number: 2005925510

ISBN 10: 0-387-25889-2
ISBN 13: 987-0387-25889-8

Printed on acid-free paper.

Printed in the United States of America.   (BS/MVY)

9 8 7 6 5 4 3 2 1

springeronline.com

Foreword

As the director of training programs in biomedical informatics, first at Stanford and now at Columbia, I have found that one of the most frequent inquiries from graduate students is, "Although I am happy with my research focus and the work I have done, how can I design and carry out a practical evaluation that proves the value of my contribution?" Informatics is a multifaceted interdisciplinary field with research that ranges from theoretical developments to projects that are highly applied and intended for near-term use in clinical settings. The implications of "proving" a research claim accordingly vary greatly depending on the details of an individual student's goals and thesis statement. Furthermore, the dissertation work leading up to an evaluation plan is often so time consuming and arduous that attempting the "perfect" evaluation is frequently seen as impractical or as diverting students from central programming or implementation issues that are their primary areas of interest. They often ask what compromises are possible so they can provide persuasive data in support of their claims without adding two to three years to their graduate-student life.

Our students at Stanford clearly needed help in dealing more effectively with such dilemmas, and it was therefore fortuitous when, in the autumn of 1991, we welcomed two superb visiting professors to our laboratory. We had known both Chuck Friedman and Jeremy Wyatt from earlier visits and professional encounters, but it was coincidence that offered them sabbatical breaks in our laboratory during the same academic year. Knowing that each had strong interests and skills in the areas of evaluation and clinical trial design, I hoped they would enjoy getting to know one another and would find that their scholarly pursuits were both complementary and synergistic. To help stir the pot, we even assigned them to a shared office that we try to set aside for visitors, and within a few weeks, they were putting their heads together as they learned about the evaluation issues that were rampant in our laboratory.

The on-site contributions by Drs. Friedman and Wyatt during that year were marvelous, and I know that they continue to have ripple effects at Stanford to this day. They served as local consultants as we devised evaluation plans for existing projects, new proposals, and student research. By the Spring, they had identified the topics and themes that needed to be understood better by those in our laboratory, and they offered a well-received seminar course on evaluation methods for medical information systems. It was out of the class notes formulated for that course that the present volume evolved. Its availability since publication of the first edition allowed the Stanford program to rejuvenate and refine the laboratory's knowledge and skills in the area of evaluating medical information systems. It has had a similar impact in diverse biomedical informatics training environments both in the U.S. and abroad, so the publication of this revised second edition has been eagerly awaited.

This book fills an important niche that is not effectively covered by other biomedical informatics textbooks or by the standard volumes on evaluation and clinical trial design. I know of no other writers who have the requisite knowledge of statistics and cognition, coupled with intensive study of biomedical informatics and an involvement with creation of applied systems as well. Drs. Friedman and Wyatt are scholars and educators, but they are also practical in their understanding of the world of clinical medicine and the realities of system implementation and validation in settings that defy formal controlled trials. Thus, the book is not only of value to students of biomedical informatics, but will continue to be a key reference for all individuals involved in the implementation and evaluation of basic and applied systems in biomedical informatics.

Edward H. Shortliffe, MD, PhD FACMI, MACP
Department of Biomedical Informatics
College of Physicians and Surgeons
Columbia University in the City of New York
February 2005

Series Preface

This series is directed to healthcare professionals who are leading the transformation of health care by using information and knowledge. Launched in 1988 as *Computers in Health Care*, the series offers a broad range of titles: some addressed to specific professions such as nursing, medicine, and health administration; others to special areas of practice such as trauma and radiology. Still other books in the series focus on interdisciplinary issues, such as the computer-based patient record, electronic health records, and networked healthcare systems.

Renamed *Health Informatics* in 1998 to reflect the rapid evolution in the discipline now known as health informatics, the series will continue to add titles that contribute to the evolution of the field. In the series, eminent experts, serving as editors or authors, offer their accounts of innovations in health informatics. Increasingly, these accounts go beyond hardware and software to address the role of information in influencing the transformation of healthcare delivery systems around the world. The series also will increasingly focus on "peopleware" and organizational, behavioral, and societal changes that accompany the diffusion of information technology in health services environments.

These changes will shape health services in the new millennium. By making full and creative use of the technology to tame data and to transform information, health informatics will foster the development of the knowledge age in health care. As coeditors, we pledge to support our professional colleagues and the series readers as they share advances in the emerging and exciting field of health informatics.

Kathryn J. Hannah, PhD, RN
Marion J. Ball, EdD

Preface:
Still Counting the Steps on Box Hill

The brief anecdote that began the preface to the first edition of this volume seems just as pertinent today. We therefore include it here again, and then introduce the pedagogical goals and target audience for this textbook. The preface concludes with a summary of changes incorporated into this second edition.

In February 1995, during a visit by the American coauthor of this volume to the home of the Wyatt family in the United Kingdom, one afternoon's activity involved a walk on Box Hill in Surrey. In addition to the coauthors of this volume, Jeremy's wife Sylvia and the two Wyatt children were present. We walked down a steep hill. As we began ascending the hill, the group decided to count the number of earthen steps cut into the path to make the climbing easier. When we arrived at the top, each of us had generated a different number.

There ensued a lively discussion of the reasons the numbers differed. Clearly, one or more of us may have lost attention and simply miscounted, but there emerged on analysis three more subtle reasons for the discrepancies.

- First, not all of the steps on our return trip went upward. Do the downward steps count at all toward the total; and if so, do they add or subtract from the count? *We realized that we had not agreed to all of the rules for counting because we did not know in advance all of the issues that needed to be taken into account.*
- Second, the path was so eroded by heavy rain that it was not always easy to distinguish a step from an irregularity. What counts as a step? In a few instances along the way, we had discussions about whether a particular irregularity was a step, and apparently we had disagreed. *It is not clear if there is any verifiably right answer to this question unless there existed plans for the construction of the steps. Even then, should a step now eroded almost beyond recognition still count as a step?*
- Third and finally, one of the children, having decided in advance that there were 108 steps, simply stopped counting once she had reached this

number. She wanted there to be no more steps and made it so in her own mind. *Beliefs, no matter how they develop, are real for the belief holders and must be taken seriously.*

Even an apparently simple counting task led to disagreements about the results. Each of us thought himself or herself perfectly correct, and we realized there was no way to resolve our differences without one person exerting power over the others by dictating the rules or arbitrating the results of our disagreements.

It struck us in 1995 that this pleasant walk in the country had raised several key dilemmas confronting anyone designing, conducting, or interpreting an evaluation. These dilemmas seemed no less pertinent in 2005 as we completed the second edition of this volume. Themes of anticipation, communication, measurement, and belief raised in this anecdote distinguish evaluation, and what should be covered in a textbook on evaluation, from what might be addressed in works addressing empirical research methods more generally. So this anecdote and the issues it raises remain a point of departure for this book and direct much of its organization and content. We continue to trust that anyone who has performed a rigorous data-driven evaluation can see the pertinence of the Box Hill counting dilemma. We hope that anyone reading this volume will in the end possess both a framework for thinking about these issues and a set of methods for addressing them.

More specifically, we have attempted to address in this book the major questions relating to evaluation in informatics.

1. Why should information resources be studied? Why is it a challenging process?
2. What are all the options for conducting such studies? How do I decide what to study?
3. How do I design, carry out, and interpret a study using a particular set of techniques: for objectivist (quantitative) studies as well as subjectivist (qualitative) studies?
4. How do economic factors play into evaluations?
5. How do I communicate study designs and study results?

When drafting the first edition, we set out to create a volume useful to several audiences: those training for careers in informatics who as part of their curricula must learn to perform evaluation studies; those actively conducting evaluation studies who might derive from these pages ways to improve their methods; and those responsible for information systems in biomedical or health settings who may wish to understand how well their services are working and how to improve them. These audiences remain the primary audiences for the second edition as well. As such, this book can alert investigators to evaluation questions they might ask, the answers they might expect, and how to obtain and understand them.

This volume is intended to be germane to all biomedical professions and professionals. The first edition employed the word "medical" in the title, and we slightly modified the title of the second edition, using instead the word "biomedical" to emphasize this intended breadth. The first edition's dual emphasis on both quantitative (what we call "objectivist") methods and qualitative ("subjectivist") methods remains in the second edition. A reader may not choose to become proficient in both of these Grand Approaches to evaluation, but we continue to see an appreciation of both as essential. Subjectivist approaches have continued to gain traction in the world of informatics evaluation since the first edition was published.

This volume is designed to serve as a textbook for a graduate level course, although we hope and intend that the work will also prove useful as a general reference. The subject matter of this volume has been the basis of graduate courses offered by us at the University of North Carolina 1993–1996, the University of Pittsburgh since 1997, and University College London from 1998 onward. Someone reading the book straight through should experience a logical development of the subject, as it addresses most of the important concepts, and develops several key methodological skill areas. To this end, "self-test" exercises with answers and "food for thought" questions have been added to many chapters. With this goal of continuity in mind, we wrote 10 of the 12 chapters of this volume ourselves and then collaborated with expert contributing authors in crafting the two chapters that stretched our own knowledge a bit too thinly.

In our view, evaluation is different from an exercise in applied statistics. This work is therefore intended to complement, not replace, basic statistics courses offered at most institutions. (We assume our readers to have only a basic knowledge of statistics.) The reader will find in this book material derived from varying methodological traditions including psychometrics, statistics and research design, ethnography, clinical epidemiology, health economics, organizational behavior, and health services research–as well as the literature of informatics itself. We have found it necessary to borrow terminology, in addition to methods, from all of these fields. Because these different fields tend to employ different labels for similar concepts, we have deliberately chosen one specific term to represent each important concept in this volume and have tried to employ our choice consistently through-out. But as a result, some readers may find the book using an unfamiliar term to describe what, for them, is a familiar idea.

Several chapters also develop in some detail examples taken from the informatics literature or from unpublished studies. The example studies were chosen because they illustrate key issues and because they are works with which we are familiar through present or past collaboration. This prox-imity gave us access to the raw data and other materials from these studies, which allowed us to generate pedagogic examples often differing in empha-sis from the published literature about them. Information resources forming the basis of these examples include the Hypercritic system developed at

Erasmus University in the Netherlands, the TraumAID system developed at the Medical College of Pennsylvania and the University of Pennsylvania, and the T-HELPER system developed at Stanford University. We have retained these examples in the second edition. Even though these information resources have aged technologically, the evaluation challenges raised by their development and deployment are no less salient.

We consciously did *not* write this book for software developers or engineers who are primarily interested in formal methods of software verification. In the classic distinction between validation and verification, this book is more directed at validation, but also goes beyond validation in the sense that software engineers use this term. Nor did we write this book for professional methodologists who might expect to read about contemporary advances in the methodological areas from which much of this book's content derives. Nonetheless, we hope that this book will prove useful to individuals from a broad range of professional backgrounds—and especially those interested in applying well-established evaluation techniques specifically to problems in biomedical informatics.

The second edition of this volume entails both major and minor changes. The major changes include a complete revision of the chapter on subjectivist methods. This is Chapter 10 in the numbering system of the second edition, corresponding to Chapter 9 in the first edition. The new numbering system resulted from another change: the division of the first edition's Chapter 7 into two revised chapters on design and analysis of quantitative studies. The second edition also includes a completely new Chapter (11) on economic aspects of evaluation. This new chapter addresses what we saw as a major content deficiency of the first edition. Chapter 3 underwent a major facelift to establish more clearly how the general methods of evaluation apply to the world of informatics, and to assist readers more directly in the formulation of evaluation studies. In the numbering scheme of the second edition, chapters 1, 2, 4–6, 9, and 12 were significantly revised based on our own further thinking as well as thoughts shared with us by many readers of the first edition. We elected to delete the chapter on organizational issues in evaluation (Chapter 11 in the first edition) from this revised volume. We took this action in large part because the new Chapter 10 contained many of the methodological points of the earlier chapter. We intend to make some of the material from the deleted chapter, as well as new material about evaluation as we accumulate it, available on the Web site that will accompany the book. This resource can be found at http://springeronline.com/0-387-25889-2.

The evaluation methods presented in this volume are generic and should apply to all informatics domains including biological research as well as health care and education. We have also made some changes in this edition to reflect the emergence of bioinformatics, but the examples in the volume remain weighted toward clinical information resources and health care. We expect to develop and make available in the future more examples addressing bioinformatics via the book's Web site.

In conclusion, we would like to acknowledge the many colleagues and collaborators whose contributions have made this work possible. They include contributing chapter authors Joan Ash, Mark Roberts, Allen Smith and Zoë Stavri. We continue to be indebted to Ted Shortliffe and the members of the Section on Medical Informatics at Stanford University for their support and ideas during our sabbatical leaves there in 1991–1992, when the original ideas for this book took shape. We also continue to be grateful to colleagues Johan van der Lei, Mark Musen, John Clarke, and Bonnie Webber for the volume's specific examples that derive from their own research. George Hripcsak provided comprehensive feedback that was very helpful in guiding the creation of the second edition.

Chuck specifically thanks his students at Pitt, UNC, Duke, NIH, and Woods Hole for challenging him repeatedly both in and out of class. Chuck also thanks Stuart Bondurant, Dean of the UNC School of Medicine from 1979 to 1994, for his unfailing support, which made this volume possible. He thanks Thomas Detre and Arthur Levine, Senior Vice Chancellors at the University of Pittsburgh, for their mentorship and counsel from 1996 to the present day. And he thanks Milton Corn of the National Library of Medicine for being a wonderful source of advice and support during his recent tenure there. Three MIT physicists Chuck has been very fortunate to know and work with—the late Nathaniel Frank, the late Jerrold Zacharias, and Edwin Taylor—taught him the importance of meeting the needs of students who are the future of any field. Chuck's son Nathaniel, the best writer Chuck knows, is an inspiration to be both interesting and clear; son Andrew helped Chuck appreciate the importance of bioinformatics. Finally, Chuck wishes to thank his special friend and colleague, Patti Abbott, for putting sunshine into every day, including those many days that were largely devoted to this second edition.

Jeremy acknowledges the useful insights gained from many coworkers during collaborative evaluation projects, especially from Doug Altman (CRUK Centre for Statistics in Medicine, Oxford) and David Spiegelhalter (MRC Biostatistics Unit, Cambridge). The UK Medical Research Council funded the traveling fellowship that enabled Jeremy to spend a year at Stanford in 1991–1992. Students on masters courses and others at University College London, City University and the Academic Medical Centre, Amsterdam have also helped him clarify many of the ideas expressed in this book. Finally, Jeremy thanks his family, Sylvia, David, and Jessica and his parents Moira and Selwyn for their patience and support during the long gestation of this book and its second edition.

Charles P. Friedman, PhD
Pittsburgh, PA, and Bethesda, MD, USA

Jeremy C. Wyatt, MD
Dundee, UK

Contents

Contributors

Joan S. Ash, PhD
Associate Professor, Division of Medical Informatics and Outcomes Research, Oregon Health and Science University School of Medicine, Portland, OR 97201, USA

Mark S. Roberts, MD, MPP
Associate Professor of Medicine, Health Policy and Management, Industrial Engineering; Chief of the Section of Decision Sciences and Clinical Systems Modeling, Division of General Medicine, University of Pittsburgh, Pittsburgh, PA 15260, USA

Allen C. Smith III, PhD
Associate Dean for Student and Academic Affairs, Northeastern Ohio Universities College of Medicine, Rootstown, OH 44272, USA

P. Zoë Stavri, PhD, MLS
Assistant Professor, Oregon Health and Science University, Portland, OR 97201; Visiting Assistant Professor, Health Sciences Informatics, School of Medicine, The Johns Hopkins University, Baltimore, MD 21205, USA

1
Challenges of Evaluation in Biomedical Informatics

This chapter develops, in a general and informal way, the many topics that are explored in more detail in later chapters of this book. It gives a first definition of evaluation, describes why evaluation is needed, and notes some of the problems of evaluation in biomedical informatics that distinguish it from evaluation in other areas. In addition, it lists some of the many types of information systems and resources, the questions that can be asked about them, and the various perspectives of those concerned.

First Definitions

Most people understand the term "evaluation" to mean measuring or describing something, usually to answer questions or help make decisions. Whether we are choosing a holiday destination or a web browser, we evaluate the options and how well they fit key objectives or personal preferences. The form of the evaluation differs widely according to what is being evaluated and how important the decision is. Therefore, in the case of holiday destinations, we may ask our friend which Hawaiian island she prefers, and why, before searching for more specific information about hotels. For a web browser, we may focus on more technical details, such as the time to open a web site or its compatibility with our disability. Thus, the term "evaluation" describes a range of data-collection activities designed to answer questions ranging from the casual "What does my friend think of Maui?" to the more focused "Is web browser *A* quicker than web browser *B* on my computer?"

In biomedical informatics, we study the collection, processing, and communication of information related to health care, research, and education. We build "information resources," usually consisting of computer hardware and software, to facilitate these activities. For healthcare applications, such information resources include systems to collect, store, and communicate data about specific patients (e.g., clinical workstations and electronic patient records) and systems to assemble, store, and reason using medical knowledge (e.g., medical knowledge bases and decision-support systems). For basic and clinical research applications, information resources include genomic and proteomic databases, tools to analyze these data and correlate genotypes with phenotypes, and methods for identifying patients eligible for clinical trials.* In health education, there are Internet-based programs for distance learning and virtual reality simulations for learning medical procedures. There is clearly a range of biomedical information and communication resources to evaluate.

To further complicate the picture, each information resource has many aspects that can be evaluated. The technically minded might focus on inherent characteristics, asking such questions as: "How many columns are there per database table?" or "How many probability calculations per second can this resource sustain?" Clinicians, researchers, and students might ask more pragmatic questions, such as: "Is the information in this resource completely up-to-date?" or "How much time must I invest in becoming proficient with this resource, and will it do anything to help me personally?" Those with a broader perspective might wish to understand the impact of these resources on organization or management, asking questions such as: "How well does this electronic patient record support clinical audit?" or "Will sophisticated educational simulations change the role of the faculty in teaching?" Thus, evaluation methods in biomedical informatics must address not only a range of different types of information resources, but also a range of questions about them, from the technical characteristics of specific systems to their effects on people and organizations.

In this book, we do not exhaustively describe how each possible evaluation method can be used to answer each kind of question about each kind of information resource. Instead, we describe the range of techniques available and focus on those that seem most useful in biomedical informatics. We introduce, in detail, methods, techniques, study designs, and analysis methods that apply across a range of evaluation problems. The methods introduced in this volume are applicable to the full range of information resources directed at health care, biomedical research, and education. The examples we introduce and discuss will come primarily from clinical and educational application. While there is a great deal of interest in a rapidly developing set of information resources to support bioinformatics and clinical research, there is relatively little experience with the evaluation of these tools.

In the language of software engineering, our focus is much more on software validation than software verification. Validation means checking that the "right" information resource was built, which involves both determining that the original specification was right and that the resource is per-

---

* In this volume, the term "bioinformatics" will be used to refer to the use of information resources in support of biological research. In this parlance, bioinformatics is a subset of the broader domain of biomedical informatics.

forming to specification. By contrast, verification means checking whether the resource was built to specification. As we introduce evaluation methods in detail, we will distinguish the study of software functions from the study of their impact or effects on users and the wider world. Although software verification is important, this volume will only summarize some of the relevant principles in Chapter 3 and refer the reader to general computer science and software-engineering texts.

Reasons for Performing Evaluations

Like any complex, time-consuming activity, evaluation can serve multiple purposes. There are at least five major reasons why we evaluate biomedical information resources.[1]

1. *Promotional:* To encourage the use of information resources in biomedicine, we must be able to reassure clinicians, patients, researchers, and educators that these resources are safe and bring benefit to persons, groups, and institutions through improved cost-effectiveness or safety, or perhaps by making activities possible that were not possible before.

2. *Scholarly:* If we believe that biomedical informatics exists as a discipline or scientific field, ongoing examination of the structure, function, and impact of biomedical information resources must be a primary method for identifying and confirming the principles that lie at the foundation of the field.[2] In addition, some developers of information resources carry out evaluations from different perspectives out of basic curiosity in order to see if the resources are able to perform functions that were not in the original specifications.

3. *Pragmatic:* Without evaluating the resources they create, developers can never know which techniques or methods are more effective, or why certain approaches failed. Equally, other developers are not able to learn from previous mistakes and may reinvent a square wheel.

4. *Ethical:* Before using an information resource, clinicians, researchers, educators, and administrators must be satisfied that it is functional and be able to justify its use in preference to alternative information resources and the many other innovations that compete for the same budget.

5. *Medicolegal:* To reduce the risk of liability, developers of an information resource should obtain accurate information to allow them to label it correctly[3] and assure users that it is safe and effective. Users need evaluation results to enable them to exercise their professional judgment before using these resources, thus helping the law regard each user as a "learned intermediary." An information resource that treats the users merely as automatons, without allowing them to exercise their skills and judgment, risks being judged by the strict laws of product liability instead of the more lenient principles applied to provision of professional services.[4]

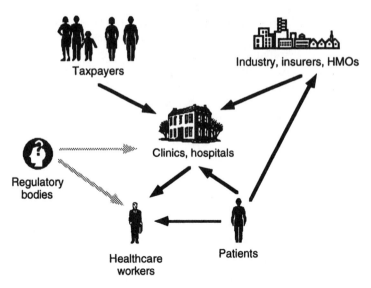

FIGURE 1.1. Actors involved in health care delivery and regulation.

Every evaluation study should be motivated by one or more of these factors; otherwise, it risks being what has been called a "triple blind study," in which neither evaluators, participants, nor readers of the report can fathom why it was done.[†] Awareness of the major reason for conducting an evaluation often helps frame the major questions to be addressed and avoids any disappointment that may result if the focus of the study is misdirected. We return in Chapter 3 to the problem of deciding how much to emphasize each of the many questions that arise in most evaluation studies.

Who Is Involved in Evaluation and Why?

We have already mentioned the range of perspectives in biomedical informatics, from the technical to the organizational. With specific regard to the clinical domain, Figure 1.1 shows some of the actors involved in paying for (solid arrows) and regulating (shaded arrows) the healthcare process. Any of these actors may be affected by a biomedical information resource, and each may have a unique view of what constitutes benefit. More specifically, in a typical clinical information resource project, the key "stakeholders" are the developer, the user, the patients whose management may be affected, and the person responsible for purchasing and maintaining the information resource. Each of these individuals or groups may have different questions

---

[†] Personal communication with Peter Branger, 2000.

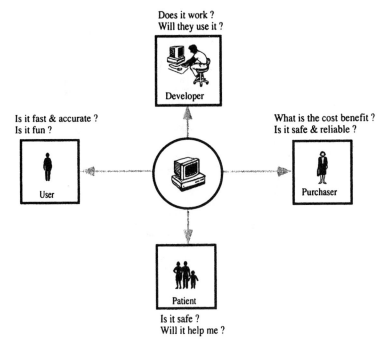

FIGURE 1.2. Differing perspectives on a clinical information resource.

to ask about the same information resource (Figure 1.2). Thus, whenever we design evaluation studies, it is important to consider the perspectives of all stakeholders in the information resource. Any one study usually satisfies only some of them. A major challenge for evaluators is to distinguish those persons who must be satisfied from those whose satisfaction is optional.

What Makes Evaluation So Difficult?

Evaluation, as defined earlier, is a general investigative activity applicable to many fields. Many thousands of evaluation studies have been performed, and much has been written about evaluation methods. Why, then, write a book specifically about evaluation in biomedical informatics?

The evaluation of biomedical information resources lies at the intersection of three areas, each notorious for its complexity (Figure 1.3): biomedicine as a field of human endeavor, computer-based information systems, and the general methodology of evaluation itself. Because of the complexity of each area, any work that combines them necessarily poses serious challenges. These challenges are discussed in the sections that follow.

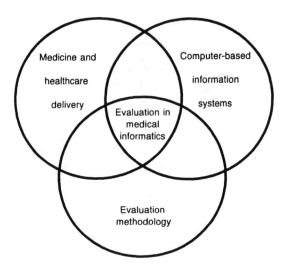

FIGURE 1.3. Complexity of evaluation in biomedical informatics.

Problems Deriving from Biomedicine as a Field of Human Endeavor

The goal of this section is to introduce readers unfamiliar with this domain to some of the complexities of biomedicine, and perhaps to introduce even those familiar with the domain to some of the implications of this complexity for evaluating biomedical information resources.

Donabedian informed us that any healthcare innovation might influence three aspects of a health care system:[5]

1. *Structure* of the healthcare system, including the space it occupies, equipment available, financial resources required, and the number, skills, and inter-relationships of staff.
2. *Processes* that take place during healthcare activity, such as the number and appropriateness of diagnoses, investigations, or therapies administered.
3. *Outcomes* of health care for both individual patients and the community, such as quality of life, complications of procedures, and average length of survival.

Donabedian's analysis, which focused primarily on the provision of health care, actually applies to all of biomedicine. Thus, the impact of an information resource directed at health care, biomedical research, or health-related education can be seen in relation to relevant aspects of structure, process, or outcome. Complexity arises because an information resource may lead to an improvement in one area (patient outcomes, for example) accompanied by deterioration in another (the costs of running the service perhaps). In education, introduction of extensive simulation techniques may improve learning outcomes, but may also require significant renovation of classroom space and equipment installation. Extensive use of new computer-based tools in biological research has led to questions about staffing. These include whether "bioinformatics" specialists, expert at using computer-based tools, should be hired by each laboratory, or whether they should be hired at the institutional level and perhaps be located in the health sciences library.

Biomedical domains are characterized by varying degrees of professional autonomy and contrasting local culture, with strong implications for the deployment and use of information resources. In clinical settings, the roles of nursing and other personnel are well-defined and hierarchical in comparison to those in many other professions. This means that information resources designed for one specific group of professionals, such as a residents' information system designed for one hospital,[6] may hold little benefit for others. Despite the obvious hierarchy, it often comes as a surprise to those developing information systems that junior physicians cannot be obliged by their senior counterparts to use a specific information resource, as is the case in the banking or airline industries where these practices became "part of the job." The culture of biomedical research is often more pro-innovation than the culture of health care. However, in academic institutions, persons who are pro-information technology (IT) in their research roles can be equally anti-IT in their clinical roles. Thus, the local acceptance and use of information resources by professionals, especially healthcare workers, may be a limiting factor in evaluation studies.

Because it is a safety-critical area, there is a strong tradition of demanding evidence prior to adoption of innovations in health care and in the education of professionals who provide health care. Because there may be more skeptics among healthcare providers than in other professions, more rigorous proof of safety and effectiveness is required when evaluating information resources here than in areas such as retail sales or manufacturing. Clinicians are rightly skeptical of innovative technology, but may be unrealistic in their demand for evidence of benefit if the innovation threatens their current practice. Because we humans are usually more skeptical of new practices than existing ones, we tend to compare an innovation with an idealization of what it is replacing. The standard required for proving the effectiveness of computer-based information resources may be inflated beyond that required for existing methods of handling information, such as the paper medical record.

Complex regulations apply to those developing or marketing clinical therapies or investigational technology. It is becoming increasingly clear that these regulations will apply to all computer-based information resources, not only to those that manage patients directly, without a human intermediary.[7] Serious consequences, financial and otherwise, may follow from failure by software developers to adequately evaluate their products.

For example, one large laboratory information system company saw $90 million wiped off its market value in 2003, when the Food and Drug Administration (FDA) published a warning about a fault in their product on the FDA home page.[8] Developers of these resources will need to increasingly comply with a comprehensive schedule of testing and monitoring procedures, which may form an obligatory core of evaluation methods in the future.

Biomedicine is well known to be a complex domain, with students spending a minimum of seven years to gain professional certification in medicine. It is not atypical for a graduate student in molecular biology to spend five years in pursuit of a PhD and follow this with a multi-year postdoctoral training experience. In the United States, professional training in other fields, such as nursing and pharmacy, has lengthened in recognition of the nature and complexity of what is to be learned. For example, a single internal medicine textbook contains approximately 600,000 facts,[9] and practicing medical experts have as many as two million to five million facts at their fingertips.[10] Medical knowledge itself[9] and methods of healthcare delivery and research change rapidly, so the goal posts for a biomedical information resource may move significantly during the course of an evaluation study.

The problems that biomedical information resources assist in solving are complex, highly variable, and difficult to describe. Patients often suffer from multiple diseases, which may evolve over time and at differing rates, and they may undergo a number of interventions over the course of the study period. Two patients with the same disease can present with very different sets of clinical signs and symptoms. There is variation in the interpretation of patient data among medical centers. What may be regarded as an abnormal result or an advanced stage of disease in one setting may pass without comment in another because it is within their laboratory's normal limits or is an endemic condition in their population. Thus, simply because an information resource is safe and effective when used in one center on patients with a given diagnosis, one is not entitled to prejudge the results of evaluating it in another center or in patients with a different disease profile.

Biological researchers have largely solved the very complex problem of understanding genome structure, but now they face an even more complex problem in understanding genome function: how gene expression affects health and disease and the implications of person-to-person variation in genetic structure. Biomedical information resources are challenged to help scientists manage the enormous amounts of data—three billion DNA base-pairs in the genome, and approximately 30,000 genes whose structure can vary across billions of people—that are now of fundamental interest to biological research. In education, the challenges encountered by students striving to be clinicians and researchers are both profound and idiosyncratic. The subject matter itself is sophisticated and changing rapidly. What a person can learn is largely determined by what that person already knows and can do, so information resources that aid learning must respond to individual learner needs.[11]

The causal links between introducing a biomedical information resource and achieving improvements in the outcomes of interest are long and complex, even in comparison with other biomedical interventions such as drug therapy. In part, this is because the functioning of an information resource and its impact may depend critically on how healthcare workers or patients actually interact with the resource (Figure 1.4, shaded arrows), if they use it at all. These concerns are increasingly relevant with the advent of eHealth and consumer health informatics. In the clinical domain especially, it is probably unrealistic to look for quantifiable changes in outcomes following the introduction of many information resources until one has first documented the resulting changes in the structure or processes of health care delivery. For example, MacDonald and colleagues showed during the 1980s that the Regenstrief healthcare information system affected clinical decisions and actions with its alerts and reminders.[12] Almost 10 years later, clear evidence of a reduction in the length of stay was obtained.[13] In Chapter 3, we discuss circumstances in which it may be sufficient, within the realm of biomedical informatics, to evaluate the effects of an information resource on a clinical process, such as the proportion of patients with heart attacks who are given a clot-dissolving drug. We believe it is the role of the field of health services research to carry out primary or secondary research

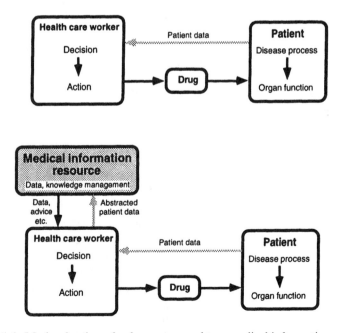

FIGURE 1.4. Mode of action of a drug compared to a medical information resource.

in order to demonstrate the causal link between changes in clinical practice and changes in patient outcome.

In some cases, changes in work processes resulting from introduction of an information resource are difficult to interpret because the resulting improved information management or decision-taking merely clears one log jam and reveals another. An example of this situation occurred during the evaluation of the ACORN (Admit to CCU OR Not) chest pain decision-aid, designed to facilitate more rapid and accurate diagnosis of patients with acute ischemic heart disease in the emergency room.[14] Although ACORN allowed emergency room staff to rapidly identify patients requiring admission to the cardiac care unit (CCU), it uncovered an existing problem: the lack of beds in the CCU and delays in transferring other patients out of them.[15]

In the clinical domain, the processes of decision-making are complex and have been studied extensively.[16,17] Clinicians make many kinds of decisions—including diagnosis, monitoring, choice of therapy, and prognosis—using incomplete and fuzzy data, some of which are appreciated intuitively and not recorded in the clinical notes. If an information resource generates more effective management of both patient data and medical knowledge, it may intervene in the process of medical decision-making in a number of ways; consequently, it may be difficult to decide which component of the resource is responsible for the observed changes. Often this does not matter, but if one component is expensive or hard to create, understanding why and how the resource brings benefit becomes important. Understanding why a resource brings benefit can be much more difficult than determining the magnitude of this benefit.

Data about individual patients typically are collected at several locations and over periods of time ranging from an hour to decades. Unfortunately, clinical notes usually contain only a subset of what was observed and seldom contain the reasons why actions were taken.[18] Because reimbursement agencies often have access to clinical notes, the notes may even contain data intended to mislead chart reviewers or conceal important facts from the casual reader.[19,20] Thus, evaluating an electronic medical record system by examining the accuracy of its contents may not give a true picture.

There is a general lack of "gold standards" in health care. For example, diagnoses are rarely known with 100% certainty, partly because it is unethical to do all possible tests in every patient, or even to follow up patients without good cause, and partly because of the complexity of the human biology. When attempting to establish a diagnosis or the cause of death, even if it is possible to perform a postmortem examination, correlating the observed changes with the patients' symptoms or findings before death may prove impossible. Determining the "correct" management for a patient is even harder, as there is wide variation even in so-called consensus opinions,[21] which is reflected in wide variations in clinical practice even in neighboring areas. An example is the use of endotracheal intubation in patients with severe head injuries, which varied from 15% to 85% among teaching hospitals, even within California.** In addition, getting busy physicians to give their opinions about the correct management of patients for comparison with a decision support system's advice may take as much as a full year.[22]

Healthcare providers practice under strict legal and ethical obligations to give their patients the best care available, to them no harm, keep them informed about the risks of all procedures and therapies, and maintain confidentiality. These obligations often impinge on the design of evaluation studies. For example, because healthcare workers have imperfect memories and patients take holidays and participate in the unpredictable activities of real life, it is impossible to impose a strict discipline for data recording, and study data are often incomplete. Before any field studies of an information resource can be undertaken, healthcare workers and patients are entitled to a full explanation of the possible benefits and disadvantages of the resource. Even if it is a randomized trial, since half the patients or healthcare workers will be allocated randomly to the intervention group, all need to be counseled and give their consent prior to being enrolled in the study. Similar challenges to evaluation apply to the educational domain. For example, students in professional schools are in a "high-stakes" environment where grades and other measures of performance can shape the trajectory of their future careers. Students will be understandably attracted to information resources they perceive as advantageous to learning and averse to those they perceive to offer little or no benefit at a great expenditure of time. Randomization or other means of arbitrary assignment of students to groups, for purposes of evaluative experiments, may be seen as anathema. Similar feelings may be seen in biological research, where competitiveness among laboratories may mitigate against controlled studies of information resources deployed in these settings.

Problems Deriving from the Complexity of Computer-Based Information Resources

From a computer-science perspective, an important goal of evaluating an information resource is to verify that the program code faithfully performs those functions it was designed to perform. One approach to this goal is to try to predict the resource's function and impact from knowledge of the program's structure. However, although software engineering and formal methods for specifying, coding, and testing computer programs have become more sophisticated, programs of even modest complexity challenge these techniques. Since we cannot logically or mathematically derive a program's function from its structure, we often are left with exhaustive "brute-force" techniques for program verification.

** Personal communication with Bryan Jennett, 1990.

The task of verifying a program (obtaining proof that it performs all and only those functions specified) using brute-force methods increases exponentially according to the program's size and the complexity of the tasks it performs. This is an "NP-hard" problem (see glossary). Put simply, to verify a program using brute-force methods requires application of every combination of possible input data items and values for each in all possible sequences. This entails at least n factorial trials of the program, where n is the number of input data items.

A range of computer-based information resources has been applied to biomedicine (Table 1.1), each with different target users, input data, and goals. Even though they are increasingly commonplace, computer-based information resources remain a relatively novel technology in biomedicine, with a legacy of 30 to 40 years. With any relatively new technology, novel challenges arise. For example, practitioners may not use a decision support system until it has been shown to be valuable, but persons need to use the system in order to demonstrate its value. We call this phenomenon the "evaluation paradox." Moreover, many information resources do not reach their maximum impact until they are fully integrated with other information resources that operate in the same work environment and until they become part of routine work practice.[23]

In some projects, the goals of the new information resource are not precisely defined. Developers may be attracted by technology and produce applications of it without first demonstrating the existence of a clinical, scientific, or educational problem that the application is designed to address.[15] An example was a conference entitled "Medicine Meets Virtual Reality: *Discovering Applications* for 3D Multimedia" [our italics]. The lack of a clear need for the information resource makes some biomedical informatics projects difficult or impossible to evaluate, and we will see in later chapters that understanding the need for a proposed information resource is often the driving question of an evaluation study.

TABLE 1.1. Range of computer-based information resources in medicine.

Clinical data systems	Clinical knowledge systems
Clinical databases	Computerized textbooks (e.g., *Scientific American Medicine* on CD-ROM)
Communications systems (e.g., picture archiving and communication systems)	Teaching systems (e.g., interactive multimedia anatomy tutor)
On-line signal processing (e.g., 24-hour ECG analysis system)	Patient simulation programs (e.g., interactive active acid-base metabolism simulator)
Alert generation (e.g., ICU monitor, drug interaction system)	Passive knowledge bases (e.g., MEDLINE bibliographic system)
Laboratory data interpretation	Patient-specific advice generators (e.g., MYCIN antibiotic therapy advisor)
Medical image interpretation	Medical robotics

Most information resources are deliberately configured or tailored to a given institution as a necessary part of their deployment. Hence, it may be difficult to compare the results of one evaluation with a study of the same information resource conducted in another location. It is even reasonable to ask whether two variants of the "same" basic software package configured for two different environments should be considered the same package. In addition, the notoriously rapid evolution of computer hardware and software means that the time course of an evaluation study may be greater than the lifetime of the information resource itself. While this problem is often exaggerated and used by some as a reason not to invest in evaluation, it nonetheless is an important factor shaping how evaluation studies in biomedical informatics should be designed and conducted.

Biomedical information resources often contain several distinct components, including interface, database, reasoning, and maintenance programs, as well as data, knowledge, business logic, and dynamic inferences about the user and the current activity of the user. Such information resources may perform a range of functions for users. This means that if evaluators are to answer questions such as, "What part of the information resource is responsible for the observed effect?" or "Why did the information resource fail?," they must be familiar with each component of the information resource, their functions, and their potential interactions.[14]

Problems of the Evaluation Process Itself

Evaluation studies, as envisioned in this book, do not focus solely on the structure and function of information resources; they also address their impact on persons who are customarily users of these resources and on the outcomes of users' interactions with them. To understand users' actions, investigators must confront the gulf between peoples' private opinions, public statements, and actual behavior. What is more, there is clear evidence that the mere act of studying human performance changes it, a phenomenon usually known as the Hawthorne effect.[24] Finally, humans vary widely in their responses to stimuli, from minute to minute and from one person to another. Thus, evaluation studies of biomedical information resources require analytical tools from the behavioral and social sciences, biostatistics, and other scientific fields dedicated to "human" problems where high variability is the rule rather than the exception.

Many evaluation studies are performed in the laboratory, before an information resource is deployed. These studies require "test material" (clinical cases, scientific problems) and information resource users (e.g., clinicians, scientists, students, patients). Both are often in shorter supply than the study design requires. In clinical research, the availability of patients is usually overestimated, sometimes by a factor of ten—Lasagna's Law.* Planners of

---

* Personal communication with Douglas Altman, 1991.

TABLE 1.2. Possible questions that may arise during evaluation of a medical information resource.

Questions about the resource	Questions about the impact of the resource
Is there a clinical need for it?	Do people use it?
Does it work?	Do people like it?
Is it reliable?	Does it improve users' efficiency?
Is it accurate?	Does it influence the collection of data?
Is it fast enough?	Does it influence users' decisions?
Is data entry reliable?	For how long do the observed effects last?
Are people likely to use it?	Does it influence users' knowledge or skills?
Which parts cause the effects?	Does it help patients?
How can it be maintained?	Does it change use of healthcare facilities?
How can it be improved?	What might ensue from widespread use?

evaluations can readily fall prey to the same delusion. In addition, it may be unclear what kind of test material or users to include in such a study. Often study designers are faced with trade-offs between selecting test material or users with high fidelity to the real-world practice—those who can help achieve adequate experimental control in the study and those who are available and willing to participate. Finally, one of the more important determinants of the results of an evaluation study is the manner in which test material is abstracted and presented to users. For example, one would expect differing results in a study of an information resource's accuracy depending on whether the test data were abstracted by the resource developer or by the intended users.

There are many reasons for performing evaluations, ranging from assessing a student's mastery of new subject matter to making national health policy decisions or understanding the implications of a technical change on resource performance. There are inevitably many actors in evaluation studies (see Figure 1.1), including information resource developers, users, and patients, all of whom may have different perspectives on which questions to ask and how to interpret the answers. Table 1.2 lists some sample questions that may arise about the resource itself and its impact on users, patients, and the healthcare system. The multiplicity of possible questions creates challenges for the designers of evaluation studies. Any one study inevitably fails to address some questions and may fail to answer adequately some questions that are explicitly addressed.

Addressing the Challenges of Evaluation

No one could pretend that evaluation is easy. This entire book describes ways that have been developed to solve the many problems discussed in this chapter. First, evaluators should recognize that a range of evaluation approaches are available and that they should adopt a specific "evaluation mindset" (described in Chapter 2). This mindset includes the awareness that every study is to some extent a compromise. To help overcome the many potential difficulties, evaluators require knowledge and skills drawn from a range of disciplines, including statistics, measurement theory, psychology, sociology, and anthropology. To avoid committing excessive evaluation resources at too early a stage, the intensity of evaluation activity should be titrated to the stage of development of the information resource: It is clearly inappropriate to subject to a multicenter randomized trial a prototype information resource resulting from a three-month student project.[25] This does not imply that evaluation can be deferred to the end of a project. Evaluation plans should be appropriately integrated with system design and development from the outset, as further discussed in Chapter 3.

If the developers are able to enunciate clearly the aims of an information resource, defining the questions to be answered by an evaluation study becomes easier. As will be seen in later chapters, evaluators should also watch for adverse or unexpected effects. Life is easier for evaluators if they can build on the work of their predecessors; for example, many studies require reliable and valid quantitative ways to measure relevant attitudes, work processes, or relevant outcomes. If these measurement tools already exist, evaluators should use them in their studies rather than developing new measures, which would have to undergo a time-consuming process of thorough validation. One valuable role evaluators may play is to dampen the often-unbridled enthusiasm of developers for their own systems, focusing the developers' attention on a smaller number of specific benefits it is reasonable to expect.

As illustrated above, there are many potential problems when evaluating biomedical information resources, but evaluation is possible, and many hundreds of useful evaluations have already been performed. For example, Hunt and colleagues[26] reviewed the results of 68 randomized controlled trials of decision support systems studying the care given to over 87,000 patients and concluded that most showed clear evidence of an impact on clinical processes and a smaller number showed improved patient outcomes. Designing formal experiments to detect changes in patient outcome due to the introduction of an information resource is possible, as will be discussed in a later chapter. It is not our wish to deter evaluators, merely to open their eyes to the complexity of this area.

The Place of Evaluation Within Informatics

Biomedical informatics is a complex, derivative field. Informatics draws its methods from many disciplines and from many specific lines of creative work within these disciplines.[27] Some of the fields underlying informatics are what may be called basic. They include, among others, computer science,

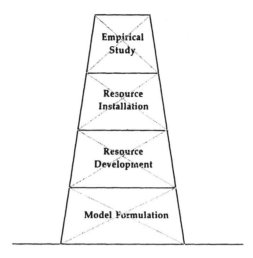

FIGURE 1.5. Tower model. (Adapted from ref. 28 the *Journal of the American Medical Informatics Association*, with permission.)

information science, cognitive science, decision science, statistics, and linguistics. Other fields supporting informatics are applied more in their orientation, including software and computer engineering, clinical epidemiology, and evaluation itself. One of the strengths of informatics has been the degree to which individuals from these different disciplinary backgrounds, but with complementary interests, have learned not only to coexist, but also to collaborate productively.

However, this diverse intellectual heritage for informatics can make it difficult to define creative or original work in the field.[28] The "tower" model, shown in Figure 1.5, asserts that creative work in informatics occurs at four levels that build on one another. Projects at every level of the tower can be found on the agenda of professional meetings in informatics and published in journals within the field. The topmost layer of the tower embraces empirical studies of information resources (systems) that have been developed using abstract models and perhaps installed in settings of ongoing health care or education. Because informatics is so intimately concerned with the improvement of health care, the value or worth of resources produced by the field is a matter of significant ongoing interest.[29] Studies occupy the topmost layer because they rely on the existence of models, systems, and settings where the work of interest is underway. There must be *something* to study. As will be seen later, studies of information resources usually do not await the ultimate installation or deployment of these resources. Even conceptual models may be studied empirically, and information resources themselves can be studied through successive stages of development.

Studies occupying the topmost level of the tower model are the focus of this book. Empirical studies include measurement and observations of the performance of information resources and the behavior of people who in

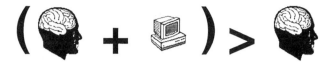

FIGURE 1.6. A "Fundamental Theorem" of biomedical informatics.

some way use these resources, with emphasis on the interaction between the resources and the people and the consequences of these interactions. Included under empirical studies are activities that have traditionally been called "evaluation." The term "evaluation" has been included in the title of this book instead of "empirical methods" because the former term is most commonly used in the field. The importance of evaluation and, more generally, empirical methods is becoming recognized by those concerned with information technology. In addition to articles reporting specific studies using the methods of evaluation, books on the topic, apart from this one, have appeared.[30–32]

Another way to look at the role of evaluation in biomedical informatics is to consider the "inequality" illustrated in Figure 1.6. This inequality has been proposed as a "Fundamental Theorem" of biomedical informatics.[33] The theorem suggests that the goal of informatics is to deploy information resources that help persons (i.e., clinicians, students, scientists, patients) do whatever they do "better" than would be the case without support from these information resources. Most individuals who work with information technology in biomedicine believe that the theorem will hold in most cases when the information resources have been properly designed and implemented. Seen in this light, evaluation studies examine whether the fundamental theorem is satisfied. When it is not, studies can suggest helpful modifications in technology or the way in which it is used.

Finally, if abstract principles of biomedical informatics exist,[2,34] then evaluating the structure, function, and impact of biomedical information resources should be one of our primary methods for uncovering these principles. Without evaluation, biomedical informatics becomes a diffuse, impressionistic, anecdotal field, with little professional identity or chance of making progress toward greater scientific understanding and more effective clinical systems. Thus, overcoming the problems described in this chapter to evaluate a range of resources in various clinical settings has intrinsic merit and contributes to the development of biomedical informatics as a field. Evaluation is not merely a possible, but a necessary component of biomedical informatics activity.[34]

Food for Thought

1. Choosing any alternative area of biomedicine as a point of comparison (e.g., drug development), list as many factors as you can that make studies in biomedical informatics more difficult to conduct successfully than

in your chosen area. Given these difficulties, is it worthwhile to conduct empirical studies in biomedical informatics, or should we use intuition or the marketplace as the primary indicator of the value of an information resource?

2. Many writers on the evaluation of clinical information resources believe that the evaluations that should be done should be closely linked to the stage of development of the resource under study (see reference 25 in this chapter). Do you believe this position is reasonable? What other logic or criteria may be used to help decide what studies should be performed in any given situation?

3. Suppose you were running a philanthropic organization that supported biomedical informatics. When investing the scarce resources of your organization, you might have to choose between funding system/resource development and empirical studies of resources already developed. Faced with this decision, what weight would you give to each? How would you justify your decision?

4. To what extent is it possible to ascertain the effectiveness of a biomedical informatics resource? What are the most important criteria of effectiveness?

References

1. Wyatt J, Spiegelhalter D. Evaluating medical expert systems: what to test, and how? Med Inf (Lond) 1990;15:205–217.
2. Heathfield H, Wyatt J. The road to professionalism in medical informatics: a proposal for debate. Methods Inf Med 1995;34:426–433.
3. Rigby M, Forsström J, Roberts R, Wyatt J. Verifying quality and safety in health informatics services. BMJ 2001;323:552–556.
4. Brahams D, Wyatt J. Decision-aids and the law. Lancet 1989;2:632–634.
5. Donabedian A. Evaluating the quality of medical care. Millbank Mem Q 1966; 44:166–206.
6. Young D. An aid to reducing unnecessary investigations. BMJ 1980;281: 1610–1611.
7. Brannigan V. Software quality regulation under the Safe Medical Devices Act, 1990: Hospitals are now the canaries in the software mine. In: Clayton P, ed. *Proceedings of the 15th Symposium on Computer Applications in Medical Care.* New York: McGraw-Hill; 1991:238–242.
8. Wray R. FDA move costs Misys £60m. The Guardian 14-10-03. Available at: http://www.guardian.co.uk/business/story/0,3604,1062395,00.html. Accessed April 1, 2005.
9. Wyatt J. Use and sources of medical knowledge. Lancet 1991;338:1368–1373.
10. Pauker S, Gorry G, Kassirer J, Schwartz W. Towards the simulation of clinical cognition: taking a present illness by computer. Am J Med 1976;60:981–996.
11. Friedman CP, Ozbolt JG, Masys DR. Toward a new culture for biomedical informatics: report of the 2001 ACMI symposium. J Am Med Inform Assoc 2001;8(6):519–526.

12. McDonald CJ, Hui SL, Smith DM, et al. Reminders to physicians from an introspective computer medical record: a two-year randomized trial. Ann Intern Med 1984;100:130–138.
13. Tierney WM, Miller ME, Overhage JM, McDonald CJ. Physician order writing on microcomputer workstations. JAMA 1993;269:379–383.
14. Wyatt J. Lessons learned from the field trial of ACORN, an expert system to advise on chest pain. In: Barber B, Cao D, Qin D, eds. *Proceedings of the Sixth World Conference on Medical Informatics, Singapore.* Amsterdam, North Holland: 1989:111–115.
15. Heathfield HA, Wyatt J. Philosophies for the design and development of clinical decision-support systems. Methods Inf Med 1993;32:1–8.
16. Elstein A, Shulman L, Sprafka S. *Medical Problem Solving: An Analysis of Clinical Reasoning.* Cambridge, MA: Harvard University Press; 1978.
17. Evans D, Patel V, eds. *Cognitive Science in Medicine.* London: MIT Press; 1989.
18. Van der Lei J, Musen M, van der Does E, in't Veld A, van Bemmel J. Comparison of computer-aided and human review of general practitioners' management of hypertension. Lancet 1991;338:1504–1508.
19. Musen M. The strained quality of medical data. Methods Inf Med 1989;28:123–125.
20. Wyatt JC. Clinical data systems. Part I. Data and medical records. Lancet 1994;344:1543–1547.
21. Leitch D. Who should have their cholesterol measured? What experts in the UK suggest. BMJ 1989;298:1615–1616.
22. Gaschnig J, Klahr P, Pople H, Shortliffe E, Terry A. Evaluation of expert systems: issues and case studies. In: Hayes-Roth F, Waterman DA, Lenat D, eds. *Building Expert Systems.* Reading, MA: Addison-Wesley; 1983.
23. Wyatt J, Spiegelhalter D. Field trials of medical decision-aids: potential problems and solutions. In: Clayton P, ed. *Proceedings of the 15th Symposium on Computer Applications in Medical Care, Washington.* New York: McGraw-Hill; 1991:3–7.
24. Roethligsburger F, Dickson W. *Management and the Worker.* Cambridge, MA: Harvard University Press; 1939.
25. Stead W, Haynes RB, Fuller S, et al. Designing medical informatics research and library projects to increase what is learned. J Am Med Inform Assoc 1994;1:28–34.
26. Hunt DL, Haynes RB, Hanna SE, Smith K. Effects of computer-based clinical decision support systems on physician performance and patient outcomes: a systematic review. JAMA 1998;280:1339–1346.
27. Greenes RA, Shortliffe EH. Medical informatics: an emerging academic discipline and institutional priority. JAMA 1990;263:1114–1120.
28. Friedman CP. Where's the science in medical informatics? J Am Med Inform Assoc 1995;2:65–67.
29. Clayton P. Assessing our accomplishments. Symp Comput Applications Med Care 1991;15:viii–x.
30. Anderson JG, Aydin CE, Jay SE, eds. *Evaluating Health Care Information Systems.* Thousand Oaks, CA: Sage; 1994.
31. Cohen P. *Empirical Methods for Artificial Intelligence.* Cambridge, MA: MIT Press; 1995.

32. Jain R. *The Art of Computer Systems Performance Analysis*. New York: Wiley; 1991.
33. Friedman C. The fundamental theorem of medical informatics. Invited presentation at: the University of Washington, Seattle; October 21, 2000; Seattle, WA.
34. Wyatt JC. Medical informatics: artifacts or science? Methods Inf Med 1996;35:197–200.

2
Evaluation as a Field

The previous chapter should have succeeded in convincing the reader that evaluation in biomedical informatics, for all its potential benefits, is difficult in the real world. The informatics community can take some comfort in the fact that it is not alone. Evaluation is difficult in any field of endeavor. Fortunately, many good minds—representing an array of philosophical orientations, methodological perspectives, and domains of application—have explored ways to address these difficulties. Many of the resulting approaches to evaluation have met with substantial success. The resulting range of solutions, the field of evaluation itself, is the focus of this chapter.

If this chapter is successful, the reader will begin to sense some common ground across all evaluation work while simultaneously appreciating the range of tools available. This appreciation is the initial step in recognizing that evaluation, though difficult, is possible.

Evaluation Revisited

For decades, behavioral and social scientists have grappled with the knotty problem of evaluation. As it applies to biomedical informatics, this problem can initially be expressed as the need to answer a basic set of questions. To the inexperienced, these questions might appear deceptively simple.

- An information resource is developed. Is the resource performing as intended? How can it be improved?
- Subsequently, the resource is introduced into a functioning clinical, scientific or educational environment. Again, is it performing as intended, and how can it be improved? Does it make any difference in terms of clinical, scientific or educational practice? Are the differences it makes beneficial? Are the observed affects those envisioned by the developers or different effects?

Note that we can append "why or why not?" to each of these questions. In actuality, there are many more potentially interesting questions than have been listed here.

Out of this multitude of possible questions comes the first challenge for anyone planning an evaluation: to select the best or most appropriate set

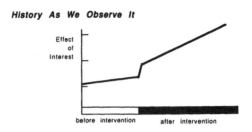

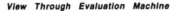

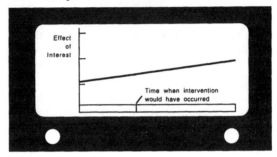

FIGURE 2.1. Hypothetical "evaluation machine."

of questions to explore in a particular situation. This challenge was introduced in Chapter 1 and is reintroduced here. The issue of what can and should be studied is the primary focus of Chapter 3. The questions to study in any particular situation are not inscribed in stone and would probably not be miraculously handed down from On High if one climbed a tall mountain in a thunderstorm. Many more questions can be stated than can be explored, and it is often the case that the most interesting questions reveal their identity only after a study has been commenced. Further complicating the situation, evaluations are inextricably political. There are legitimate differences of opinion over the relative importance of particular questions. Before any data are collected, those conducting an evaluation may find themselves in the role of referee between competing views and interests as to what questions should be on the table.

Even when the questions can be stated in advance, with consensus that they are the "right" questions, they can be difficult to answer persuasively. Some would be easy to answer if a unique kind of time machine, which might be called an "evaluation machine," were available. As shown in Figure 2.1, the evaluation machine would enable us to see how the work environment would appear if our resource had never been introduced.* By com-

---

* Readers familiar with methods of epidemiology may recognize the "evaluation machine" as an informal way of portraying the counterfactual approach to the study of cause and effect. More details about this approach may be found in a standard epidemiology text, such as Rothman and colleagues.[1]

paring real history with the fabrication created by the evaluation machine, accurate conclusions can potentially be drawn about the effects of the resource. Even if there was an evaluation machine, however, it could not solve all our problems. It could not tell us why these effects occurred or how to make the resource better. To obtain this information, we would have to communicate directly with many of the actors in our real history in order to understand how they used the resource and their views of the experience. There is usually more to evaluation than demonstrations of effects.

In part because there is no evaluation machine, but also because ways are needed to answer additional important questions for which the machine would be of little help, there can be no single solution to the problem of evaluation. There is, instead, an interdisciplinary field of evaluation with an extensive methodological literature.[2-4] This literature details many diverse approaches to evaluation, all of which are currently in use. These approaches will be introduced later in the chapter. The approaches differ in the kinds of questions that are seen as primary, how specific questions get onto the agenda, and the data-collection methods ultimately used to answer these questions. In informatics, it is important that such a range of methods is available because the questions of interest can vary dramatically—from the focused and outcome-oriented (Does implementation of this resource affect morbidity and/or mortality?) to the practical, and market-oriented questions, such as those frequently stated by Barnett:[†]

1. Is the system used by real people with real patients?
2. Is the system being paid for with real money?
3. Has someone else taken the system, modified it, and claimed they developed it?

Evaluation is challenging in large part because there are so many options and there is almost never an obvious best way to proceed. The following points bear repeating:

1. In any evaluation setting, there are many potential questions to address. What questions are asked shapes (but does not totally determine) what answers are generated.
2. There may be little consensus on what constitutes the best set of questions.
3. There are many ways to address these questions, each with advantages and disadvantages.
4. There is no such thing as a perfect evaluation.

Individuals conducting evaluations are in a continuous process of compromise and accommodation. At its root, the challenge of evaluation is to

---

[†] These questions were given to the authors in a personal communication on December 8, 1995. A slightly different version of these questions is found on page 286 of Blum.[5]

collect and communicate useful information while acting in this spirit of compromise and accommodation.

Deeper Definitions of Evaluation

Not surprisingly, there is no single accepted definition of evaluation. A useful goal for the reader may be to evolve a personal definition that makes sense, can be concisely articulated, and can be publicly defended without obvious embarrassment. The reader is advised not to settle firmly on a definition now. It is likely to change many times based on later chapters of this book and other experiences. To begin development of a personal definition, three discrete definitions from the evaluation literature are offered, along with some analysis of their similarities and differences. All three of these definitions have been modified to apply specifically to biomedical informatics.

Definition 1 (adapted from Rossi and Freeman[2]): Evaluation is the systematic application of social science research procedures to judge and improve the way information resources are designed and implemented.

Definition 2 (adapted from Guba and Lincoln[3]): Evaluation is the process of describing the implementation of an information resource and judging its merit and worth.

Definition 3 (adapted from House[4]): Evaluation is a process leading to a settled opinion that something about an information resource is the case, usually—but not always—leading to a decision to act in a certain way.

The first definition of evaluation is probably the most mainstream. It ties evaluation to the quantitative empirical methods of the social sciences. How restrictive this definition is depends, of course, on one's definition of the social sciences. The authors of this definition would certainly believe that it includes experimental and quasi-experimental methods that result in quantitative data. Judging from the contents of their book, the authors probably would not see the more qualitative methods derived from ethnography and social anthropology as highly useful in evaluation studies.** Their definition further implies that evaluations are carried out in a planned, orderly manner, and that the information collected can engender two types of results: improvement of the resource and some determination of its value.

The second definition is somewhat broader. It identifies descriptive questions (How is the resource being used?) as an important component of evaluation while implying the need for a complete evaluation to result in some type of judgment. This definition is not as restrictive in terms of the methods

---

** The authors have stated (p. 265) that "assessing impact in ways that are scientifically plausible and that yield relatively precise estimates of net effects requires data that are quantifiable and systematically and uniformly collected."

used to collect information. This openness is intentional, as these authors embrace the full gamut of methodologies, from the experimental to the anthropologic.

The third definition is the least restrictive and emphasizes evaluation as a process leading to deeper understanding and consensus. Under this definition, an evaluation could be successful even if no judgment or action resulted, so long as the study resulted in a clearer or better-shared idea by some significant group of individuals regarding the state of affairs surrounding an information resource.

When shaping a personal definition, the reader should keep in mind something implied by the above definitions, but not explicitly stated: that evaluation is an empirical process. Data of varying shapes and sizes are always collected. It is also important to view evaluation as an applied or service activity. Evaluations are tied to and shaped by the specific information resource(s) under study. Evaluation is useful to the degree that it sheds light on issues such as the need for, function of and utility of those information resources.

The Evaluation Mindset: Distinction Between Evaluation and Research

The previous sections probably make evaluation look like a difficult thing to do. If scholars of the field disagree in fundamental ways about what evaluation is and how it should be done, how can relative novices proceed at all, much less with confidence? To address this dilemma, a mindset for evaluation is introduced, a general orientation that anyone conducting any kind of evaluation might constructively bring to the undertaking. As several important characteristics of this mindset are introduced, some of the differences and similarities between evaluation and research should also come into clearer focus.

1. *Tailor the study to the problem.* Every evaluation is made to order. Evaluation differs profoundly from mainstream views of research in that an evaluation derives importance from the needs of an identified set of "clients" (those with the "need to know") rather than the open questions of an academic discipline. Many evaluations also contribute new knowledge of general importance to an academic discipline. While such contributions are always desirable, they should be viewed as a serendipitous by-product of evaluation.

2. *Collect data useful for making decisions.* As discussed previously, there is no theoretical limit to the questions that can be asked and, consequently, to the data that can be collected in an evaluation study. What is done is primarily determined by the decisions that ultimately need to be made and the information seen as useful to inform these decisions. Evaluators must

be sensitive to the distinction between what is necessary (to inform key decisions) versus what is "merely" interesting.[5]

3. *Look for intended and unintended effects.* Whenever a new information resource is introduced into an environment, there can be many consequences. Only some of them relate to the stated purpose of the resource. During a complete evaluation, it is important to look for and document effects that were anticipated, as well as those that were not, and continue the study long enough to allow these effects to manifest. The literature of innovation is replete with examples of unintended consequences. During the 1940s, rural farmers in Georgia were trained and encouraged to preserve their vegetables in jars in large quantities to ensure they would have a balanced diet throughout the winter. The campaign was so successful that the number of jars on display in the farmers' homes became a source of prestige. Once the jars became a prestige factor, however, the farmers were disinclined to consume them, so the original purpose of the training was subverted.[6] On a topic closer to home, the QWERTY keyboard became a universal standard even though it was actually designed to *slow* typing out of concern about jamming the keys of a manual typewriter, a mechanical device that has long since vanished.[7]

4. *Study the resource while it is under development and after it is deployed.* In general, the decisions evaluation can facilitate are of two types. *Formative* decisions are made for the purpose of improving an information resource. These decisions usually are made while the resource is under development, but they can also be made after the resource is deployed. *Summative* decisions made after a resource is deployed in its envisioned environment deal explicitly with how effectively the resource performs in that environment. It can take many months, and sometimes years, for a deployed resource to stabilize within an environment. Before conducting the most useful summative studies, it may be necessary for investigators to allow this amount of time to pass.

5. *Study the resource in the laboratory and in the field.* Completely different questions arise when an information resource is still in the laboratory and when it is in the field. *In vitro* studies, conducted in the developer's laboratory, and *in situ* studies, conducted in an ongoing clinical or educational environment, are both important aspects of evaluation.

6. *Go beyond the developer's point of view.* The developers of an information resource usually are empathic only up to a point and often are not predisposed to be detached and objective about *their* system's performance. Those conducting the evaluation often see it as part of their job to get close to the end-users and portray the resource as the users experience it.[8]

7. *Take the environment into account.* Anyone who conducts an evaluation study must be, in part, an ecologist. The function of an information resource must be viewed as an interaction between the resource, a set of "users" of the resource, and the social/organizational/cultural "context,"

which does much to determine how work is carried out in that environment. Whether a new resource functions effectively is determined as much by its goodness-of-fit with its environment as by its compliance with the resource designers' operational specifications as measured in the laboratory.

8. *Let the key issues emerge over time.* Evaluation studies are a dynamic process. The design for an evaluation, as it might be stated in a project proposal, is typically just a starting point. Rarely are the important questions known with total precision or confidence at the outset of a study. In the real world, evaluation designs must be allowed to evolve as the important issues come into focus. As will be seen later in this chapter, some approaches to evaluation are more conducive to such evolution than are others.

9. *Be methodologically Catholic and eclectic.* It is necessary to derive data-collection methods from the questions to be explored, rather than bringing some predetermined methods or instruments to a study. Some questions are better addressed with qualitative data collected through open-ended interviews and observation. Others are better addressed with quantitative data collected via structured questionnaires, patient chart audits, or logs of user behavior. For evaluation, quantitative data are not clearly superior to qualitative data. Most comprehensive studies use data of both types. Accordingly, those who conduct evaluations must know rigorous methods for collection and analysis of both types.

This evaluator's mindset is different from that of a traditional researcher. The primary difference is in the binding of the evaluator to a "client," who may be one or two individuals, a large group, or several groups who share a "need to know" but may be interested in many different things. What these clients want to know—not what the evaluator wants to know—largely determines the evaluation agenda. By contrast, the researcher's allegiance is usually to a focused question or problem. In research, a question with no immediate impact on what is done in the world can still be important. Within the evaluation mindset, this is not the case. Although many important scientific discoveries have been accidental, researchers as a rule do not actively seek out unanticipated effects. Evaluators often do. Whereas researchers usually value focus and seek to exclude from a study as many extraneous variables as possible, evaluators usually seek to be comprehensive. A complete evaluation of a resource focuses on developmental as well as in-use issues. In research, laboratory studies often carry more credibility because they are conducted under controlled circumstances and they can illuminate cause and effect relatively unambiguously. During evaluation, field studies often carry more credibility because they illustrate more directly (although perhaps less definitively) the utility of the resource. Researchers can afford to, and often must, lock themselves into a single data-collection paradigm. Even within a single study, evaluators often employ many paradigms.

Anatomy of Evaluation Studies

Despite the fact that there are no a priori questions and a plethora of approaches, there are some structural elements that all evaluation studies have in common. As stated above, evaluations are guided by the need to know of some individual or group. No matter who that someone is—the development team, funding agency, or other individuals and groups—the evaluation must begin with a process of negotiation to identify the questions that will be a starting point for the study. The outcomes of these negotiations are a mutual understanding of why and how the evaluation is to be conducted, usually stated in a written contract or agreement, as well as an initial expression of the questions the evaluation seeks to answer. The next element of the study is investigation, the collection of data to address these questions, and, depending on the approach selected, possibly other questions that arise during the study. The modes of investigation are numerous, ranging from the performance of the resource on a series of benchmark tasks to observation of users working with the resource.

The next element is a mechanism for reporting the information back to those individuals with the need to know. The format of the report must be in line with the stipulations of the contract; the content of the report follows from the questions asked and the data collected. The report is most often a written document, but it does not have to be. The purposes of some evaluations are well served by oral reports or live demonstrations. It is the evaluator's obligation to establish a process through which the results of his or her study are communicated, thus creating the potential for the study's findings to be put to constructive use. No investigator can guarantee a constructive outcome for a study, but there is much that can be done to increase the likelihood of a salutary result. In addition, note that a salutary result of a study is not necessarily one that casts in a positive light the resource under study. A salutary result is one where the "stakeholders" learn something important from the study findings.

The diagram of Figure 2.2 may seem unnecessarily complicated to students or researchers who are building their own information resource and

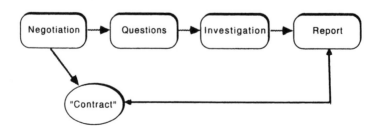

FIGURE 2.2. Anatomy of an evaluation study.

wish to evaluate it in a preliminary way. To these individuals, a word of caution is offered. Even when they appear simple and straightforward at the outset, evaluations have a way of becoming complex. Much of this book deals with these complexities and how they can be anticipated and managed.

Philosophical Bases of Evaluation

Several authors have developed classifications (or "typologies") of evaluation methods or approaches. Among the best was that developed in 1980 by Ernest House.[4] A major advantage of House's typology is that each approach is elegantly linked to an underlying philosophical model, as detailed in his book. This classification divides current practice into eight discrete approaches, four of which may be viewed as "objectivist" and four as "subjectivist." This distinction is important. Note that these approaches are *not* entitled "objective" and "subjective," as those words carry strong and fundamentally misleading connotations: of scientific precision in the former case and of imprecise intellectual voyeurism in the latter.

The objectivist approaches derive from a logical–positivist philosophical orientation—the same orientation that underlies the classical experimental sciences. The major premises underlying the objectivist approaches are as follows.

- Information resources, the people who use them, and the processes they affect, all have attributes that can be measured. All observations of these attributes will ideally yield the same results. Any variation in these results would be attributed to measurement error. It is also assumed that an investigator can measure these attributes without affecting how the resource under study functions or is used.
- Rational persons can and should agree on what attributes of a resource are important to measure and what results of these measurements would be identified as a most desirable, correct, or positive outcome. If a consensus does not exist initially among these rational persons, they can be brought to consensus over time.
- While it is possible to disprove a well-formulated scientific hypothesis, it is never possible to fully prove one; thus, science proceeds by successive disproof of previously plausible hypotheses.
- Because numerical measurement allows precise statistical analysis of performance over time or performance in comparison with some alternative, numerical measurement is *prima facie* superior to a verbal description. Qualitative data may be useful in preliminary studies to identify hypotheses for subsequent, precise analysis using quantitative methods.

- Through these kinds of comparisons, it is possible to prove beyond reasonable doubt that a resource is superior to what it replaced or to some competing resource.

Chapters 4 through 8 of this book explore these issues and address objectivist methods in detail.

Contrast the above with a set of assumptions that derive from an "intuitionist–pluralist" worldview that gives rise to a set of subjectivist approaches to evaluation.

- What is observed about a resource depends in fundamental ways on the observer. Different observers of the same phenomenon might legitimately come to different conclusions. Both can be "objective" in their appraisals even if they do not agree. It is not necessary that one is right and the other wrong.
- It does not make sense to speak of the attributes of a resource without considering its context. The value of a resource emerges through study of the resource as it functions in a particular patient-care scientific or educational environment.
- Individuals and groups can legitimately hold different perspectives on what constitutes desirable outcomes of introducing a resource into an environment. There is no reason to expect them to agree, and it may be counterproductive to try to lead them to consensus. An important aspect of an evaluation would be to document the ways in which they disagree.
- Verbal description can be highly illuminating. Qualitative data are valuable in and of themselves and can lead to conclusions as convincing as those drawn from quantitative data. Therefore, the value of qualitative data goes far beyond that of identifying issues for later "precise" exploration using quantitative methods.
- Evaluation should be viewed as an exercise in argument, rather than demonstration, because any study, as House[4] points out (p. 72), appears equivocal when subjected to serious scrutiny.

The approaches to evaluation that derive from this subjectivist philosophical perspective may seem strange, imprecise, and "unscientific" when considered for the first time. This stems in large part from widespread acceptance of the objectivist world-view in biomedicine. The importance and utility of subjectivist approaches to evaluation are emerging, however. Within biomedical informatics, there is growing support for such approaches.[8–10] As has been stated previously, the evaluation mindset includes methodological eclecticism. It is important for those trained in classical experimental methods at least to understand, and possibly even to embrace, the subjectivist worldview if they are going to conduct fully informative evaluation studies. Chapters 9 and 10 of this book address subjectivist approaches in detail.

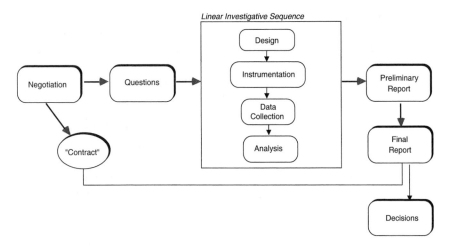

FIGURE 2.3. Specific anatomy of objectivist studies.

The General Anatomy Revisited

Having described a general anatomy of all evaluation studies, and then divided the universe of studies into two groups, it is reasonable to ask how this general anatomy differs across the groups before proceeding to describe all eight approaches in House's typology. Figure 2.3 illustrates the typical anatomy of an objectivist study, and Figure 2.4 does the same for a subjectivist study. The differences are seen primarily in the "investigation" aspect of the process.

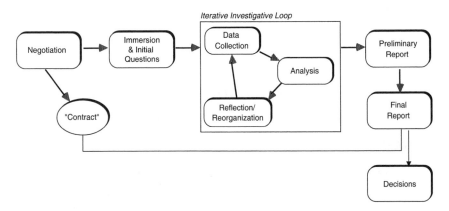

FIGURE 2.4. Specific anatomy of subjectivist studies.

The investigation aspect of objectivist studies can be seen as a *Linear Investigative Sequence* proceeding from detailed design of the study, to the development of instruments for collection of quantitative data, and then to the collection and subsequent analysis of these data. In principle, at least, the investigators go through this investigative sequence once and proceed from there to report their findings.

By contrast, the subjectivist investigation is organized along the lines of an *Iterative Investigative Loop*. The investigation proceeds through cycles of primarily qualitative data collection and analysis of these data, followed by a stage of reflection on what has been learned and reorganization of the investigators beliefs. Because of the investigators' reflection and reorganization within each cycle of the loop, it is possible for entirely new evaluation questions to arise for exploration in subsequent cycles. In later chapters, it will be seen that knowing when to exit from the loop is a major methodological issue for subjectivist investigations. The subjectivist approaches also include, as a key step, a period of "immersion" into the environment under study—the process of becoming familiar with, and familiar to, those in the environment.

Multiple Approaches to Evaluation

House[3] classified evaluation into eight archetypal approaches, four of which can be viewed as objectivist and four as subjectivist. Although most evaluation studies conducted in the real world can be unambiguously tied to one of these approaches, some studies exhibit properties of several approaches and cannot be cleanly classified. The label "approach" has been deliberately chosen, so it is not confused with "methods." In later chapters, methods will be referred to specifically as the procedures for collecting and analyzing data, whereas an evaluation approach is a broader term, connoting the strategy directing the design and execution of an entire study. Following this exposition of eight approaches is an exercise for the reader to classify each of a set of evaluation studies in biomedical informatics into one of these categories.

Approaches Rooted in Objectivist Assumptions

The first four approaches derive from the objectivist philosophical position.

Comparison-Based Approach

The comparison-based approach employs experiments and quasi-experiments. The information resource under study is compared to a control condition, a placebo, or a contrasting resource. The comparison is based on a relatively small number of "outcome variables" that are assessed in all groups. This approach thus seeks to simulate the "evaluation machine" using randomization, controls, and statistical inference to argue that the information resource was the cause of any differences observed. Examples of comparison-based studies include the work of McDonald and colleagues on physician reminders,[11] the studies from Stanford on rule-based diagnostic systems,[12] and the work of Evans and colleagues on decision support in antibiotic prescribing.[13] The controlled trials of medical decision support systems, first reviewed systematically by Johnson and colleagues,[14] and later by Hunt and colleagues,[15] fall under the comparison-based approach. The Turing test[16] can be seen as a specific model for a comparison-based evaluation.

Objectives-Based Approach

The objectives-based approach seeks to determine if a resource meets its designers' objectives. Ideally, such objectives are stated in detail. This minimizes the ambiguity faced by evaluators when developing procedures to measure the degree of attainment of these objectives. These studies are comparative only in the sense that the observed performance of the resource is viewed in relation to stated objectives. The concern is whether the resource is performing up to expectations, not if the resource is outperforming what it replaced. The objectives that are the benchmarks for these studies are typically stated at an early stage of resource development. Although clearly suited to laboratory testing of a new resource, this approach can also be applied to testing a deployed resource as well. Consider the example of a resource to provide advice to emergency room physicians.[17] The designers might set as an objective that the system's advice be available within 10 minutes of the time the patient is first seen. An objectives-based evaluation study would measure the time for this advice to be delivered and compare it to the pre-stated objective.

Decision-Facilitation Approach

With the decision-facilitation approach, evaluation seeks to resolve issues important to developers and administrators, so these individuals can make decisions about the future of the resource. The questions posed are those that the decision-makers state, although those conducting the evaluation may help the decision-makers frame these questions so they are more amenable to empirical study. The data-collection methods follow from the questions posed. These studies tend to be "formative" in focus. The results of studies conducted at the early stages of resource development are used to chart the course of further development, which in turn generates new questions for further study. A systematic study of alternative formats for computer-generated advisories, conducted while the resource to generate the advisories is still under development, provides a good example of this approach.[18]

Goal-Free Approach

With the three approaches described above, the evaluation is guided by a set of goals for the information resource. Therefore, any study is polarized by these manifest goals and is much more sensitive to anticipated rather than unanticipated effects. With the "goal-free" approach, those conducting the evaluation are purposefully blinded to the intended effects of an information resource and pursue whatever evidence they can gather to enable them to identify all the effects of the resource, regardless of whether or not these are intended.[19] This approach is rarely applied in practice, but it is useful to individuals designing evaluations to remind them of the multiplicity of effects an information resource can engender.

Approaches Rooted in Subjectivist Assumptions

There are four subjectivist approaches to evaluation.

Quasi-Legal Approach

The quasi-legal approach establishes a mock trial, or other formal adversary proceeding, to judge a resource. Proponents and opponents of the resource offer testimony and may be examined and cross-examined in a manner resembling standard courtroom procedure. Based on this testimony, a jury witness to the proceeding can then make a decision about the merit of the resource. As in a debate, the issue can be decided by the persuasive power of rhetoric, as well as the persuasive power of that which is portrayed as fact. There are few published examples of this technique formally applied to informatics, but the technique has been applied to facilitate difficult decisions in other biomedical areas.[20]

Art Criticism Approach

The art criticism approach relies on formal methods of criticism and the principle of "connoisseurship."[21] Under this approach, an experienced and respected critic, who may or may not be trained in the domain of the resource but has a great deal of experience with resources of this generic type, works with the resource over a period. She or he then writes a review highlighting the benefits and shortcomings of the resource. Within informatics, the art criticism approach may be of limited value if the critic is not expert in the subject-matter domain of the biomedical information resource under review. For example, if the resource provides advice to users or automates a task that was heretofore performed manually, a critic without domain knowledge could offer useful insights about the resource's general functioning and ease of use, but would be unable to judge whether the automated task was carried out properly or whether the advice provided was clinically or scientifically valid. Because society does not routinely expect critics to agree, the potential lack of interobserver agreement does not invalidate this approach. Although they tend to be more informal and tend to reflect less direct experience with the resource than would be the case in a complete "art criticism" study, software reviews that routinely appear in technical journals and magazines are examples of this approach in common practice.

Professional Review Approach

The professional review approach is the well-known "site visit" approach to evaluation. It employs panels of experienced peers who spend several days in the environment where the resource is deployed. Site visits often are directed by a set of guidelines specific to the type of project under study but sufficiently generic to accord the reviewers a great deal of control over the conduct of any particular visit. They are generally free to speak with whomever they wish and to ask of these individuals whatever they consider important to know. They may request documents for review. Over the course of a site visit, unanticipated issues may emerge. Site visit teams frequently have interim meetings to identify these emergent questions and generate ways to explore them. As a field matures, it becomes possible to articulate formal review criteria that could be the focus of site visits, supporting application of the professional review approach. In biomedical informatics, the evolving evaluation criteria for computer-based patient records[22] is one example of such guidelines.

Responsive/Illuminative Approach

The responsive/illuminative approach seeks to represent the viewpoints of those who are users of the resource or an otherwise significant part of the environment where the resource operates.[23] The goal is understanding, or "illumination," rather than judgment. The methods used derive largely from ethnography. The investigators immerse themselves in the environment where the resource is operational. The designs of these studies are not rigidly predetermined. They develop dynamically as the investigators' experience accumulates. The study team begins with a minimal set of orienting questions; the deeper questions that receive thorough ongoing study evolve over time. Many examples of studies using this approach can be found in the literature of biomedical informatics.[24-27]

Self-Test 2.1

The answers to these exercises appear at the end of this chapter.

1. Associate each of the following hypothetical studies with a particular approach to evaluation. For each, try to identify a single approach that is a "best fit."
   a. A comparison of different user interfaces for a genomic sequencing tool, conducted while the resource is under development, to help the tool designers create the optimal interface.
   b. A site visit by the U.S. National Library of Medicine's Biomedical Informatics and Library Review Committee to the submitters of a competing renewal of a research grant.
   c. Inviting a noted consultant on intelligent tutoring system design to spend a day on campus to offer suggestions regarding the prototype of a new system.
   d. Conducting patient chart reviews before and after introduction of an information resource, without telling the reviewer anything about the nature of the information resource or even that the intervention was an information resource.
   e. Videotaping attending rounds on a hospital service (ward) where an information resource has been implemented and periodically interviewing members of the ward team.
   f. Determining if a new version of a proteomics database executes a standard set of performance tests at the speed the designers projected.
   g. Randomizing patients so their medical records are maintained, either by a new computer system or standard procedures, and then seeking to determine if the new system influences clinical protocol recruitment and compliance.
   h. Staging a mock debate at a health-sciences library staff retreat to decide whether the library should suspend paper subscriptions to 500 biomedical journals next year or not at all.

Why Are There So Many Approaches?

From the above examples, it should be clear that it is possible to employ almost all of these approaches to evaluation in biomedical informatics. Why, though, are there so many approaches to evaluation? The intuitive appeal—at least to those schooled in experimental science—of the comparison-based approach seems unassailable. Why do it any other way if we can demonstrate the value of an information resource, or lack thereof, definitively with a controlled study?

The goal-free approach signals one shortcoming of comparison-based studies that employ classical experimental methods. Although these studies can appear definitive when proposed, they inevitably rely on intuitive, arbitrary, or even a political choice of questions to explore or outcomes to measure. What is measured is often what *can be* measured with the kind of quantitative precision the philosophical position underlying this approach demands. It is often the case that the variables that are most readily obtainable and most accurately assessed (e.g., length of hospital stay), and which therefore are employed as outcome measures in studies, are difficult to relate directly to the effects of a biomedical information resource because there are numerous intervening or confounding factors. Studies may have null results, not because there are no effects but because these effects are not manifest in the outcome measures pursued. In other circumstances, outcomes cannot be unambiguously assigned a positive value. For example, if use of a computer-based tutorial program is found to raise medical students' national licensure examination scores, which are readily obtained and highly reliable, it usually does not settle the argument about the value of the tutorial program. Instead, it may only kindle a new argument about the validity of the examination used as an outcome measure. In the most general case, a resource produces several effects: some positive and some negative. Unless the reasons for these mixed effects can somehow be explored further, the impact of a resource cannot be comprehensively understood, or it may be seriously misestimated. When there are mixed results, oftentimes the resource is judged entirely by the single result of most interest to the group holding the greatest power. A resource that actually improves nursing care may be branded a categorical failure because it proved to be more expensive than anticipated.

Comparison-based studies are also limited in their ability to explain differences that are detected or to shed light on why, in other circumstances, no differences are found. Consider, for example, a resource developed to identify "therapeutic misadventures"—problems with drug therapy of hospitalized patients—before these problems can become medical emergencies.[28] Such a resource would employ a knowledge base encoding rules of proper therapeutic practice and would be connected to a hospital information system containing the clinical data about in-patients. When the resource detected a difference between the rules of proper practice and the data about a specific patient, it would issue an advisory to the clinicians responsible for the care of that patient. If a comparison-based study of this system's effectiveness employed only global outcome measures, such as length of stay or morbidity and mortality, and the study yielded null results, it would not be clear what to conclude. It may be that the resource is having no beneficial effect, but it also may be that a problem with the implementation of the system—which, if detected, can be rectified—is accounting for the null results. The failure of the system to deliver the advisories in a visible place in a timely fashion could account for an apparent failure of the resource. In this case, a study using the decision-facilitation approach or the responsive/illuminative approach might reveal the problem with the resource and, from the perspective of the evaluator's mindset, be a much more valuable study.

The existence of multiple alternatives to the comparison-based approach also stems from features of biomedical information resources and from the challenges, as discussed in Chapter 1, of studying these resources specifically. First, biomedical information resources are frequently revised; the system may change in significant ways for legitimate reasons before there is time to complete a comparison-based study. Second, alternative approaches are well suited to developing an understanding of how the resource works within a particular environment. The success or failure may be attributable more to match or mismatch with the environment than intrinsic properties of the resource itself. Without such understanding, it is difficult to know how exportable a particular resource is and what factors are important to explore as the resource is considered for adoption by a site other than the place of its development. Third, there is a need to understand how users employ biomedical information resources, which requires an exercise in description, not judgment or comparison. If the true benefits of information and knowledge resources emerge from interaction of person and machine, approaches to evaluation that take the nature of human cognition into account must figure into a complete set of investigative activities.[29] Finally, alternative approaches offer a unique contribution in their ability to help us understand *why* something happened in addition to *that* something happened. The results of a comparison-based study may be definitive in demonstrating that a resource had a specific impact on research, education, or patient care; but these results may tell us little about what aspect of the resource made the difference or the chain of events through which this effect was achieved.

The arguments above should be interpreted as another plea for catholicism, for open-mindedness, in evaluation. We are suggesting that a mode of study from which something important can be learned is a mode of study worth pursuing. In evaluation, the methods should follow from the questions and the context in which the evaluation is set. It is wrong to give any particular method of study higher status than the problem under study.

Roles in Evaluation Studies

Another important way to see the complexity in evaluation is via the multiple roles that are played in the conduct of each study. A review of these roles is useful to help understand the process of evaluation and to help those planning studies to anticipate everything that needs to be done. At the earliest stage of planning a study, and particularly when the evaluation contract is being negotiated, attention to these roles and their interworkings helps ensure that the contract will be complete and will serve well in guiding the conduct of the study.

These roles and how they interrelate are illustrated in Figure 2.5. It is important to note from the outset of this discussion that the same individual may play multiple roles, and some roles may be shared by multiple indi-

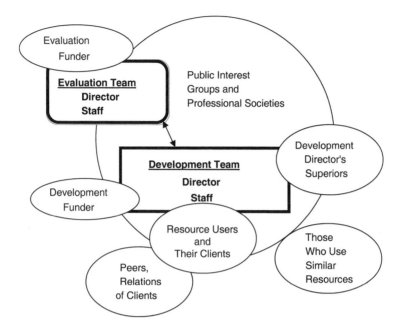

FIGURE 2.5. Roles in an evaluation study.

viduals. In general, the smaller the scale of the study, the greater the overlap in roles.

The first set of roles relates to the individuals who conduct the study. These individuals include the director of the evaluation, who is the person professionally responsible for the study, and any staff members who might work for the director. As soon as more than one person is involved in the conduct of a study, interpersonal dynamics among members of this group become an important factor contributing to the success or failure of the study.

There is a separate set of roles related directly to the development of the resource under study. Those who fulfill these roles include the director of the resource's development team, his or her staff, the users of the resource, and their clients. For an information resource supporting health care, the resource users are typically healthcare professionals and their clients are the patients receiving care.

The third set of roles includes individuals or groups (or both) who, although they are not developing the resource or otherwise direct participants in the study, nonetheless may have a profound interest in the study's outcome. In the jargon of evaluation, these individuals are generally known as "stakeholders." These individuals or groups include those who fund the development of the resource, those who fund the evaluation (who may be different from those who fund the resource), supervisors of the director of resource development, those who use similar resources in other settings, peers and relations of the clients, and a variety of public interest groups and professional societies. Each of these groups, possibly to varying extents, might have interests in the information resource itself and the effects resulting from its deployment.

At the first stage of planning a study, it is an excellent idea to make a list of these roles and indicate which individuals or groups occupy each one. Sometimes this exercise requires a few educated guesses, but it should still be undertaken at the outset.

Self-Test 2.2

Below is a description of the evaluation plan for the T-HELPER project at Stanford University.[30,31] This description is intentionally incomplete for purposes of constructing a practice exercise. After reading the description, answer each of the following questions. (Answers to questions 1 and 2 are found at the end of this chapter.)

1. Indicate who, in this study, played each of the roles discussed above and depicted in Figure 2.3.
2. The project evaluation focuses on two questions relating to protocol enrollment and user attitudes. If you were designing an evaluation to address these questions, what approach(es) would you consider using?
3. What other evaluation questions, not addressed in the study, might have been of interest for this project?

Case Study: T-HELPER: Computer Support for
Protocol-Directed Therapy

This project developed computer-based techniques for clinical data and knowledge management in the area of acquired immunodeficiency syndrome (AIDS) therapy. It also was developed to implement those methods in a system that can be used for patient care and that can be evaluated in clinical settings. Clinicians used the new system, called THERAPY-HELPER (or simply T-HELPER) to review and maintain the records of patients receiving protocol-directed therapy for human immunodeficiency virus (HIV). The entire effort was supported by a five-year grant to Stanford University from the Agency for Health Care Policy and Research (now the Agency for Healthcare Research and Quality).

The project was conducted in four stages:

1. T-HELPER I was developed to facilitate a data-management environment for patients with HIV infection. T-HELPER I provided a graphical medical record that allowed healthcare workers to review past data and to enter new information while perusing textual information regarding those protocols under which the patient is being treated or for which the patient might be eligible.

2. T-HELPER II, an enhanced version of T-HELPER I, incorporated active decision support capabilities to encourage enrollment in and compliance with protocol-based therapy.

3. T-HELPER I and T-HELPER II were installed at two large county-operated AIDS clinics in northern California: the Immunocompromised Host Clinic at ABC Medical Center and the XYZ AIDS program.

4. A rigorous evaluation of the T-HELPER systems was undertaken. The studies explored the effect of each version of the system on (i) the rate of patient enrollment in clinical trial protocols, and (ii) physician satisfaction with the T-HELPER system. The study design allowed assessment of the incremental value of the decision support functions provided in T-HELPER II.

I. *Development group*: The project was divided into three general areas of effort: (i) system development (supervised by Dr. M); (ii) system installation and user training (supervised by Dr. F); and (iii) system evaluation (supervised by Dr. C). The project was under the overall supervision of Dr. M. Several research staff members and graduate students were employed over the five years on various aspects of the project.

II. *Trial/evaluation sites*: ABC Medical Center is a 722-bed facility and a teaching hospital of the Stanford University School of Medicine. At the outset of the project, six HIV-related protocols from the California Cooperative Treatment Group (CCTG) were operative at this center. In addition, a number of privately sponsored protocols were in progress. Twenty-eight percent of HIV-infected residents in its home county seek care at ABC, a group that is estimated to be 22% Hispanic, 8% African American, 9% female, and 14% intravenous (IV) drug users. At the project outset, the XYZ AIDS clinic provided care to an estimated 377 HIV-infected patients annually. The patient population was approximately 33% African American, 16% Hispanic, 24% women, and 36% IV drug users.

III. *System installation*: Full utilization of the T-HELPER system required three main logistical requirements: (i) installing appropriate networks in the two clinics, (ii) interfacing with the registration systems at each clinic, and (iii) arranging for laboratory data connections. The networking is necessary to allow healthcare providers to use the system in multiple locations throughout the clinic: in each examination room, in each provider workroom, and in the nursing and registration work areas. Registration data connections were necessary to simplify the importing of demographic data into T-HELPER and provide data about which patients are active in the clinic at a particular time. Laboratory data were required to provide input to the decision support modules and give additional clinical information to providers that would help attract users to the workstation to complete their work. Each installation site expressed concerns about patient data confidentiality. This concern meant that the network installations had to be stand-alone and would not have any connectivity to other networked environments. Furthermore, because of differences in networking technology, it was not practical to directly link the T-HELPER network with the existing computer systems at each site. Instead, special-purpose point-to-point links were made to the registration and laboratory systems at ABC and XYZ.

IV. *System evaluation*: The primary goal of the evaluation was to determine if the T-HELPER II system increased the rate of accrual of eligible and potentially eligible patients to clinical protocols. In addition, the evaluation group examined physicians' knowledge and acceptance of the computer as an adjunct to patient care and in collaborative research. It then correlated these attitudes with use of and compliance with the T-HELPER systems.

Why It May Not Work Out as the Books Suggest

If we did possess the "evaluation machine", described earlier in this chapter, life would be easier, but not perfect. We would design and implement our information resources, let the machine tell us what would have happened had the resources not been implemented, and then compare the two scenarios. The difference would, of course, be a measure of the "effect" of the resource; but there may be many other factors, not detectable by the machine, that are important to investigate. It has been shown throughout this chapter how the unavailability of the evaluation machine, and other factors, have led many creative individuals to devise an assortment of evaluation approaches. Because of the richness and diversity of these approaches, it is safe to say that an informative study probably can be designed to address any question of substantive interest in informatics.

However, even the best-designed studies do not work out as planned. One of the worst failure scenarios occurs when apparently meritorious studies—studies of important issues and that are well designed—are not carried out. Resistance to the conduct of a study can develop either before the study is actually begun or during its progress. There are two principal reasons why this occurs. In both cases, it can be seen that attention to the roles in an evaluation (Figure 2.5) and the importance of advance negotiation of an evaluation contract can both signal problems and help the study designers navigate through them.

- *Sometimes we would rather not know* or *"fear of the clear"*: Some, perhaps many, resource developers believe they have more to lose than to gain from a thorough ongoing study of their information resource. This belief is more likely to occur in the case of a resource perceived to be functioning very successfully or in the case of a resource that generates a great deal of interest because of some novel technology it employs. There are three logical counterarguments to those who might resist a study under these circumstances: (1) the perception of the resource's success will likely be confirmed by the study; (2) the study, if it supports these perceptions, can show how and perhaps why the resource is successful; and (3) a study would generate information leading to improvement of even the most successful resource. With reference to Figure 2.5, stakeholders outside the development team can bring pressure on the resource developers to support or tolerate a study, but studies imposed under these circumstances tend to progress with great difficulty because trust does not exist between the evaluation team and the development team.

- *Differences in values*: Performance of an evaluation adds an overhead to any information technology project. It often requires the resource developers to engage in tasks they would not otherwise undertake (such as programming the resource to function in several different ways; at a minimum, it usually requires some modifications in the project's implementation timeline). If the development group does not value the information they obtain from a study, they may, for example, be unwilling to await the results of a study before designing some aspect of the resource that could be shaped by these results, or they may be reluctant to freeze production version of a system long enough for a study to be completed. Underlying differences in values also may be revealed as a form of perfectionism. The resource developers or other stakeholders may argue that less-than-perfect information is of no utility because it cannot be trusted. ("Indeed, if all evaluations are equivocal when subjected to serious scrutiny, why bother?") Because everyone on earth makes important decisions based on imperfect information every day, such a statement should not be taken literally. It is more likely revealing an underlying belief that the effort entailed in a study will not be justified by the results that will be generated. Some of these differences in belief between evaluators and resource developers can be reconciled; others cannot.

The potential for these clashes of values to occur underscores the importance of the negotiations leading to an evaluation contract. If these negotiations come to a complete halt over a specific issue, it may be indicative of a gap in values that cannot be spanned, making the study impossible. In that case, all parties are better off if this is known early. For their part, evaluators must respect the values of the developers by designing studies that have minimal detrimental impact on the project's developmental activities and timeline. It must be stressed that it is the responsibility of the evaluation team and study director to identify these potential value differences and initiate a collaborative effort to address them. The evaluation team should not expect the system developers to initiate such efforts, and under no circumstances should they defer resolution of such issues in the interest of getting a study started. When the development and evaluation teams overlap, the problem is no less sticky and requires no less attention. In this case, individuals and groups may find themselves with an internal conflict unless they engage in conversations among themselves, alternating between the developers and the evaluators' positions, about how to resolve value differences imposed by the conduct of a study in the context of resource development.

When evaluation works well, as it often does, the development and evaluation teams perceive each other as part of a common enterprise, with shared goals and interests. Communication is honest and frequent. Because no evaluation contract can anticipate every problem that may arise during the conduct of a study, problems are resolved through open discussion, using the evaluation contract as a basis. Most problems are resolved through compromise.

Conclusion

Evaluation, like biomedical informatics itself, is a derivative field. What is done—the specific questions asked and the data collected to illuminate these questions—derives from what interested individuals want to know. In Chapter 3, a catalog of evaluation questions will be presented that are pertinent to biomedical informatics in order to give enhanced shape and substance to our often-repeated claim about the large numbers of questions that exist. A classification of the "kinds" of studies people in informatics tend to undertake also will be presented. These catalogs and typologies are too general to offer more than a first level of guidance to designers of a study. The significant issues to investigate are specific to the resource in question and the environment, current or projected, in which the resource is or will be deployed.

Food for Thought

To deepen your understanding of the concepts presented in this and the previous chapter, you may wish to consider the following questions:

1. Are there any a priori evaluation questions in biomedical informatics, or questions that must be a part of every evaluation?

2. In your opinion, what is the difference between research and evaluation in biomedical informatics?

3. Do you believe that independent, unbiased observers of the same behavior or outcome should agree on the *quality* of that outcome?

4. Many of the evaluation approaches assert that a single unbiased observer is a legitimate source of information during an evaluation,

even if that observer's data or judgments are unsubstantiated by others. Can you offer some examples in our society where we vest important decisions in a single experienced and presumed impartial individual?

5. Do you agree with the statement that all evaluations appear equivocal when subjected to serious scrutiny?

Answers to Self-Tests

Self-Test 2.1

Question 1

a. Decision-facilitation
b. Professional review
c. Art criticism
d. Goal-free
e. Responsive/illuminative
f. Objectives-based
g. Comparison-based
h. Quasi-legal

Self-Test 2.2

1. *Evaluation funder*: Agency for Health Care Policy and Research (now AHRQ). *Evaluation team*: Director was Dr. C with unnamed staff. *Development funder*: Agency for Health Care Policy and Research. *Development team*: Director was Dr. M. (subdivided into two groups under Dr. M and Dr. F). *Clients*: The care providers at ABC and XYZ, as well as the patients with HIV, who use these facilities. *Development director's superiors*: Unnamed individuals at Stanford University who direct the center or department in which the project was based. *Peers, relations of clients*: Friends and relatives of HIV patients and care providers at the two clinics. *Those who use similar resources*: The community of care providers who work with HIV patients who are on clinical protocols. *Public-interest groups and professional societies*: The full gamut of patient support and advocacy groups, as well as professional societies, relating to AIDS/HIV.

2. The first evaluation question, as stated, seems best suited to a comparison-based approach. The second question also could be addressed by the comparison-based approach, but it would also be well served by a subjectivist, responsive/illuminative approach. Note that, because this study was federally sponsored, the professional review approach also may have been used, as it is not unusual for a project of this duration and extent to be site visited at some point.

References

1. Rothman KJ, Greenland S. *Modern Epidemiology*. Philadelphia, PA: Lippen-cott-Raven; 1998.
2. Rossi PH, Freeman HE. *Evaluation: A Systematic Approach*. Newbury Park, CA: Sage; 1989.
3. Guba EG, Lincoln YS. *Effective Evaluation*. San Francisco, CA: Jossey-Bass; 1981.
4. House ER. *Evaluating with Validity*. Beverly Hills, CA: Sage, 1980.
5. Miller PL, Sittig DF. The evaluation of clinical decision support systems: what is necessary versus what is interesting. Med Inform 1990;15:185–190.
6. Rogers EM, Shoemaker FF. *Communication of Innovations*. New York: Free Press; 1971.
7. Blum BI. *Clinical Information Systems*. New York: Springer-Verlag; 1986.
8. Forsythe DE, Buchanan BG. Broadening our approach to evaluating biomed-ical information systems. Symp Comput Applications Med Care 1992;16:8–12.
9. Anderson JG, Aydin CE, Jay SJ, eds. *Computers in Health Care: Research and Evaluation*. Newbury Park, CA: Sage; 1995.
10. Sackett DL, Wennberg JE. Choosing the best research design for each question: It's time to stop squabbling over the "best" methods. BMJ 1997;315:16–36.
11. McDonald CJ, Hui SL, Smith DM, et al. Reminders to physicians from an intro-spective computer medical record: a two-year randomized trial. Ann Intern Med 1984;100:130–138.
12. Yu VL, Fagan LM, Wraith SM, et al. Antimicrobial selection by computer: a blinded evaluation by infectious disease experts. JAMA 1979;242:1279–1282.
13. Evans RS, Pestotnik SL, Classen DC, Clemmer TP, Weaver LK, Orme JF Jr, Lloyd JF, Burke JP. A computer-assisted management program for antibiotics and other antiinfective agents. N Engl J Med 1998 Jan 22;338(4):232–238.
14. Johnston ME, Langton KB, Haynes RB, Matthieu D. A critical appraisal of research on the effects of computer-based decision support systems on clinician performance and patient outcomes. Ann Intern Med 1994;120:135–142.
15. Hunt DL, Haynes RB, Hanna SF, Smith K. Effects of computer-based clinical decision support systems on physician performance and patient outcomes: a sys-tematic review. JAMA 1998;280:1339–1346.
16. Turing AM. Computing machinery and intelligence. Mind Q Rev Psychol Philos 1950;59:433–460.
17. Wyatt J. Lessons learned from the field trial of ACORN, an expert system to advise on chest pain. In: Barber B, Cao D, Qin D, eds. *Proceedings of the Sixth World Conference on Medical Informatics, Singapore*. Amsterdam: North Holland; 1989:111–115.
18. De Bliek R, Friedman CP, Speedie SM, Blaschke TF, France CL. Practitioner preferences and receptivity for patient-specific advice from therapeutic moni-toring system. Symp Comput Applications Med Care 1988;12:225–228.
19. Scriven M. Goal free evaluation. In: House ER, ed. *School Evaluation*. Berke-ley, CA: McCutchan; 1973.
20. Smith R. Using a mock trial to make a difficult clinical decision. BMJ 1992;305:284–287.
21. Eisner EW. *The Enlightened Eye: Qualitative Inquiry and the Enhancement of Educational Practice*. New York: Macmillan; 1991.

22. CPR Systems Evaluation Work Group. CPR Project Evaluation Criteria (version 2.1), The Nicholas E. Davies Recognition Program. Schaumberg, IL; 1996.
23. Hamilton D, MacDonald B, King C, Jenkins D, Parlett M, eds. *Beyond the Numbers Game.* Berkeley, CA: McCutchan; 1977.
24. Kaplan B, Duchon D. Combining qualitative and quantitative methods in information systems research: a case study. MIS Q 1988;4:571–586.
25. Fafchamps D, Young CY, Tang PC. Modelling work practices: input to the design of a physician's workstation. Symp Comput Applications Med Care 1991;15:788–792.
26. Forsythe D. Using ethnography to build a working system: rethinking basic design assumptions. Symp Comput Applications Med Care 1992;16:505–509.
27. Ash JS, Gorman PN, Lavelle M, Payne TH, Massaro TA, Frantz GL, Lyman JA. A cross-site qualitative study of physician order entry. J Am Med Inform Assoc 2003;10:188–200.
28. Speedie SM, Skarupa S, Oderda L, et al. MENTOR: continuously monitoring drug therapy with an expert system. MEDINFO 1986:237–239.
29. Patel V, Kaufman D. Medical informatics and the science of cognition. J Am Med Inform Assoc 1998;5:493–502.
30. Musen MA, Carlson RW, Fagan LM, Deresinski SC, Shortliffe EH. T-HELPER: automated support for community-based clinical research. Symp Comput Applications Med Care 1992;16:719–723.
31. Musen MA. Computer Support for Protocol-Directed Therapy. Final Report of AHCPR Grant HS06330, August 1995.

3
Determining What to Study

In Chapter 1, the challenges of conducting evaluations in biomedical informatics were introduced, and the specific sources of complexity that give rise to these challenges were discussed. In Chapter 2, the range of approaches that can be used to conduct evaluations in biomedical informatics and across many areas of human endeavor was introduced. Chapter 2 also stressed that the investigator can address many of these challenges by viewing each evaluation study as anchored by specific purposes. Each study is conducted for some identifiable client group, often to inform specific decisions that must be made by members of that group. The work of the investigator is made possible by focusing on the specific purposes the particular study is designed to address, often framing them as a set of questions, and choosing the approach or approaches best suited to those purposes. A study is successful if it provides credible information to help members of an identified audience make decisions.

In this chapter, the focus returns to informatics per se as we explore the specific purposes of evaluation studies of information resources in biomedical settings. The emphasis changes from *how* to study to *what* to study. Whereas, in Chapter 2, a tour of the various evaluation approaches was provided, in this chapter a tour of evaluation purposes is provided that ranges from validation of the need for an information resource to exploration of its impact on healthcare or research outcomes after it is deployed. The specific characteristics of information resources that can be studied will also be introduced. Although discussion in this chapter is largely weighted toward clinical information resources, much of what follows also applies to resources that support biomedical research, education, and administration.

The approach in Chapter 2, and to a significant degree that of this chapter, is to provide a comprehensive listing of what is possible in designing and conducting evaluations. By alerting the reader to all of the options and breaking them down into logical groupings, this "cataloging" approach can simplify the study design process by allowing the investigator to choose designs and methods from a list rather than having to invent them. This strategy also helps ensure that important options for conducting a study are not overlooked. To provide somewhat more-detailed guidance about choosing what to study (and with what methods) in particular situations, four typical evaluation scenarios will be introduced later in this chapter, along with an explanation of how to employ these as examples. These scenarios will illustrate general strategies employed by experienced investigators to identify specific evaluation questions.

Even experienced investigators wrestle with the problem of deciding what to study and how. There is, unfortunately, no formula, and every evaluation, to some significant degree, must be custom designed. In the end, decisions about what evaluation questions to pursue and how to pursue them are exquisitely sensitive to each study's special circumstances and constrained by the resources that are available for it. Evaluation is very much the art of the possible. Later in this chapter (page 73), the formal technique of "option appraisal" will be introduced, accompanied by an explanation of how this method can sometimes be used to help unravel the difficult decision for investigators about what priority to give to each of the many evaluation questions that usually arise as candidates for study.

However, before even thinking about the range of evaluation questions that can be asked, the first issue we need to address is: why worry about defining evaluation questions at all.

The Importance of Identifying Questions

Figure 3.1, first introduced in Chapter 2 but repeated here, can be used as a framework for planning all evaluation studies. The first stage in any study is negotiation—identifying the broad aim and objectives of the study, what kind of deliverables are required, who has interests in or otherwise will be concerned about the study results, where the study personnel will be based, the resources available (including timeline for deliverables), and any constraints on what can be studied. This negotiation process also will usually

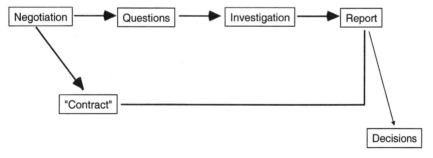

FIGURE 3.1. A framework for planning evaluation studies (repeated here from Chapter 2).

establish the broad scope of the study: Does it encompass technical issues (e.g., the reliability of the hardware that powers the resource), issues relating to people (such as user attitudes)—or more far-reaching issues such as the cost and efficiency of work within the organization?

Once the study's scope has been established, the next step is to convert the perspectives of the concerned parties, and what these individuals or groups want to know, into a finite set of questions. It is important to recognize that, for any evaluation setting that is interesting enough to merit formal evaluation, the number of potential questions is infinite. The essential step of identifying a tractable number of questions has a number of benefits:

- It helps to crystallize thinking of both investigators and key members of the audience who are the "stakeholders" in the evaluation.
- It guides the investigators and clients through the critical process of assigning priority to certain issues, thus productively narrowing the focus of a study.
- It converts broad statements of aim (e.g., "to evaluate a new order communications system") into specific questions that can potentially be answered (e.g., "What is the impact of the order communications system on how clinical staff spend their time, the rate and severity of adverse drug events, and length of patient stay?").
- It allows different stakeholders in the evaluation process—patients, professional groups, managers—to see the extent to which their own concerns are being addressed and to ensure that these feed into the evaluation process.
- Most important, perhaps, it is hard, if not impossible, to develop investigative methods without first identifying questions, or at least focused issues, for exploration. The choice of methods follows from the evaluation questions, not from the novel technology powering the information resource or the type of resource being studied. Some investigators choose to apply the same set of the methods to any study, irrespective of the questions to be addressed, or choose to emphasize evaluation questions compatible with the methods they prefer. This approach is not endorsed by the authors.

It is also important to distinguish between informal evaluations, which people undertake continuously as they make choices as part of their everyday personal or professional lives, from the formal evaluations that conform to the architecture of Figure 3.1. In these formal evaluations, the questions that are addressed are those that survive a narrowing process that begins with discussions involving stakeholder groups and conclusions that are ratified by those paying for the study or otherwise in a position of authority. Therefore, when starting a formal evaluation, a major decision is whom to consult to establish the questions that will get "on the table," how to log and analyze their views, and what weight to place on each of these views.

There is always a range of potential players in any evaluation (see Chapter 2), and there is no formula directing whom to consult or in what order. The investigators will apply their common sense and learn to follow their instincts; it is often useful to establish a steering group to advise on whose concerns are most relevant.

Through discussions with various stakeholder groups, the hard decisions regarding the scope of the study are made. A significant challenge for investigators is the risk of being swamped in detail created by the multiplicity of questions that can be asked in any study. To manage through the process, it is useful to reflect on the major issues identified after each round of discussions with stakeholders and then identify the questions that address these issues. Where possible, it is helpful to keep questions at the same level of granularity. Some investigators find tools for issue tracking, such as white boards, Post-It notes, or mind-mapping software, useful. What is important at this stage is to keep a sense of perspective, distinguishing the issues as they arise and organizing them into some kind of hierarchy; for example, with low-, medium-, and high-level issues. Inter-dependencies should be noted and care should be taken to avoid intermingling global issues with more focused issues. For example, when evaluating an electronic lab notebook system for researchers, it is important to distinguish focused, low-level issues such as the time taken for users to enter data from global issues such as the impact of the resource on research productivity.

To help investigators in their study planning, the full range of what can potentially be studied will be listed, as well as what can be derived from this and a catalogue of nine study types relevant to evaluation across all of biomedical informatics. To both ensure that the most important questions do get "on the table" and to help eliminate the less-important ones, it can be useful to start with such a comprehensive list.

The Full Range of What Can Be Formally Studied

In relation to biomedical settings, there are five major aspects of an information resource that can be studied:

1. Need for the resource: Investigators study the status quo *absent* the resource, including the nature of problems the resource is intended to address and how frequently these problems arise.
2. Design and development process: Investigators study the skills of the resource development team and the development methodologies employed by the team to understand if the resulting resource is likely to function as intended.
3. Resource static structure: Here, the focus of the evaluation includes specifications, flow charts, program code, and other representations of the resource that can be inspected without actually running it.

4. Resource usability and dynamic functions: The focus is on the usability of the resource and how it performs when it is used in studies prior to full deployment.
5. Resource effect and impact: Finally, after deployment, the focus switches from the resource itself to its effects on users, patients, and healthcare organizations.

In a theoretically "complete" evaluation, sequential studies of a particular resource might address all of these aspects over the life cycle of the resource. In the real world, however, it is difficult, and rarely necessary, to be so comprehensive. Over the course of its development and deployment, a resource may be studied many times, with the studies in their totality touching on many or most of these aspects. Some aspects of an information resource will be studied informally using anecdotal data collected via casual methods. Other aspects will be studied more formally in ways that are purposefully designed to inform specific decisions and that involve systematic collection and analysis of data. Distinguishing those aspects that will be studied formally from those left for informal exploration is a major goal of negotiations conducted with the stakeholders.

Nine Study Types

By bringing into consideration some additional factors that shape evaluation studies, these five foci for evaluation can be expanded into nine important evaluation study types, described below and summarized in Table 3.1. Each study type is likely to appeal to certain stakeholders in the evaluation process, as suggested in the rightmost column of the table. Both objectivist and subjectivist evaluation methods can be used to answer the questions embraced by all nine study types.

Table 3.1 is generated with an emphasis on the purpose of the study (the "what") as opposed to the approaches or methods of investigation (the "how") that were discussed in Chapter 2. The reader may wish to read across each row of the table to obtain an understanding of the contrasts among these study types. Table 3.2, later in this chapter, follows a similar pattern, but portrays the study type with the version of the resource needed, the setting in which it occurs, who uses the resource during the study, the kinds of tasks for which the resource is employed, and the kinds of measures that need to be made during the study. The paragraphs that follow, along with the four evaluation scenarios and Self-Test 3.1, provide an opportunity to explore these contrasts in more detail.

Needs Assessment

Needs assessment seeks to clarify the information problem the resource is intended to solve, as discussed further in Scenario 1 (page 62). These studies take place before the resource is designed. They usually take place in the

TABLE 3.1. Classification of generic study types by broad study questions and the stakeholders most concerned.

Study type	Aspect studied	Broad study question	Audience/stakeholders primarily interested in results
1. Needs assessment	Need for the resource	What is the problem?	Resource developers, funders of the resource
2. Design validation	Design and development process	Is the development method in accord with accepted practices?	Funders of the resource; professional and governmental certification agencies
3. Structure validation	Resource static structure	Is the resource appropriately designed to function as intended?	Professional indemnity insurers, resource developers; professional and governmental certification agencies
4. Usability test	Resource dynamic usability and function	Can intended users navigate the resource so it carries out intended functions?	Resource developers, users
5. Laboratory function study	Resource dynamic usability and function	Does the resource have the potential to be beneficial?	Resource developers, funders, users, academic community
6. Field function study	Resource dynamic usability and function	Does the resource have the potential to be beneficial in the real world?	Resource developers, , funders users
7. Lab user effect study	Resource effect and impact	Is the resource likely to change user behavior?	Resource developers and funders, users
8. Field user effect study	Resource effect and impact	Does the resource change actual user behavior in ways that are positive?	Resource users and their clients, resource purchasers and funders
9. Problem impact study	Resource effect and impact	Does the resource have a positive impact on the original problem?	The universe of stakeholders

setting where the resource is to be deployed, although simulated settings may sometimes be used to study problems in communication or decision-making, as long as the potential users of the resource are included. Ideally, these potential users will be studied while they work with real problems or cases to clarify how information is used and communicated, as well as identify the causes and consequences of inadequate information flows. The investigator seeks to understand users' skills, knowledge, and attitudes, as well as how they make decisions or take actions. To ensure that developers and funders have a clear model of how a proposed information resource will fit with working practices and structures, evalutors also may need to study health care or research processes, team functioning or relevant aspects of the larger organization in which work is done. Finally, the consequences of the current problems may be quantified in terms of costs or adverse outcomes.

Design Validation

Design validation focuses on the quality of the processes of information resource design and development; for example, by asking an expert to review these processes. The expert may review documents, interview the development team, compare the suitability of the software-engineering methodology and programming tools used to others available, and generally apply his/her expertise to identify potential flaws in the approach used to develop the software, as well as constructively suggest how these might be corrected.

Structure Validation

Structure validation addresses the static form of the software, usually after a first prototype has been developed. This type of study is most usefully performed by an expert or a team of experts with experience in developing software for the problem domain and concerned users. For these purposes, the investigators need access to both summary and detailed documentation about the system architecture, the structure and function of each module, and the interfaces between them. The expert might focus on the appropriateness of the algorithms that have been employed and check that they have been correctly implemented. Experts might also examine the data structures (e.g., whether they are appropriately normalized) and knowledge bases (e.g., whether they are evidence-based, up-to-date, and modeled in a format that will support the intended analyses or reasoning). Most of this will be done by inspection and discussion with the development team, without actually running the software.

Note that the study types listed up to this point do not require a functioning information resource. However, beginning with usability testing below, the study types require the existence of at least a functioning prototype.

Usability Testing

Usability testing focuses on system function and addresses whether intended users could actually operate or navigate the software to determine whether the resource has the potential to be helpful. In this type of study, use of a prototype by typical users informs further development and should improve its usability, as described in detail under Scenario 2 later in this chapter. It usually entails installing the software in a laboratory or classroom setting; introducing users to it, then allowing them to either navigate at will and provide unstructured comments or to attempt to complete some scripted tasks. Data can be collected by the computer itself, the user, an observer, via audio or video tape, or by more sophisticated technical methods, such as eye-tracking tools. Many software developers have usability testing labs equipped with one-way mirrors and sophisticated measurement systems staffed by experts in human–computer interaction to carry out these studies—an indication of the importance increasingly attached to this type of study.

Laboratory-Function Studies

Laboratory-function studies go beyond usability to explore more specific aspects of the information resource, such as the quality of data captured, the speed of communication, the validity of the calculations carried out, or the appropriateness of advice given. These functions relate less to the basic usability of the resource and more to how the resource performs in relation to what it is trying to achieve for the user or the organization. When carrying out any kind of function testing, the results (speed of processing, accuracy of output, etc.) will depend crucially on any data input, so it is important to match the tasks employed in these studies as closely as possible to those to which the resource will be applied in real working life. If there is likely to be some skilled element in extracting the data from the tasks (e.g., for a diagnostic decision support system, taking an accurate history and recording the key physical findings from a patient) or in selecting specific analytical approaches to be employed by the resource, representatives of the intended user population need to be employed in these studies.

Field-Function Studies

Field-function studies are a variant of laboratory-function testing. In these studies the resource is "pseudo-deployed" in a real work place and employed by real users, up to a point. However, in field-function tests, although the resource is used by real users with real tasks, there is no immediate access by the users to the output or results of interaction with the resource that might influence their decisions or actions, so no effects on these can occur. The output is recorded for later review by the evaluators, and perhaps by the users themselves.

Studies of the effect or impact of information resources on users and problems are in many ways the most demanding. As an information resource matures and the focus of study moves from its functions to its possible effects on clinical practice, basic research, or educational practice, the observations that need to be made become more complex.

Laboratory-User Effect Studies

In laboratory-user effect studies, simulated user actions are studied. Practitioners employ the resource and are asked what they would "do" with the results or advice that the resource generates, but no action is taken. Laboratory-user impact studies are conducted outside the practice environment with prototype or released versions of the resource. Although such studies involve individuals who are representative of the "end-user" population, the primary results of the study derive from simulated actions so the care of patients or conduct of research is not affected by a study of this type.

The subtle differences between the questions addressed by usability, laboratory-function and laboratory impact studies are illustrated using the well-known PubMed interface to the Medline database of biomedical literature:

- Usability study: Can the user enter search terms?
- Laboratory function study: Can the user conduct a search that yields relevant references as judged by others?
- Laboratory impact study: Given a research or clinical problem, can the users conduct a search that alters their assessment of the problem?

Field-User Effect Studies

In field-user effect studies, real actions involving the care of patients or other modes of practice are studied. This requires a resource that is robust and usable by a broad spectrum of users, restricting this kind of study to information resources that can be deployed for routine use. This type of study provides an opportunity to test whether the resource is actually used by the intended users, whether they obtain accurate and useful information from it, and whether this use affects their decisions and actions in significant ways. In user effect studies, the emphasis is on the behaviors and actions of users, and not the consequences of these behaviors. There are many rigorous studies of carefully developed information resources revealing that the information resource is either not used, despite its seeming potential, or that when used, no decisions or actions are improved as a result.[1,2] These findings demonstrate that, however promising the result of previous levels of evaluation, an information resource with the potential to add cost or risk to patient care or research requires an impact study to determine its ultimate effects once it is rolled out into routine practice.

Problem Impact Studies

Problem impact studies are similar to field-user effect studies in many respects, but differ profoundly in what is being explored. Problem impact studies examine whether the original problem or need that motivated creation or deployment of the information resource have been addressed in a satisfactory way. This often requires an investigation that looks beyond the actions of care providers, researchers, or patients to examine the consequences of these actions. For example, an information resource designed to reduce medical errors may affect the behavior of some clinicians who employ the resource, but for a variety of reasons, leave the error rate unchanged. The causes of errors may be multi-factorial and the changes induced by the information resource may address only some of these factors. In other domains, an information resource may be widely used by researchers to access biomedical information, as determined by a user effect study, but a subsequent problem impact study may or may not reveal effects on scientific productivity. New educational technology may change the ways students learn, but may or may not increase their performance on standardized examinations. Fully comprehensive problem impact studies will also be sensitive to unintended consequences. Sometimes, the solution to the target problem creates other unintended and unanticipated problems that can affect perceptions of success. As email became an almost universal mode of communication, almost no one anticipated the problem of "spam".

Factors Distinguishing the Nine Study Types

Table 3.2 further distinguishes the nine study types, as described above, using a set of key factors that are discussed in detail in the paragraphs that follow.

The Setting in Which the Study Takes Place

Studies of the design process, the resource structure, and many resource functions are typically conducted outside the active practice environment, in a "laboratory" setting. Studies to elucidate the need for a resource and studies of its impact on users would usually take place in ongoing practice settings—known generically as the "field"—where healthcare practitioners, researchers, students, or administrators are doing real work in the real world. The same is true for studies of the impact of a resource on persons and organizations. These studies can take place only in a setting where the resource is available for use at the time and where professional activities occur and/or important decisions are made. To an investigator planning studies, an important consideration that determines the kind of study possible is the degree of access to real users in the field setting. If, as a practical matter, access to the field setting is very limited, then several study types listed in Tables 3.1 and 3.2 are not possible and the range of evaluation questions that can be addressed is limited accordingly.

The Version of the Resource Used

For some kinds of studies, a prototype version of the resource may be sufficient, whereas for studies in which the resource is employed by intended

TABLE 3.2. Factors distinguishing the nine generic study types.

Study type	Study setting	Version of the resource	Sampled users	Sampled tasks	What is observed
1. Needs assessment	Field	None, or pre-existing resource to be replaced	Anticipated resource users	Actual tasks	User skills, knowledge, decisions, or actions; care processes, costs, team function or organization; patient outcomes
2. Design validation	Development lab	None	None	None	Quality of design method or team
3. Structure validation	Lab	Prototype or released version	None	None	Quality of resource structure, components, architecture
4. Usability test	Lab	Prototype or released version	Proxy, real users	Simulated, abstracted	Speed of use, user comments, completion of sample tasks
5. Laboratory function study	Lab	Prototype or released version	Proxy, real users	Simulated, abstracted	Speed and quality of data collected or displayed; accuracy of advice given, etc.
6. Field function study	Field	Prototype or released version	Proxy, real users	Real	Speed and quality of data collected or displayed; accuracy of advice given, etc.
7. Lab user effect study	Lab	Prototype or released version	Real users	Abstracted, real	Impact on user knowledge, simulated/pretend decisions or actions
8. Field user effect study	Field	Released version	Real users	Real	Extent and nature of resource use. Impact on user knowledge, real decisions, real actions
9. Problem impact study	Field	Released version	Real users	Real	Care processes, costs, team function, cost effectiveness

users to support real decisions and actions, a fully robust and reliable version is needed.

The Sampled Resource Users

Most biomedical information resources are not autonomous agents that operate independently of users with biomedical domain expertise. More typically, information resources function through interaction with one or more such "users" who often bring to the interaction their own domain knowledge and knowledge of how to operate the resource. In some types of evaluation studies, the users of the resource are not the end users for whom the resource is ultimately designed, but are members of the development or evaluation teams, or other individuals who can be called "proxy users" who are chosen because they are conveniently available or because they are affordable. In other types of studies, the users are sampled from the end-users for whom the resource is ultimately designed. The type of users employed gives shape to a study and can affect its results profoundly. For example, domain knowledge and skill often are needed in laboratory function tests to determine whether resource functions are indeed accurate or appropriate. With a decision support system, it often is hard to know if a suggested action is correct in a specific case, let alone likely to be useful to users. Therefore, in this case, a committee of expert practitioners may be needed to rate the resource's output and determine its quality.

The Sampled Tasks

For function-and-effect studies, the resource is actually "run." The users included in the study actually interact with the resource. This requires tasks, typically clinical or scientific cases or problems, for the users to undertake. These tasks can be invented or simulated; they can be abstracted versions of real cases or problems, shortened to suit the specific purposes of the study, or they can be live cases or research problems as they present to resource users in the real world. Clearly, the kinds of tasks employed in a study have serious implications for the study results and the conclusions that can be drawn from them.

The Observations That Are Made

All evaluation studies entail observations that generate data that are subsequently analyzed to make decisions. As seen in Table 3.2, many different kinds of observations* can be made.

---

* The term "observations" is used here very generically to span a range of activities that includes watching someone work with an information resource, as well as highly instrumented tracking or measurement.

In the paragraphs above, the term "sampling" has been introduced for both tasks and users. The technical issues of sampling will not be discussed here; however, it is important to establish that, in real evaluation studies, tasks and users are always sampled from some real or hypothetical population. Sampling occurs, albeit in different ways, in both subjectivist and objectivist studies. Sampling of users and tasks are major challenges in evaluation study design. It is never possible, practical, or desirable to try to study everyone doing everything possible with an information resource. Choosing representative samples of users and tasks will challenge the resource with a reasonable spectrum of what is expected to occur in normal practice. Under some circumstances, it is also important to know what will happen to the resource's usability, functions, or impact if the resource encounters extremes of user ability, data quality, disease incidence, or task structure. For these purposes, modeling techniques can sometimes be used to simulate what might happen under these extremes; or extreme atypical circumstances can be deliberately created by the investigator to provide a stress test of the resource. Sampling issues and their implications will be returned to on several occasions in Chapters 4 through 8.

It is perhaps extreme to state that every evaluation approach, of the eight listed in Chapter 2, can apply to all of the nine study types introduced in Tables 3.1 and 3.2. There is certainly potential to use both objectivist and subjectivist approaches across the spectrum of study types. At the two extremes, for example, both "need validation" studies and "healthcare impact" studies provide many opportunities to apply both subjectivist and objectivist approaches. Some study types are predisposed toward specific approaches. For example, design validation studies invite use of the professional review approach. The following sections of this chapter expand on a selected set of the study types presented in Tables 3.1 and 3.2.

Self-Test 3.1

For each of the following hypothetical evaluation scenarios, list which of the nine types of studies listed in Table 3.1 they include. Some scenarios may include more than one type of study.

1. An order communications system is implemented in a small hospital. Changes in laboratory workload are assessed.

2. The developers of the order communications system recruit five potential users to help them assess how readily each of the main functions can be accessed from the opening screen and how long it takes users to complete them.

3. A study team performs a thorough analysis of the information required by psychiatrists to whom patients are referred by a community social worker.

4. A biomedical informatics expert is asked for her opinion about a Ph.D. project. She requests copies of the student's code and documentation for review.

5. A new intensive care unit system is implemented alongside manual paper charting for a month. At the end of this time, the quality of the computerized data and data recorded on the paper charts is compared. A panel of intensivists is asked to identify, independently, episodes of hypotension from each data set.

6. A biomedical informatics professor is invited to join the steering group for a clinical workstation project in a local hospital. The only documentation available to critique at the first meeting is a statement of the project goal, a description of the planned development method, and the advertisements and job descriptions for team members.

7. Developers invite educationalists to test a prototype of a computer-aided learning system as part of a user-centered design workshop.

8. A program is devised that generates a predicted 24-hour blood glucose profile using seven clinical parameters. Another program uses this profile and other patient data to advise on insulin dosages. Diabetologists are asked to prescribe insulin for the patient given the 24-hour profile alone, and then again after seeing the computer-generated advice. They also are asked their opinion of the advice.

9. A program to generate alerts to prevent drug interactions is installed in a geriatric clinic that already has a computer-based medical record system. Rates of clinically significant drug interactions are compared before and after installation of the alerting program.

Four Evaluation Scenarios

In this section, four scenarios are introduced that collectively capture many of the dilemmas facing readers of the book.

1. A health problem or opportunity has been identified that seems amenable to an information/communication resource, but there is a need to define the problem in more detail.
2. A prototype information resource has been developed, but its usability and potential for benefit need to be assessed prior to deployment.
3. A locally developed information resource has been deployed within an organization, but no one really knows how useful it is proving to be.
4. A commercial resource has been deployed across a large enterprise, and there is need to understand what impact it has on users, as well as on the organization.

These scenarios do not address the full scope of evaluations in biomedical informatics, but they cover much of what people do. For each, sets of evaluation questions that frequently arise will be provided and the dilemmas that investigators face in the design and execution of evaluation studies will be examined.

Scenario 1: A Healthcare Problem or Opportunity That Seems Amenable to an Information or Communication Resource Has Been Identified, But There Is a Need to Define the Problem in More Detail

The emphasis here is clearly on understanding the nature and cause of a problem, and particularly whether the problem is due to poor information collection, management, processing, analysis, or communication. An information resource is unlikely to help if the cause lies elsewhere. It is likely that careful listening to those who have identified or "own" the problem will be necessary, as will some observation of the problem when it occurs, interviews with those who are affected, and assessment of the frequency and severity of the problem and its consequences to patients, professionals, students, organizations, and others. The emphasis will be on assessing needs as perceived across a range of constituencies, studying potential resource users in the field, assessing user skills, knowledge, decisions, or actions, as well as work processes, costs, team function, or organizational productivity. If there are existing information resources in the setting, studies of their use and the quality of data they hold can provide further valuable insights into the nature of the problem and reason it occurs. If no information problem is revealed by a thorough needs assessment, there is probably no need for a new information resource, irrespective of how appealing the notion may seem from a technical point of view.

Typical Evaluation Questions

This evaluation scenario typically raises some specific questions that can be addressed using a variety of evaluation methods. These questions include:

- What is the problem, why does it matter, and how much effort is the organization likely to devote to resolving it?
- What is the history of the problem, and has anyone ever tackled it before? How, and with what outcome?
- Where, when, and how frequently does the problem occur? What are the consequences for staff, other people, and the organization?
- Is the problem independent of other problems, or is it linked to, or even a symptom of, other problems somewhere else?
- What are all the factors leading to the problem, and how much might improvements in information handling ameliorate it?

- Who might generate better information to help others resolve the problem; how do these alternative information providers perceive the problem and their potential part in resolving it?
- What kinds of information need to be obtained, processed, and communicated for the information resource users and others concerned in solving the problem? From where, to where, when, how, and to whom?
- What other information resources exist or are planned in the environment?
- What quality and volume of information are required to ameliorate the problem enough to justify the effort involved?
- How, in general, can these information/communication needs be met? What specific functions should be built into an information resource to meet the identified needs?
- Is there anything else that a potential resource developer would like to know before spending their time on this problem?

The Case for Needs Assessments

The success of any biomedical information resource depends on how well it fulfills a healthcare, research, or teaching need, assuming there is one.[3] Usually, before developers begin the design of an information resource, someone (often a representative of the potential user community) has identified a problem amenable to a solution via improved utilization of biomedical information or knowledge. Sometimes, however, and particularly for information resources employing cutting-edge technology, the project is initiated by the developers without careful conceptualization of the professional practice problem the resource is intended to address. Often, a suitable demonstration site for such projects can be located, but equally often, the project deteriorates from this point as the developer tries to persuade the increasingly mystified professionals in that site of the potential of a "breakthrough" that is, in fact, a solution in search of a problem. Thus, defining the need for an information resource before it is developed is an important precursor to any developmental effort.

Let us say, for the sake of argument, that a clinician notices that the postoperative infection rate on a certain ward is high, and that, for unknown reasons, patients may not be receiving the prophylactic antibiotics that are known to be effective. The clinicians uncovering the problem may merely note it, or they may try to define and understand it more, in which case the investigation becomes an evaluation study. In increasing order of complexity, the "investigators" may discuss the problem with colleagues, conduct a staff survey to explore the nature and extent of the perceptions of the problem, collect actual healthcare data to document the problem, and perhaps compare the locally collected data with published results based on data collected elsewhere. Such careful study would require a definition of what constitutes a postoperative infection (e.g., does it include chest infections as well as wound infections?) and then conducting an audit of postoperative infections and the drugs prescribed before and after surgery.

Defining the problem is always necessary to guide the choice of a specific solution. While professionals in informatics may be prone to believe that all problems can be addressed with advanced information- or knowledge-based technologies, problems and potentially effective solutions to address them come in many shapes and sizes. For example, the root cause of the example problem above may be that handwritten orders for antibiotics are misread by clerks and the wrong drug is administered. Particularly in the short term, this etiology recommends a very different kind of solution from what would be obtained if the source of the problem were out-of-date antibiotic knowledge on the part of the physicians themselves. Once the mechanisms of the problem are uncovered, it may prove most efficient to address them with educational sessions, wall posters, or financial incentives instead of new information technology. If an information resource is the chosen solution, the resource users and developers need to choose the appropriate kind of information to provide (advice to prescribe an appropriate antibiotic from the formulary), the appropriate time it is to be delivered (6 hours before to 2 hours after surgery), and the appropriate mode of delivery (incorporation into an order set, advice on-screen to the resident or intern, or a printed reminder affixed to the front of the case record).

Efforts to define the need for an information resource before commencing development work are complicated by the fact that users typically cannot articulate how they use information to perform day-to-day tasks (the "paradox of expertise") and often are unable to imagine how computer-based techniques might improve the quality or availability of this information. In some projects, resource development is based directly on classical systems analysis in which users are first interviewed about their requirements, then sign off a lengthy requirements document.[†] The requirements are then translated into system specification documents, and finally into the finished system. When classical systems analysis is conducted, users are typically unable to understand the written requirements documentation to visualize what is being proposed; they have neither the time nor the experience to imagine what the functioning software will look and feel like. An increasingly functional prototype is often much more useful in helping them formulate their specific requirements.[4,5] It is for this reason that much software development now follows a "prototype and test" method, with empha-

---

[†] Systems analysis can be seen as a distinct cluster of methods that focus on analyzing and modeling data structures, data flows, workflows, and tasks, but it is outside of the scope of this book. The result of the systems analysis process is specifications of an information resource that can be turned into an information resource prototype.

sis on building prototypes of the resource, testing them with users, and revising them to rectify identified deficiencies.[6] The reader is referred to the sections on capturing and defining user requirements in standard software-engineering texts through techniques such as rapid prototyping and user-centered design workshops[7,8] for further details.

Scenario 2: A Prototype Information Resource Has Been Developed, But Its Usability and Potential for Benefit Need to Be Assessed Prior to Deployment

The primary evaluation issue here is the upcoming decision to continue with the development of the prototype information resource. Validation of the design and structure of the resource will have been conducted, either formally or informally, but not yet a usability study. If this looks promising, a laboratory evaluation of key functions also is advised before making the substantial investment required to turn a promising prototype into a system that is stable and likely to bring more benefits than problems to users in the field. Here, typical questions will include:

- Who are the target users, and what are their background skills and knowledge?
- Does the resource make sense to target users?
- Following a brief introduction, can target users navigate themselves around important parts of the resource?
- Can target users select relevant tasks in reasonable time and with reasonable accuracy using the resource?
- What user characteristics correlate with the ability to use the resource and achieve fast, accurate performance with it?
- What other kinds of people can use it safely?
- How to improve the screen layout, design, wording, menus, etc.
- Is there a long learning curve? What user training needs are there?
- How much ongoing help will users require once they are initially trained?
- What concerns do users have about the system—usability, accuracy, privacy, effect on their jobs, other side effects?
- Based on the performance of prototypes in users' hands, does the resource have the potential to meet user needs?

These questions fall within the scope of the usability and laboratory-function testing approaches listed in Table 3.1. A range of techniques—borrowed from the human–computer interaction field and employing both objectivist and subjectivist approaches—can be used, including:

- Seeking the views of potential users after both a demonstration of the resource and a hands-on exploration. Methods such as focus groups may be very useful to identify not only immediate problems with the software and how it might be improved, but also potential broader concerns and unexpected issues that may include user privacy and long-term issues around user training and working relationships.

- Studying users while they carry out a list of predesigned tasks using the information resource. Methods for studying users include watching over their shoulder; video observation (sometimes with several video cameras per user); think out-loud protocols (asking the user to verbalize their impressions as they navigate and use the system); and automatic logging of keystrokes, navigation paths, and time to complete tasks.[9]
- Use of validated questionnaires to capture user impressions, often before and after an experience with the system, with one example being the Telemedicine Preparedness questionnaire.[10]
- Specific techniques to explore how users might improve the layout or design of the software. For example, to help understand what users think of as a "logical" menu structure for an information resource, investigators can use the card-sorting technique. This entails listing each function available on all the menus on a separate card and then asking users to sort these cards into several piles according to which function seems to go with which.[11]

Depending on the aim of a usability study, it may suffice to employ a small number of potential users. Nielsen has shown that, if the aim is only to identify major software faults, the proportion identified rises quickly up to about five or six users, then much more slowly to plateau at about 15 to 20 users.[11,12] Five users will often identify 80% of software problems. However, investigators conducting such small studies, useful though they may be for software development, cannot then expect to publish them in a scientific journal. The achievement in this case is having found answers to a very specific question about a specific software prototype. This kind of local reality test is unlikely to appeal to the editors or readers of a journal. By contrast, the results of formal laboratory function studies, which typically employ more users, are more amenable to journal publication.

Scenario 3: A Locally Developed Information Resource Has Been Deployed Within an Organization, But No One Really Knows How Useful It Is Proving to Be

The situation here is quite different from the preceding scenario. Here, the system is already deployed in one part of the organization, so it has already moved well beyond the prototype stage. The key issues are whether the resource is being used, by whom, whether this usage is appropriate, and what benefits the resource use is bringing to the organization. With reference to Tables 3.1 and 3.2, this scenario typically calls for field-user effect studies.

Typical evaluation questions here might include:

- Is the resource being used at all; if so, by whom?
- Are these the intended users, and if not, why not?
- Is the information being captured or communicated by the resource of good quality (accurate, timely)?
- What are users' attitudes and beliefs about using the resource in day-to-day work? Do these beliefs depend on the users' background, work assignments, or role in the organization?
- Does the information resource appear to be causing any problems? What are these problems, and how often do they occur?
- Do there appear to be benefits from the use of the resource? What are they?
- Do the benefits of the resource derive from features unique to a limited set of users or the specific areas where it has been deployed?

The evaluation approach under this scenario can employ a mixture of study types using a mix of methods. Subjectivist studies could be useful to get an initial impression about who uses the resource and what they perceive as its benefits and problems. These studies may identify focused areas for further more-detailed study; or if the objectives of the study are limited, subjectivist studies may be an end in themselves. If the usage or likely impact (positive or negative) of the resource is of interest, further studies can be conducted using either objectivist or subjectivist methods to answer in greater detail questions about the resource for the organization. Studies of usage rates may be important if there is evidence of limited user effect, and could be followed by usability studies and both lab and field-based studies of resource function to identify where the resource needs improvement. If the results of effect studies are promising, it may be beneficial to study whether the need for the resource exists in other parts of the organization where it is currently not available or is not being used. If these needs assessment studies are positive, widespread deployment of the system across the organization can take place, whereas if the results of these studies are less promising, the resource may have only limited utility.

Scenario 4: A Commercial Resource Has Been Deployed Across a Large Enterprise, and There Is Need to Understand Its Impact on Users as Well as on the Organization

The type of evaluation questions that arise here include:

- In what fraction of occasions when the resource could have been used was it actually used?
- Who uses it, why, are these the intended users, and are they satisfied with it?

- Does using the resource improve influence information quality or communication?
- Does using the resource influence user knowledge or skills?
- Does using the resource improve their work?
- For clinical information resources, does using the resource change outcomes for patients?
- How does the resource influence the whole organization and relevant subunits?
- Do the overall benefits and costs or risks differ for specific groups of users, departments, and the whole organization?
- How much does the resource really cost the organization?
- Should the organization keep the resource as it is, improve it, or replace it?
- How can the resource be improved, at what cost, and what benefits would result?

To each of the above questions, one can add "Why or why not?" to get a broader understanding of what is happening because of use of the resource.

This evaluation scenario, suggesting a problem impact study, is often what people think of first when the concept of evaluation is introduced. However, it has been shown in this chapter that it is one of many evaluation scenarios, arising relatively late in the life cycle of an information resource. When these impact-oriented evaluations are undertaken, they usually result from a realization by stakeholders who have invested significantly in an information resource, that the benefits of the resource are uncertain and there is a need to justify recurring costs. These stakeholders usually vary in the kind of evaluation methods that will convince them of the impacts that the resource is or is not having. Many such stakeholders will wish to see quantified indices of benefits or harms stemming from the resource—for example, the number of users and daily uses, the amount the resource improves productivity or reduces costs, or perhaps other benefits such as reduced waiting times to perform key tasks or procedures, lengths of hospital stay, or occurrence of adverse events. Such data are collected through the kind of objectivist studies discussed in Chapters 7 and 8 and the relevant economic methods described in Chapter 11. Other stakeholders may prefer to see evidence of perceived benefit and positive views of staff, in which case staff surveys, focus groups, and unstructured interviews may prove the best evaluation methods. Often, a combination of many methods is necessary to extend the goal of the investigation from understanding what impact the resource has to why this impact occurs—or fails to occur.

If the investigator is pursuing objectivist methods, deciding which of the possible effect variables to include in an impact study and developing ways to measure them can be the most challenging aspect of an evaluation study design. (These and related issues receive the attention of five full chapters of this book.) Investigators usually wish to limit the number of effect measures employed in a study, for many reasons: to make optimal use of limited evaluation resources, to minimize manipulation of the practice environment, and to avoid statistical analytical problems that result from a large number of measures. Appendix A lists some potential measures of the impact of various information resources on health care itself, providers of care, and organizations.

As will be seen in Chapters 9 and 10, effect studies can use subjectivist approaches to allow the most relevant "effect" issues to emerge over time and with increasingly deep immersion into the study environment. This emergent feature of subjectivist work obviates the need to decide in advance which effect variables to explore, and is considered by proponents of subjectivist approaches to be among their major advantages.

In health care particularly, every intervention carries some risk, which must be judged in comparison to the risks of doing nothing or of providing an alternative intervention. It is difficult to decide whether an information resource is an improvement unless the performance of the current decision-takers is also measured[13,14] in a comparison-based evaluation. For example, if physicians' decisions are to become more accurate following introduction of a decision support tool, the resource needs to be "right" when the user would usually be "wrong." This could mean that the tool's error rate is lower than that of the physician, its errors are in different cases, or they should be of a different kind or less serious than those of the clinician.

For effect studies, it is often important to know something about how the practitioners carry out their work prior to the introduction of the information resource. Suitable measures include the accuracy, timing, and confidence level of their decisions and the amount of information they require before making a decision. Although data for such a study can sometimes be collected by using abstracts of cases or problems in a laboratory setting, these studies inevitably raise questions of generalization to the real world. One of many trade-offs that occur in the design of evaluation studies can be observed here. Although control over the mix of cases possible in a laboratory study can lead to a more precise estimate of practitioner decision-making, it ultimately may prove better to conduct a baseline study while the individuals are doing real work in a real practice setting. Often, this audit of current decisions and actions provides useful input to the design of the information resource[3,4] and provides a reference against which resource performance may later be compared.

When conducting problem impact studies in healthcare settings, investigators can sometimes save themselves much time and effort without sacrificing validity by measuring effect in terms of certain healthcare processes rather than patient outcomes.[15] For example, measuring the mortality or complication rate in patients with heart attacks requires data collection from hundreds of patients, as complications and death are (fortunately) rare events. However, as long as large, rigorous trials or meta-analyses have determined that a certain procedure (e.g., giving heart-attack patients streptokinase within 24 hours) correlates closely with the desired patient outcome, it is perfectly valid to measure the rate of performing this procedure as a valid "surrogate" for the desired outcome. Mant and Hicks demonstrated that measuring the quality of care by quantifying a key process in this way might require one-tenth as many patients as measuring outcomes.[15]

Why Are Formal Evaluation Studies Needed?

At this point, some readers of this volume may be questioning why elaborate empirical studies of information resources are needed at all. Why is it not possible, for example, to model the performance of information resources, and thus save much time and effort? The answer lies, largely, in the nature of computational artifacts. For some disciplines, specification of the structure of a device allows one to predict how it will function, and engineers can even design new objects with known performance characteristics directly from functional requirements. Examples of such devices are elevators and conventional road bridges: The principles governing the behavior of materials and of civil and mechanical engineering are sufficiently well understood that a new elevator or bridge can be designed to a set of performance characteristics with the expectation that it will perform as predicted. Testing of models of these devices is rarely needed. Field testing of the artifact, once built, is conducted to reveal relatively minor anomalies, which can be rapidly remedied, or to tune or optimize performance. However, when the object concerned is a computer-based resource, and not a bridge, the story is different. Software designers and engineers have theories linking the structure to the function of only the most trivial computer-based resources.[7,8] Because of the lack of a comprehensive theory connecting structure and function, there is no way to know exactly how an information resource will perform until it is built and tested; similarly, there is no way to know that any revisions will bring about the desired effect until the next version of the resource is tested.

In sum, the only practical way of determining if a reasonably complex body of computer code does what it is intended to do is to test it. This testing can take many shapes and forms. The informal design, test, and revise activity that characterizes the development of all computer software is one such form of testing and results in software that usually functions as expected by the developers. More formal and exhaustive approaches to software design, verification, and testing using hazard analysis, synthetic test cases, and other approaches help to guarantee that the software will do what it was designed to do.[8] Even these approaches, however, do not guarantee the success of the software when put into the hands of users. This requires evaluation studies of the types described in this book, which can be undertaken before, during, and after the initial development of an information resource. Such

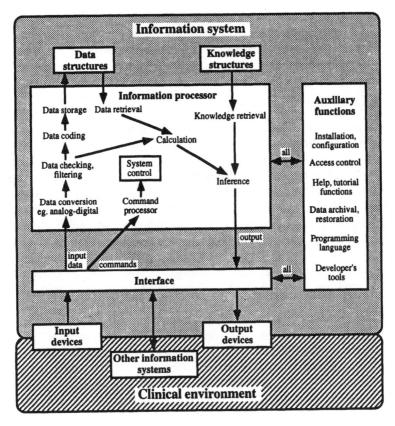

FIGURE 3.2. Components of a generic information resource.

evaluation studies can guide further development; indicate if the resource is likely to be safe for use in real patient-care, research, or educational settings; or elucidate if it has the potential to improve the professional performance of the users and disease outcomes in their clients.

As shown in Figure 3.2, information resources are built from many components, each with many functions that can be tested. A sample of the more specific functions most relevant to particular resource components or to intact biomedical information resources of different kinds is listed in Appendix B.

Many other works elaborate on the points offered here. Spiegelhalter[16] and Gaschnig and colleagues[17] discussed these phases of evaluation in more detail, drawing analogies from the evaluation of new drugs or the conventional software life cycle, respectively. Wasson and colleagues[18] discussed the evaluation of clinical prediction rules together with some useful methodological standards that apply equally to information resources. Lundsgaarde,[19] Miller,[20] Nykanen,[21] and Wyatt and Spiegelhalter[22] described, with differing emphases, the evaluation of healthcare information resources, often focusing on decision support tools that pose some of the most extreme challenges. Other books have explored more technical health technology assessment or organizational approaches to evaluation methods.[23-26]

The Special Issue of Safety

Before disseminating any biomedical information resource that stores and communicates data or knowledge and is designed to influence real-world practice decisions, it is important to check that it is safe when used as intended. In the case of new drugs, it is a statutory duty of developers to perform extensive *in vitro* testing and *in vivo* testing in animals before any human receives a dose. For information resources, equivalent safety tests might include measuring how fast the information resource functions compared to current procedures and estimating how often it corrupts or retrieves erroneous data or furnishes incorrect advice. It may be necessary to repeat these measurements following any substantial modifications to the information resource, as the correction of errors may itself generate more errors or uncover previously unrecognized problems.

Examining an information resource for safe operation is particularly important when evaluating those that attempt to directly influence the decisions made by front-line health professionals. Ensuring that such a resource is safe requires measurement of how often it gives poor advice using data representative of patients in whose management it is intended to assist and comparing the advice given with the decisions made by current decision-makers, as seen by expert judges.

The advice or output generated by most information resources depends critically on the quality and quantity of data available to it, and thus, at least partly, on the manner in which the resources are used by practitioners. Practitioners who are untrained, in a hurry, or exhausted at 3:00 am may all obtain less-reliable output because of the poor quality of data they input. Thus, to generate valid results, functional tests must put the resources in actual users' hands or in the hands of people with similar knowledge, skills, and experience if real users are not available.

Evaluation Strategy: Deciding What and How Much to Study

Matching What Is Evaluated to Decisions That Need to be Made

A recurrent and troublesome issue in many evaluation studies is not choosing what to measure, or even which methods to use in a specific study, but how to balance the often-competing demands of the different stakeholders involved in commissioning the study, as well as how to allocate resources fairly to answer the many questions that typically arise.

One way to resolve this strategic problem is to recall that, of the many reasons for performing evaluations, very often the key reason is to collect information to support a choice between two or more options: for example, to purchase commercial resource A or B or to develop interface design A or B. Therefore, the more a proposed study generates information that is interesting, but does not actually inform this choice, the lower the priority it must take. To make these determinations, however, some way is needed to distinguish between information that is necessary to the choice and information that is merely interesting.

People making real-world choices of these types—especially those with significant financial or political consequences—often formalize the process using a technique called "option appraisal."[27] In an option appraisal, the choice is made by scoring and ranking several options (e.g., to purchase resource A, B, or C), often including the null option (no purchase). The person or group responsible for the choice then selects the criteria they wish to use and how they will score them.

When option appraisal is applied as a planning tool for evaluation, the criteria used in the option appraisal are the major questions that need to be answered in the evaluation study. The score assigned against each criterion in the option appraisal depends on the results of evaluation studies that attempt to answer the relevant question for each option. Sometimes, it is very easy to assign the scores. For example, if the primary criterion is cost, the "evaluation study" may consist simply of phone calls to the suppliers of each candidate information resource. Often, however, significant evaluation and data collection is required before the score for each option can be assigned—for example, if the scoring criterion is user experience or the ratio of costs to benefits. By focusing on criteria that will be used by decision-makers in an option appraisal, investigators can usually identify the key questions that their evaluation studies need to address and how the results will be used. When criteria emerge from an option appraisal as particularly important—for example, those listed first or weighted more heavily—the investigator knows that the results of the evaluation addressing these criteria are crucial, and that extra attention to detail and a higher proportion of the evaluation budget are warranted for studies addressing these criteria.

For the reasons above, it is often useful to introduce stakeholders to the idea of option appraisal if they are not already familiar with it. The option appraisal framework is especially useful to limit the number of questions that stakeholders want answered. Any evaluation question that does not map to one of the criteria that will be used by stakeholders to choose between options contributes to an evaluation study whose results will be of no practical interest.

TABLE 3.3. Sample questions at differing levels of evaluation.

Level of evaluation	Sample question
A lab report, guideline, email or other component of the information being processed	What is the impact on lab report content of the introduction of bedside terminals?
The information resource as a whole	How long does it take for lab results to get to the bedside terminal?
A patient or case	Are patients satisfied when their nurse uses a bedside terminal?
A health professional	Are nurses satisfied when they use a bedside terminal?
A clinical team	How are communication patterns within the team influenced by the introduction of bedside terminals?
Part of a healthcare delivery organization (e.g., ward)	Is the throughput of the ICU affected by the introduction of bedside terminals?
The entire healthcare delivery organization	How has the introduction of bedside terminals affected the rate of adverse events across the hospital, and thus its indemnity position?

Choosing the Level of Evaluation

One of the fundamental choices required when planning any evaluation study is the level or scale at which to focus the study. For example, in clinical fields, this level can be one or more of the following: a lab report, guideline, email or other component of the information being processed or communicated, the resource as a whole, a patient or case, a health professional such as a nurse or physician, a multidisciplinary clinical team, or part or all of a healthcare delivery organization such as a hospital ward or the whole hospital. To illustrate this, Table 3.3 shows some sample questions that might prompt investigators to study each of these levels.

It is important to realize that logistical factors often require studies to be conducted at higher levels of scale. This occurs when individual objects such as patients or health professionals interact and thus cannot be separated out for study. An example would be studying the impact of an antenatal information kiosk by providing a password to half the women attending a clinic. Because those women without a password could either "borrow" one or look over the shoulders of women with a password using the kiosk, it would be logistically difficult to restrict usage to the intended group. Even if the "control" women failed to share passwords, women typically share their experiences and information in an antenatal clinic; therefore, it would be naïve to assume that if the kiosk were only made available to half the women, the other half would be completely ignorant of its contents. Similar arguments apply to studying the effect of an educational course for health professionals or the impact of a new set of reference databases. These interactions require that the investigator raise the level of the evaluation to focus on groups rather than individuals.

Matching What Is Evaluated to the Type of Information Resource

There are many types of information resources containing many functional components. Clearly, it is impossible to generate an exhaustive list of everything that can be studied for every kind of resource, but as previously mentioned, the appendices to this chapter provide samples of some of the issues that can be addressed for a range of information resource components and complete resources. Not all of these attributes can or should be measured for every component or resource, and it often requires much thought about the purpose of the evaluation itself to produce a relevant list of issues to pursue. Because facilities for evaluation are always limited, it may be helpful to rank the items listed in the appendices in the order of their likely contribution to answering the questions the evaluation is intended to resolve. Often, as discussed in Chapter 2, priorities are set not by the investigators, but by the stakeholders in the evaluation. The investigators' role is then to initiate a process that leads to a consensus about what the priority issues should be.

Matching How Much Is Evaluated to the Stage in the Life Cycle

Evaluation, defined broadly, takes place throughout the resource development cycle: from defining the need to monitoring the continuing impact of a resource once it is deployed. The place of evaluation in the various developmental phases is illustrated in Figure 3.3. Different issues are explored, at different degrees of intensity, at each stage of resource development.

Prior to any resource development, as discussed earlier, there may be very active formal evaluation to establish needs. During the early phases of actual resource development, informal feedback and exploration of prototypes is associated with code development and debugging. A single prototype then emerges for more formal testing, with problems being fed back to the development team. Eventually, it passes preset criteria of adequacy, and its effects on users can be tested in a more formal way—though often still under controlled "laboratory" conditions. Once safety is ensured and there is reason to believe that the information resource is likely to bring benefit, its impact can be studied in a limited field test prior to wider dissemination. Once disseminated, it is valuable to monitor the effects of the resource on the institutions that have installed it and evaluate it for potential hazards that may only come to light when it is in widespread use—a direct analogy with postmarketing surveillance of drugs for rare side effects.

Evaluation is integral to information resource development, and adequate resources must be allocated for it when time and money are budgeted for a development effort. Evaluation cannot be left to the end of a project. However, it is also clear that the intensity of the evaluation effort should be

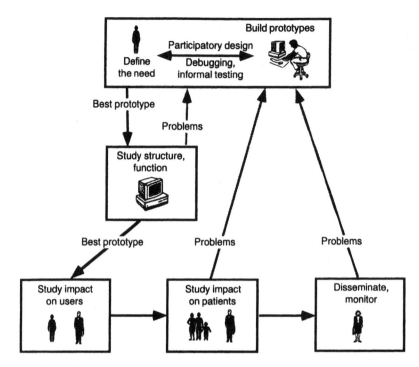

FIGURE 3.3. Changing evaluation issues during development of a health information resource.

closely matched to the resource's maturity.[28] For example, one would not wish to conduct an expensive field trial of an information resource that is barely complete, is still in prototype form, may evolve considerably before taking its final shape, or is so early in its development that it may fail because simple programming bugs have not been eliminated. Equally, once information resources are firmly established in practice settings, it may appear that no further rigorous evaluations are necessary. However, key questions may emerge only after the resource has become ubiquitous.[29,30]

Organizing Information Resource Development Projects to Facilitate Evaluation

The need for evaluation to become a pervasive component of biomedical information resource development projects has already been discussed. What follows is a list of steps that should ensure that evaluation activity proceeds hand-in-hand with the development process.

At the first stage of planning a study, it is an excellent idea to make a list of the potential project roles listed in Chapter 2, such as project funder, resource developer, users, and community representative, and indicate which stakeholders occupy each role. Sometimes this task requires educated guesses, but the exercise is still useful. This exercise will particularly serve to identify those who should be consulted during the critical early stages of designing an evaluation. Those planning development projects should be aware of the need to include a diverse and balanced membership on the evaluation team. While the "core" evaluation team may be relatively small, many evaluation projects need occasional access to the specialist skills of computer scientists, ethnographers, statisticians, health professionals and other domain experts, managers, and health economists.

Although many evaluations are carried out by the resource development team, placing some reliance on external investigators may help to uncover unexpected problems—or benefits—and is increasingly necessary for credibility. Recalling from Chapter 2 the ideal of a completely unbiased "goal-free" evaluator, it can be seen that excessive reliance on evaluation carried out by the development team can be problematic. Gary et al. recently showed that studies carried out by resource develops are three times as likely to show positive results as those published by an extend team.[31]

Parkinson's Law (tasks and organizations tend to expand to consume the resources available) can apply to resource development and evaluation activities. It is important to define the goals, time scale, and budget in advance, although it is difficult to apportion the budget between what is spent on development and what is spent on evaluation activities. A starting point for the evaluation activity should be at least five percent of the total budget, but a larger percentage is often appropriate if this is a demonstrator project or one where reliable and predictable resource function is critical to patient safety. In a closed-loop drug-delivery system, for example, a syringe containing a drug with potentially fatal effects in overdose is controlled by a computer program that attempts to maintain some body function (e.g., blood glucose, depth of anesthesia) constant or close to pre-programmed levels. Any malfunction or unexpected dependencies between the input data and the rate of drug delivery could have serious consequences. In these cases, the ratio of the budget allocated to evaluation rather than development must be larger.

As has been argued, investigators need an eclectic approach. Depending on the specific needs of the project, it may include subjectivist methods that are important to (1) elucidate problems, expectations, fears, failures, resource transferability, and effects on job roles; (2) tease out very complicated issues of cause and effect, (3) identify how to improve the resource; (4) identify unintended, as well as intended, effects; and (5) understand what else, apart from information technology, is necessary to make the information resource a success.

Finally, evaluation projects themselves do require management. Project advisory groups often are appointed to oversee the quality and progress of the overall effort from the stakeholders' perspective. Such a group typically has no direct managerial responsibility. This group should be composed of appropriate people who can advise the evaluation team about priorities and strategy, indemnify them against accusations of bias, excessive detachment or meddling in the evaluation sites, and monitor progress of the studies. Such a group can satisfy the need for a multidisciplinary advisory group and help to ensure the credibility of the study findings.

Answers to Self-Test 3.1

1. Problem impact
2. Usability test
3. Need assessment
4. Design validation
5. Field function
6. Design validation and needs assessment
7. Usability laboratory function
8. Field user effect
9. Problem impact.

References

1. Eccles M, McColl E, Steen N, Rousseau N, Grimshaw J, Parkin D, Purves I. Effect of computerized evidence based guidelines on management of asthma and angina in adults in primary care: cluster randomised controlled trial. BMJ 2002 Oct 26;325(7370):941–948.
2. Murray MD, Harris LE, Overhage JM, Zhou XH, Eckert GJ, Smith FE, Buchanan NN, Wolinsky FD, McDonald CJ, Tierney WM. Failure of computerized treatment suggestions to improve health outcomes of outpatients with uncomplicated hypertension: results of a randomized controlled trial. Pharmacotherapy 2004 Mar;24(3):324–337.
3. Heathfield HA, Wyatt J. Philosophies for the design and development of clinical decision-support systems. Methods Inf Med 1993;32:1–8.
4. Wyatt JC. Clinical data systems, Part III: Developing and evaluating clinical data systems. Lancet 1994;344:1682–1688.
5. Smith MF. Prototypically topical: software prototyping and delivery of health care information systems. Br J Health Care Comput 1993;10(6):25–27.
6. Smith MF. *Software Prototyping*. London: McGraw-Hill, 1991.
7. Sommerville I. *Software Engineering*. Reading, MA: Addison Wesley; 2002.
8. Fox J. Decision support systems as safety-critical components: towards a safety culture for medical informatics. Methods Inf Med 1993;32:345–348.
9. Staggers N, Kobus D. Comparing response time, errors, and satisfaction between text-based and graphical user interfaces during nursing order tasks. J Am Med Inform Assoc 2000 Mar–Apr;7(2):164–176.
10. Demiris G, Speedie S, Finkelstein S. A questionnaire for the assessment of patients' impressions of the risks and benefits of home telecare. J Telemed Telecare 2000;6(5):278–84.
11. Nielsen J. Card sorting. Available at: http://www.useit.com. Accessed, June 24, 2005.
12. Nielsen J, Landauer TK. A mathematical model of the finding of usability problems. In: *Proceedings of the ACM INTERCHI'93 Conference, Amsterdam, The Netherlands, 24–29 April 1993*. 206–213.

13. Wellwood J, Spiegelhalter DJ, Johannessen S. How does computer-aided diagnosis improve the management of acute abdominal pain? Ann R Col Surg Engl 1992;74:140–146.
14. de Dombal FT, Leaper DJ, Horrocks JC, et al. Human and computer-aided diagnosis of acute abdominal pain: further report with emphasis on performance of clinicians. BMJ 1974;1:376–380.
15. Mant J, Hicks N. Detecting differences in quality of care: the sensitivity of measures of process and outcome in treating acute myocardial infarction. BMJ 1995;311:793–796.
16. Spiegelhalter DJ. Evaluation of medical decision-aids, with an application to a system for dyspepsia. Stat Med 1983;2:207–216.
17. Gaschnig J, Klahr P, Pople H, Shortliffe E, Terry A. Evaluation of expert systems: issues and case studies. In: Hayes-Roth F, Waterman DA, Lenat D, eds. *Building Expert Systems*. Reading, MA: Addison Wesley; 1983.
18. Wasson JH, Sox HC, Neff RK, Goldman L. Clinical prediction rules: applications and methodological standards. N Engl J Med 1985;313:793–799.
19. Lundsgaarde HP. Evaluating medical expert systems. Soc Sci Med 1987;24: 805–819.
20. Miller PL. Evaluating medical expert systems. In: Miller PL, ed. *Selected Topics in Medical AI*. New York: Springer-Verlag; 1988.
21. Nykanen P, ed. *Issues in the Evaluation of Computer-Based Support to Clinical Decision Making. Report of SYDPOL WG5*. Denmark: SYDPOL; 1989.
22. Wyatt J, Spiegelhalter D. Evaluating medical expert systems: what to test and how? Med Inf (Lond) 1990;15:205–217.
23. Szczepura A, Kankaanpaa J. *Assessment of Health Care Technologies*. London: Wiley; 1996.
24. van Gennip EM, Talmon JL, eds. *Assessment and Evaluation of Information Technologies in Medicine*. Amsterdam: IOS Press; 1995.
25. Anderson JG, Aydin CE, Jay SJ, eds. *Evaluating Health Care Information Systems*. Thousand Oaks, CA: Sage; 1994.
26. McNair P, Brender J. Methodological and methodical perils and pitfalls within assessment studies performed on IT-based solutions in healthcare. Aalborg University, Aalborg Virtual Centre for Health Informatics; 2003. Technical report No. 03-1.
27. Perry A, Capewell S, Walker A, Chalmers J, Redpath A, Major K, Morrison CE, Craig N, Cobbe S, Smith WC. Measuring the costs and benefits of heart disease monitoring. *Heart*. 2000 Jun;83(6):651–656.
28. Stead W, Haynes RB, Fuller S, et al. Designing medical informatics research and library projects to increase what is learned. J Am Med Inform Assoc 1994;1:28–34.
29. Haynes R, McKibbon K, Walker C, Ryan N, Fitzgerald D, Ramsden M. Online access to MEDLINE in a clinical setting. Ann Intern Med 1990;112:78–84.
30. Lindberg DA, Siegel ER, Rapp BA, Wallingford KT, Wilson SR. Use of MEDLINE by physicians for clinical problem solving. JAMA 1993;269: 3124–3129.
31. Gary A, Adhikan N, McDonald H, et al. Effect of computerized clinical decision support systems on practitioner performance and patient outcomes. A systematic review. JAMA 2005;293:1223–1238.

Appendix A

Areas of Potential Information Resource Impact on Health Care, Care Providers, and Organizations

Database

Frequency of data loss, breaches of data confidentiality, downtime and its consequences, speed of response (e.g., transaction rates or time per transaction) when database is in routine use.

Data Coding/Translation Process

Accuracy of coded data following clinical input; problems when coding data (e.g., percentage of data items that users wished to enter that were successfully coded, number of new codes added by users).

Data Retrieval Process

Ease of searching, which search methods are used; time to formulate a search; user satisfaction with searches.

Data retrieval: completeness, time taken for data retrieval; degradation with number of cases stored.

Any Data Input Process

Ease of data entry, usage rate, subjective ease of data entry.

Objective accuracy of data entry, time taken, number of actions (e.g., key presses) taken to enter data items, number of errors correctly detected by the resource; variation among users, repeatability with same user; learning effect.

Speech Input System

Ease of use, accuracy in a real environment, number of repetitions needed, deliberate use of restricted subsets of vocabulary, speed of use, speaker invariance, resistance to background noise, directionality, frequency that users enter data or commands via alternate means, percentage of time used via the telephone.

Knowledge Resource (e.g., as a Full-Text Database, Part of an Advice Generator)

Users' perceptions of coverage, detail, ease of reading output, speed, how much is current, ease of using index, finding synonyms.

Searching precision, recall and speed given a citation or a specific question; recall after a fixed time spent browsing without a specific question given in advance; quality and number of references included in paragraphs on a given topic retrieved after free access to resource.

Effects on accuracy and timing of users' decisions and actions; effect on users' subjective confidence about a case; effect on users' knowledge or understanding of medicine.

Advice Generator

Users' perceptions of the length, ease of comprehension, structuring and accuracy of the advice; how well calibrated any probability estimates appear.

Effects of correct and incorrect advice on accuracy and timing of users' decisions and actions: to collect patient data, to order investigations of diagnosis or interpretation of test results, to refer or admit a patient, to give or adjust therapy, to give a prognosis.

Effect of advice on users' subjective confidence about a case; effect of advice on users' knowledge or understanding of biomedicine.

Critique Generator

Users' perceptions of length, ease of comprehension, structuring, accuracy of critique comments; influence of each critique comment on accuracy and timing of users' decisions and actions; effect of critique on users' subjective confidence about a case; effect of critique on users' knowledge or understanding of biomedicine.

Explanation Generator

Users' perceptions of length, ease of comprehension, structuring, accuracy; range of user questions it addressed; influence of explanation on user (e.g., causing them to ignore incorrect advice when their prior intention was right or to take correct advice when their prior intention was wrong); effect of explanation on users' subjective confidence about a case; effect of explanation on users' knowledge or understanding of biomedicine.

Imaging System

Users' estimate of adequacy of system; number and types of images stored and communicated; usage rates, times, and sites; times taken to review one image and to review all the images necessary for a decision; effect on accuracy of users' diagnostic, therapeutic, prognostic decisions and actions; effect on users' subjective confidence about a case; effect on users' knowledge or understanding of biomedicine.

Teaching System

Subjective response to the resource; rate and duration of use of the various components (e.g., graphics, simulation routines); total time spent by users per session; time taken to access and learn a given set of facts; accuracy of recall of learned facts, decrement over time; effect on users' diagnostic, therapeutic, prognostic decisions and actions; effect on users' subjective confidence about similar clinical cases; effect on users' knowledge or understanding of biomedicine.

Patient Simulation Package

Subjective ease of use; number of parameters adjusted by users (as a percentage of the total number); effect on users' diagnostic, therapeutic, prognostic decisions and actions; effect on users' subjective confidence about similar cases; effect on users' knowledge or understanding of biomedicine.

Patient Monitor

Users' response to the alarms and the monitor; alarm rate, false alarm rate, detection rate for true alarm conditions; how much of the time the users disable the alarm; effect on users' diagnostic, therapeutic, prognostic decisions and actions; effect on users' subjective confidence about clinical cases.

Appendix B

Specific Functions of Selected Computer-Based Information Resources

Database

Data security: methods for backing up patient data, changing user defaults/settings.
Data confidentiality: password control, file encryption.
Flexibility of file structure, ability to extend contents of data dictionary.
Reliability of hardware/software during power loss.
Maximum transaction capacity.

Data Coding/Translation Component

Use of coded data, coding accuracy, accuracy of mapping codes to another system; percent of data items possible to code; ease of extending codes.

Data-Retrieval Component

Completeness, speed of data retrieval, degradation with 10,000 cases using different search methods (query by example, Boolean, string search).

Fidelity of data output to data input (e.g., rounding errors, use of different synonyms).

Any Data-Input Component

Subjective ease, objective accuracy, time taken, number of actions (e.g., key presses) required to enter data items, number of errors correctly detected by resource.

Speech-Input Component

Accuracy, speaker invariance, resistance to background noise, directionality, ability to enter words via keyboard, accuracy when used via telephone, size of vocabulary, speed of recognition.

Knowledge Resource (Full-Text Database)

Ease of navigation, retrieval using a standardized vocabulary or synonyms, understanding contents, speed, ease of keeping knowledge up to date.

Advice Generator

Length, apparent ease of comprehension, structuring, accuracy of advice; calibration of any probability estimates.

Critique Generator

Length, ease of comprehension, structuring, accuracy of critique comments.

Explanation Generator

Length, ease of comprehension, structuring, accuracy of explanations; flexibility over domains, range of user questions it can address.

Imaging System

Spatial resolution (number of pixels, linear size), linear calibration (use of phantoms or models), contrast range, separation (influence of adjacent features), stability over time, amount of data generated per image, internal data storage capacity, time to capture one image.

Teaching System

Time to navigate to required section, accuracy compared to other sources, coverage of topic, ability to tailor to user, ease of maintenance, usage of standard vocabulary.

Patient-Simulation Package

Ease of use, accuracy compared to what happens in real cases, number of parameters that can be changed as a percentage of the total, how well the system's internal state is communicated to the user, speed, stability over time.

Patient Monitor

Resistance to electromagnetic interference or patient movement; resolution of analogue to decimal converter; sampling rate; internal storage capacity; storage format; accuracy of parameters such as amplitudes; wave duration, rates, trends, alarms; stability of baseline; calibration.

4
The Structure of Objectivist Studies

Important human and clinical phenomena are regularly omitted when patient care is
... analyzed in statistical comparisons of therapy. The phenomena are omitted either
because they lack formal expressions to identify them or because the available expres-
sions are regarded as scientifically unacceptable.[1]

This chapter begins the exploration of objectivist studies in detail. In Chapters 4 through 8, we address the design of studies, along with how to develop measurement procedures to collect data and how subsequently to analyze the data collected. The methods introduced relate directly to the comparison-based, objectives-based, and decision-facilitation approaches to evaluation described in Chapter 2. They are useful for addressing most of the purposes of evaluation in informatics, the specific questions that can be explored, and the types of studies that can be undertaken—as introduced in Chapter 3.

In this chapter, a conceptual framework for thinking about objectivist studies is developed. Some terminology is introduced that, once established, is used consistently in the chapters that follow. Much of this terminology is familiar, but some of these familiar terms are used in ways that are novel. Unfortunately, there is no single accepted terminology for describing objectivist studies. Epidemiologists, behavioral and social scientists, information scientists, statisticians, and evaluators have developed their own variations. As informatics itself reflects several fields, so must the language. It is emphasized that the terms introduced here are more than just labels. They represent concepts that are central to understanding the structure of objectivist studies and, ultimately, to one's ability to design them.

A major theme of this chapter, and indeed all five chapters on objectivist studies, is the importance of measurement. Two of the chapters in this group are explicitly devoted to measurement because such a large proportion of the major problems to be overcome in evaluation study design are, at their core, problems of measurement. Measurement issues are also stressed here because they are sometimes overlooked in research methods courses based in other disciplines.

After introducing some measurement terminology, this chapter formally establishes the distinction between *measurement studies* designed to explore with how much error "things of interest" in informatics can be measured, and *demonstration studies*, which apply these measurement procedures to answer evaluation questions of substantive and practical concern. The distinction between measurement and demonstration studies is more than academic. As they are defined here, pure measurement studies are rarely done in informatics. For example, a review of the literature on attitudes toward information technology in health care, covering 11 years, revealed only 17 articles that could be classified as reporting measurement studies.[2] In the informatics literature, it appears that measurement issues usually are embedded in, and often confounded with, demonstration issues. Although attitudes pose some notoriously difficult challenges for measurement, similar challenges exist across the full range of outcomes, as introduced in Chapter 3, that are of concern in informatics. Indeed, a more-recent review of objectivist studies of clinical information systems revealed that only three of 27 published studies paid explicit attention to measurement issues.[3] This matter is of substantial significance because deficiencies in measurement can profoundly affect the conclusions drawn from a demonstration study. The quote that begins this chapter alerts us to the fact that our ability to investigate is circumscribed by our ability to measure. Unless we possess or can develop ways to measure what is important to know about our information resources, our ability to conduct evaluation studies—at least those using objectivist approaches—is substantially limited.

This chapter, then, lays the groundwork for understanding the interplay between measurement and demonstration, a relationship that is developed more deeply in the following four chapters on objectivist studies. The next two chapters explore measurement issues in detail. The final two chapters in this group focus on the design and conduct of demonstration studies.

Measurement Process and Terminology

In this section, some ground rules, definitions, and synonyms will be discussed that relate to the process of measurement. These definitions may use some familiar words in unfamiliar ways, and the authors apologize for what may appear to be an exercise in transforming the self-evident into the obscure. The process of measurement and the interrelations of the terms to be defined are illustrated in Figure 4.1.

Measurement

Measurement is the process of assigning a value corresponding to the presence, absence, or degree of a specific attribute in a specific object. The terms

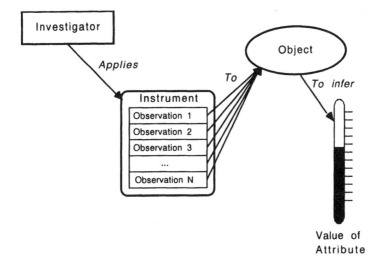

FIGURE 4.1. Process of measurement.

"attribute" and "object" are defined below. Measurement in this objectivist sense usually results in either (1) assignment of a numerical score representing the extent to which the attribute of interest is present in the object, or (2) assignment of an object to a specific category. Taking the temperature (attribute) of a patient (object) is an example of the process of measurement.

Object and Object Class

The object is the entity on which the measurement is made, the characteristics of which are being described. Every measurement process begins with the specification of a class of objects. Each act of measurement is performed on an individual object, which is a member of the class. Persons (patients, care providers, students, and researchers), information resources, practitioner or research groups, and healthcare and academic organizations are important examples of object classes in biomedical informatics on which measurements are frequently made.

The choice of object class is always important. After taking a set of measurements with a particular class of objects, an investigator can exploit the fact that these objects form natural sets to conduct analyses at a higher level of aggregation. For example, having measured the weights of individual patients who receive care in a set of community practices, a researcher can combine the measurement results for all patients seen in each practice. The result of this process, a set of average patient weights for each practice, makes the practice into an object class for purposes of measurement. However, it is impossible to go from higher to lower levels of aggregation.

If the original measurements are made with the practice as the object class, information about individual patients cannot later be retrieved or analyzed.

Attribute

An attribute is a specific characteristic of the object: what is being measured. Information resource speed, blood pressure, the correct diagnosis (of a clinical case), the number of new patient admissions per day, the number of kilobases (in a strand of DNA), and computer literacy are examples of pertinent attributes within biomedical informatics. Whereas some attributes are physical properties of objects, others are abstractions invented by researchers specifically for conducting investigations. For this reason, attributes are sometimes referred to as "constructs." Over time, each scientific field develops a set of attributes, "things worth measuring," that become part of the culture of that field. Researchers may tend to view the attributes that are part of their field's research tradition as a routine part of the landscape and fail to recognize that, at some earlier point in history, these concepts were unknown. Blood pressure, for example, had no meaning to humankind until circulation was understood. Computer literacy is a more recent construct stimulated by contemporary technological developments. Indeed, the most creative works of science propose completely new constructs, develop methods to measure them, and subsequently demonstrate their value in describing or predicting phenomena of interest.

Many studies in informatics address human behavior and the beliefs that are presumed to motivate this behavior. In such studies, the attributes of interest are usually not physical or physiological properties, but, rather, abstract concepts corresponding to presumed states of mind. Attitudes, knowledge, and performance are broad classes of human attributes that often interest biomedical informatics researchers. The behavioral, social, and decision sciences have contributed specific methods that enable us to measure such attributes.

Attribute–Object Class Pairs

Having defined an attribute as a quality of a specific object that is a member of a class, it is always possible to view a measurement process in terms of paired attributes and object classes. Table 4.1 illustrates this pairing of attributes and object classes for the examples discussed above. It is important to be able to analyze any given measurement situation by identifying the pertinent attribute and object class. To do this, certain questions might be asked. To identify the *attribute*, the questions might be: What is being measured? What will the result of the measurement be called? To identify the *object class*, the question might be: On whom or on what is the measurement made? The reader can use Self-Test 4.1, and the worked example preceding it, to test his or her understanding of these concepts.

TABLE 4.1. Attribute–object class pairs.

Attribute	Object class
Speed	Information resource
Blood pressure	Patient
Correct diagnosis	Patient
New admissions per day	Hospital ward team
Computer literacy	Person
Number of base-pairs	DNA strand

Instruments

The instrument is the technology used for measurement. The "instrument" encodes and embodies the procedures used to determine the presence, absence, or extent of an attribute in an object. For studies in biomedical informatics, instruments include self-administered questionnaires, traditional biomedical devices (e.g., an image acquisition device), tests of medical knowledge or skills, performance checklists, and the computer itself, through logging software that records aspects of resource use. It is apparent from these examples that many measurements in informatics require substantial human interpretation before the value of an attribute is inferred. A radiograph must be interpreted; performance checklists must be completed by observers. In such instances, a human "judge," or perhaps a panel of judges, may be viewed as an essential part of the instrumentation for a measurement process.

Observations

An observation is a question or other device that elicits one independent element of measurement data.* As measurement is customarily carried out, multiple independent observations are employed to estimate the value of an attribute for an object. This is because multiple independent observations produce a better estimate of the "true" value of the attribute than a single observation. Use of multiple observations also allows for the determination of how much variability exists across observations, which is necessary to estimate the error inherent in the measurement. As will be detailed in the next chapter, multiple observations sometimes are obtained by repeated measurements conducted under conditions that are as close to identical as possible. Under other circumstances, multiple observations are obtained under very carefully varied conditions. For example, the "speed" of an information resource can be assessed by calculating the average time taken to perform a range of appropriately selected computational

---

* When observations are recorded on a form, the term "item" is often used to describe a question or other probe that elicits one independent element of information on the form.

tasks. For these purposes, each task may be considered an independent observation.

Example

As part of a study of a computer-based resource for diagnosis, the investigators are interested in how reasonable the diagnoses suggested by the system are, even when these diagnoses are not exactly correct. They conduct a study where the "top-five" diagnoses generated by the resource for a sample of test cases are referred to a panel of experienced physicians for review.

Focusing on the measurement aspects of this process, it is important to name the attribute being measured and the relevant object class. It is also important to describe how this measurement process employs multiple independent observations.

To identify the attribute, the question might be: What is being measured and what should the result of the measurement be called? The result of the measurement is called something like the "reasonableness" of the top five diagnoses, so that is the attribute. To identify the object class, the question might be: On whom or on what is the actual measurement made? The measurement is made on the diagnosis set generated by the resource for each case, so the case or, more specifically, the "diagnosis set for each case" can be seen as the object class of measurement. The multiple observations are generated by the presumably independent ratings of the expert clinicians.

Self-Test 4.1

1. To determine the performance of a computer-based reminder system, a sample of alerts generated by the system (and the patient record from which each alert was generated) is given to a panel of physicians. Each panelist rates each alert on a four-point scale from "highly appropriate to the clinical situation" to "completely inappropriate." Focusing on the measurement aspects of this process, name the attribute being measured, the class of measurement objects, and the instrument used. Describe how this measurement process employs multiple independent observations.

2. The physicians in a large community hospital undergo training to use a new clinical information system. After the training, each physician completes a test, which is comprised of 30 questions about the system, to help the developers understand how much knowledge about the system has been conveyed via the training. Name the attribute being measured, the class of measurement objects, the instrument used. Describe how this measurement process employs multiple independent observations.

3. A computer-based resource is created to review patient admission notes and identify pertinent terms to "index" the cases using the institution's controlled clinical vocabulary. As part of a study of this new resource, a panel of judges familiar with the clinical vocabulary reviews a set of cases.

The set of terms identified by the system for each case is reviewed to see if the case is indexed correctly. From a measurement perspective, name the attribute and object class.

4. In studies of gene expression analysis, a DNA array (or chip) is used to detect levels of messenger ribonucleic acid (mRNA) expressed in a biological sample (e.g., normal or cancer tissue cells). The array consists of many different DNA strands of known sequence printed at defined positions; each such position has multiple copies of DNA strands that constitute a coherent spot on the array. The biological mRNA sample is "reverse transcribed" into complementary DNA (cDNA), labeled with a fluorescent dye and hybridized (joined) with the DNA on the array. Only the cDNA from the biological sample that matches the DNA strands on the chip will be hybridized. Finally, the array is scanned and the amount of fluorescence is assumed to correspond to the amount of hybridized DNA on each spot. Viewing the chip as a measurement instrument, name the attribute(s) being measured and the object class. Does this measurement process, as described, include multiple independent observations?

[Answers to these questions are found at the end of the chapter.]

Levels of Measurement

Measurement assigns the value of an attribute to an object, but not all attributes are created equal. Attributes differ according to how their values are naturally expressed or represented. Attributes such as height and weight are naturally expressed using continuous numerical values whereas attributes such as "marital status" are expressed using discrete values. An attribute's level of measurement denotes how its values can be represented. It will be seen in later chapters that an attribute's level of measurement directs the design of measurement instruments and the statistical analyses that can be applied to the results of measurements performed on samples of objects. There are four such levels of measurement.

1. *Nominal:* Measurement on a nominal attributes results in the assignment of each object to a specific category. The categories themselves do not form a continuum or have a meaningful order. Examples of attributes measured at the nominal level are ethnicity, medical specialty, and the bases comprising a nucleotide. To represent the results of a nominal measurement quantitatively, the results must be assigned arbitrary codes (e.g., 1 for "internists," 2 for "surgeons," 3 for "family practitioners"). The only aspect of importance for such codes is that they be employed consistently to represent measurement results. Their actual numerical or alphanumerical values have no significance.

2. *Ordinal:* Measurement at the ordinal level also results in assignment of objects to categories, but the categories have some meaningful order or

ranking. For example, physicians often use a "plus" system of recording clinical signs ("++ edema"), which represents an ordinal measurement. The staging of cancers is another clinical example of an ordinal measurement. The well-known (but now somewhat outdated) classification of computers as micro, mini, or mainframe is also measurement on an ordinal scale. When coding the results of ordinal measurements, a numerical code is typically assigned to each category, but no aspect of these codes except for their numerical order contains interpretable information.

Note that both nominal and ordinal measurements can be termed "categorical" and are often referenced that way. However, use of the term "categorical" as an umbrella descriptor for nominal and ordinal measures conceals the important difference between them.

3. *Interval:* Results of measurements at the interval level take on continuous numerical values that have an arbitrarily chosen zero point. The classic examples are the Fahrenheit and Celsius scales of temperature. This level of measurement derives its name from the "equal interval" assumption, which all interval measures must satisfy. To satisfy this assumption, equal differences between two measurements must have the same meaning irrespective of where they occur on the scale of possible values. On the Fahrenheit scale, the difference between 50 and 40 degrees has the same meaning, in terms of thermal energy, as the difference between 20 and 10 degrees. An "interval" of 10 degrees is interpreted identically all along the scale. Investigators often assume that the attributes employed in their studies have interval properties when, in fact, there is reason to question this belief. In biomedical informatics, the average response of a group of judges—each of whom responds using a set of ordinal options ("excellent," "good," "fair," "poor") on a rating form— is often used to produce a measured value for each object. It is typically assumed that the average of these ordinal judgments has interval properties. This assumption is controversial and is discussed in Chapter 6.

4. *Ratio:* Results of measurements at the ratio level have the additional property of a true zero point. The Kelvin scale of temperature, with a zero point that is not arbitrarily chosen, has the properties of ratio measurement, whereas the other temperature scales do not. Most physiological measures (such as blood pressure) and physical measures (such as length) have ratio properties. This level of measurement is so named because one can assign meaning to the ratio of two measurement results in addition to the difference between them.

In objectivist measurement, it is usually desirable to collect data at the highest possible level of measurement possible for the attribute of interest, with ratio measurement being the highest of the levels. In this way, the measured results contain the maximum amount of information. A common mistake of investigators is to obtain or record measurement results at a lower level than the attribute naturally allows. For example, in a survey of healthcare providers, the investigator may want to know each respondent's years of professional experience: naturally, a ratio measure. Frequently, however, such attributes are assessed using discrete response categories, each containing a range of years. Although this measurement strategy provides some convenience and possibly some sense of anonymity for the respondent (and may, in some cases, generate more complete data with fewer missing values), it reduces to ordinal status what is naturally a ratio variable, with inevitable loss of information. Even if the data are later going to be categorized when eventually analyzed and reported, collecting and storing the data at the highest level of measurement is a safer strategy. Data can always be converted from higher to lower levels of measurement, but it is not possible to go the other way.

Self-Test 4.2

Determine the level of measurement of each of the following:

1. A person's serum potassium level;
2. A health sciences center's national ranking in grant funding from the National Institutes of Health;
3. The distance between the position of an atom in a protein, as predicted by a computer model, and its actual position in the protein;
4. The "stage" of a patient's neoplastic illness;
5. The internal medicine service to which each of a set of patients is assigned;
6. A person's marital status;
7. A person's score on an intelligence test, such as an IQ test.

Importance of Measurement

Having introduced some concepts and terms, the importance of measurement in objectivist studies can be appreciated by revisiting the major premises underlying the objectivist approaches to evaluation. These premises were originally introduced in Chapter 2, but they are re-stated here in a somewhat revised form to exploit this new terminology. Like all premises, these are based on assumptions that reflect idealized views of the world and our ability to understand it through certain methods of empirical research. Readers who have difficulty accepting these assumptions might find themselves more attracted to the subjectivist approaches discussed in Chapters 9 and 10.

In objectivist studies, the following can be assumed:

- *Attributes* inhere in the *object* under study. Merit and worth are part of the object and can be measured unambiguously. An investigator can measure these attributes without affecting the object's structure or function.

- All rational persons agree (or can be brought to consensus) on what attributes of an object are important to measure and what measurement results would be associated with high merit or worth of the object. In biomedical informatics, this is tantamount to stating that a "gold standard" of practice can always be identified, and that informed individuals can be brought to consensus on what this gold standard is.

- Because numerical measurement of attributes allows precise statistical comparisons across groups and across time, numerical measurement is prima facie superior to verbal description.

- Through comparisons of measured attributes across selected groups of objects, it is possible to demonstrate at a specific level of confidence that a particular biomedical information resource is superior to what it replaced or to some alternative design of that resource.

From these premises, it follows that the proper execution of objectivist studies requires careful and specific attention to methods of measurement. It can never be assumed, particularly in informatics, that attributes of interest are measured without error. Accurate and precise measurement must not be an afterthought.[†] Measurement is of particular importance in biomedical informatics because, as a relatively young field, informatics does not have a well-established tradition of "things worth measuring" or proven instruments for measuring them. By and large, those planning studies are faced with the task of first deciding what to measure and then developing their own measurement methods. For most investigators, this task proves more difficult and more time-consuming than initially anticipated. In some cases, informatics investigators can adapt the measures used by others, but they often need to apply these measures to a different setting, where prior experience may not apply.

The choice of what to measure, and how, is an area where there are few prescriptions and where sound judgment, experience, and knowledge of methods come into play. Decisions about *what* and, above all, *how* to measure require knowledge of the study questions, the intervention and setting, and the experience of others who have done similar work. A methodological expert in measurement is of assistance only when teamed with others who know the terrain of biomedical informatics. Conversely, all biomedical informatics researchers should know something about measurement.

[†] Terms such as "accuracy" and "precision" are used loosely in this chapter. They will be defined more rigorously in Chapter 5.

Measurement and Demonstration Studies

The importance of measurement can be underscored by establishing a formal distinction between studies undertaken to develop and refine methods for making measurements, which are called *measurement studies*, and the subsequent use of these methods to address questions of direct importance in informatics, which are called *demonstration studies*. Establishing a distinction between these types of studies, and lending them approximately equal status in this textbook, are steps intended to ensure that measurement issues are not overlooked.

Measurement studies, then, seek to determine with how much error an attribute of interest can be measured in a population of objects, often also indicating how this error can be reduced. In an ideal objectivist measurement, all observers agree on the result of the measurement. Therefore, any disagreement is due to measurement error, which should be minimized. The more agreement among observations, the "better" is the measurement. It is also important that the observers are observing the intended attribute and not something different. Measurement procedures developed and vetted through measurement studies provide researchers with what they need to conduct demonstration studies. Once it is known with how much error an attribute can be measured using a particular procedure, the measured values of this attribute can be employed as a variable in a demonstration study to draw inferences about the performance, perceptions, or effects of an information resource. For example, once a measurement study has established the error inherent in measuring the speed of an information resource, a related demonstration study would explore whether a particular resource has sufficient speed—with speed measured using methods developed in the measurement study—to meet the needs of researchers and clinicians.

As this discussion unfolds, numerous relations between measurement and demonstration study design will be seen, but there are also many important distinctions. There are differences in terminology that can become somewhat confusing. For example, measurement studies are concerned with attributes and objects, whereas demonstration studies are concerned with variables and subjects. With measurement, the concern is with differences between individual objects and how accurate the measurement is for each one. With demonstration studies, the primary interest is usually at the level of the group and how accurately the mean (or some other indicator of central tendency) of a variable for that group can be estimated. Of course, the two issues are intertwined. It is impossible to conduct a satisfactory demonstration study using poorly performing measurement methods. As is seen in subsequent chapters, errors in measurement can make differences between groups more difficult to detect or can produce apparent differences when none are truly present.

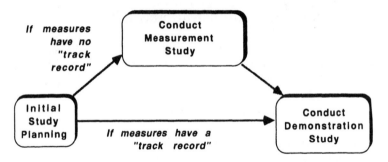

FIGURE 4.2. Measurement and demonstration studies.

The bottom line is that investigators must know that their measurement methods are adequate—"adequacy" will be defined more rigorously in the next chapter—*before* collecting data for their studies. As shown in Figure 4.2, it is necessary to perform a measurement study, usually involving data collection on a smaller scale, to establish the adequacy of all measurement procedures if the measures to be used do not have an established "track record." Even if the measurement procedures of interest have a track record in a particular health care or research environment and with a specific mix of cases and care providers, they may not perform equally well in a different environment. Therefore, measurement studies may still be necessary even when apparently tried-and-true measurement approaches are being employed. Researchers should always ask themselves—How good are my measures in this particular setting?—whenever they are planning a study and before proceeding to the demonstration phase. The importance of measurement studies for informatics was signaled in 1990 by Michaelis and colleagues.[4] References to many published measurement studies in biomedical informatics are found in the study by Cork and colleagues.[2]

Goals and Structure of Measurement Studies

The overall goal of a measurement study is to estimate with how much error an attribute can be measured for a class of objects, ultimately leading to a viable measurement process for later application to demonstration studies. In Chapter 5, a theory is developed that describes in more detail how measurement errors are estimated. In Chapter 6, building on that theory, the design of measurement studies is addressed in greater technical detail.

One specific objective of a measurement study is to determine how many independent observations are necessary to reduce error to a level acceptable for the demonstration study to follow. In most situations, the greater the number of independent observations comprising a measurement process, the smaller is the measurement error. This suggests an important trade-off because each independent observation comes at a cost. If the speed of a computer-based resource is to be tested over a range of computationally demanding tasks, each task must be carefully constructed or selected by the research team. Similarly, if the attitudes of researchers are the attributes and objects of measurement, the time required to complete a long form containing multiple items may be greater than these individuals are willing to provide. For example, a questionnaire requiring 100 answers from each respondent may be a more precise instrument than a questionnaire of half that length; however, no one, especially a busy researcher, may have the time to complete it. In this case, an investigator may be willing to trade off greater measurement error against what may be a higher rate of participation in a demonstration study. Without a measurement study conducted in advance, however, there is no way to quantify this trade-off and estimate the optimal balance point.

Another objective of measurement studies is to verify that measurement instruments are well designed and functioning as intended. Even a measurement process with an ample number of independent observations will have a high error rate if there are fundamental flaws in the way the process is conducted. For example, if human judges are involved in a rating task and the judges are not trained to use the same criteria for the ratings, the results will reveal unacceptably high error. Fatigue may be a factor if the judges are asked to do too much, too fast. Additionally, consider a computer program developed to compute a measure of medication costs automatically from a computer-based patient record. If this program has a bug that causes it to fail to include certain classes of medications, it cannot return accurate results. An appropriate measurement study can detect these kinds of problems.

The researcher designing a measurement study also should try to build into the study features that challenge the measurement process in ways that might be expected to occur in the demonstration study to follow. Only in this way is it possible to determine if the results of the measurement study will apply when the measurement process is put to actual use. For example, in the rating task mentioned above, the judges should be challenged in the measurement study with a range of cases typical of those expected in the demonstration study. An algorithm to compute medication costs should be tested with a representative sample of cases from a variety of clinical services in the hospital where the demonstration study will ultimately be conducted. A related issue is that a measurement technique may perform well with individuals from one particular culture, but perform poorly when transferred to a different culture. In informatics, this problem could arise when a study moves from a hospital that is growing and where employees have a great deal of autonomy to one where task performance is more rigidly prescribed. The same questionnaire administered in the two settings may yield different results because respondents are interpreting the questions differently. This issue, too, can be explored via an appropriately designed measurement study that includes the full range of settings where it might be used.

Measurement studies are planned in advance. The researcher conducting a measurement study creates a set of conditions, applies the measurement technique under development to a set of objects, often makes other measurements on these same objects, studies the results, and makes modifications in the measurement technique as suggested by the results. Measurement studies are conducted somewhat more informally than demonstration studies. Samples of convenience often are employed instead of systematically selected samples of objects, although there is clearly some risk involved in this practice. As a practical matter, measurement studies often are undertaken outside the specific setting where the demonstration study will later be performed. This is done because the investigator does not want to presensitize the setting in which the demonstration study will be conducted, and thus introduce bias. Also as a practical matter, in some situations where proven measurement methods do not exist, it may be impractical or impossible to conduct measurement studies in advance of the demonstration studies. In these situations, investigators use the data collected in the demonstration study as the basis for statistical analyses that are customarily done as part of a measurement study.

As an example, consider a study of a new admission–discharge–transfer (ADT) system for hospitals. The attribute of "time to process a new admission" might be important for this study. (Note that "patients" are the object class for this measurement process.) Although, on the surface, this construct might seem trivial to measure, many potential difficulties arise on closer scrutiny. To cite a few: When did the admission process for a patient begin and end? Were there interruptions, and when did each of these begin and end? Should interruptions be counted as part of processing time? In a measurement study with human observers as the instruments, three or four such observers could simultaneously observe the same set of admissions. The observers' extent of disagreement about the time to process these admissions would be used to determine how many observers (whose individual results are averaged) are necessary to obtain an acceptable error rate. If the error rate is too high, the measurement study might reveal a flaw in the form on which the observers are recording their observations, or it might reveal that the observers had not been provided with adequate instructions about how to deal with interruptions. The measurement study could be performed in the admissions suite of a hospital similar in many respects to the ones in which the demonstration study will later be performed. The demonstration study, once the measurement methods have been established, would explore whether the hospital actually processes admissions faster with the new system than with its predecessor.

Self-Test 4.3

Clarke and colleagues developed the TraumAID system[5] to advise on initial treatment of patients with penetrating injuries to the chest and abdomen. Measurement studies of the utility of TraumAID's advice required panels of judges to rate the adequacy of management of a set of "test cases"—as recommended by TraumAID and as carried out by care providers. To perform this study, case data were fed into TraumAID to generate a treatment plan for each case. The wording of TraumAID's plans was edited carefully so that judges performing subsequent ratings would have no way of knowing whether the described care was performed by a human or recommended by computer. Two groups of judges were employed in the measurement studies: one from the medical center where the resource was developed, the other a group of senior physicians from across the country.

For this measurement situation, name the attribute of interest and the object class; describe the instrumentation. List some issues that might be clarified by this measurement study.

[Answers are found at the end of the chapter.]

Gold Standards and Informatics

A final issue before leaving the topic of measurement is the often-used term "gold standard" and its relation to measurement in informatics. In biomedical informatics, the lack of so-called gold standards is often bemoaned.[6] As we embark on an exploration of objectivist methods, it is timely to ask: What exactly is a gold standard? By traditional definition, a gold standard is a composite of two notions. In the first sense, a gold standard is an expression of practice carried out perfectly: the optimal therapy for a given biomedical problem or the best differential diagnosis to be entertaining at a particular point in the evolution of a case. In the second sense, a gold standard implies complete acceptance or consensus. For a given situation, everyone qualified to render a judgment would agree to what the gold standard is. These two aspects of a gold standard are tightly interrelated. If there exists only one standard of care, it must be a standard everyone would endorse completely.

In most real-world situations of sufficient interest to merit study, perfect (gold) standards of practice do not exist. In treating patients, in conducting a high-throughput array analysis, or in the process of learning to program a computer, there is usually no unequivocal "best thing to do" at a particular point in time. Given two or more scenarios of professional practice, independent observers who are measuring the quality of this practice will not be in perfect agreement as to which scenario represents better practice. Health care, research, or education conducted with support from information technology cannot be definitively compared to practice without technology support because of the measurement problem that stems from the absence of absolute standards.

The lack of gold standards in biomedicine has led some to adopt a view that it is not useful to conduct formal empirical studies of biomedical information resources because these studies would always be tainted by the fuzziness of whatever standard is employed as the basis of comparison. Such individuals might argue further that instinctive, marketplace, or political interpretations of the value of these resources should be relied upon instead. Other, less nihilistic researchers might still conduct empirical studies, but their studies are designed to bypass the gold-standard issue. For example, instead of comparing the performance of an information resource against an imperfect standard of practice, about which there is necessarily disagreement among human experts, such studies might seek to show that the resource agrees with the experts to the same extent that experts agree with each other.[7]

In the chapters to follow, the position is taken that gold standards, even if unattainable, are worth approximating. That is, "tarnished" or "fuzzy" standards are better than no standards at all. As a theory of measurement is developed, a method for addressing the fuzziness of gold standards is developed, joining others who have engaged in similar efforts.[8,9] Perfect gold standards do not exist in biomedical informatics or in any other domain of empirical research, but the extent to which these standards are less than perfect can be estimated and expressed as forms of measurement error. Knowledge of the magnitude and origin of this error enables the researcher, in many cases, to consider the error in statistical analyses, thereby drawing stronger conclusions than otherwise would be possible. Although zero measurement error is always the best situation, a good estimate of the magnitude of the error is sufficient to allow rigorous studies to be conducted. Studies comparing the performance of information resources against imperfect standards, so long as the degree of imperfection has been estimated, represent a stronger approach than studies that bypass the issue of a standard altogether.

With this position as a backdrop (and with apologies for a colorfully mixed metaphor), the gold standard becomes a sort of red herring. More pragmatically, any standard employed in a study can be viewed as a *measured* value of a chosen attribute, which can expediently be *accepted* as a standard, knowing that it approximates but is not necessarily equal to the true "gold standard." For example, a patient's discharge diagnosis might be the imperfect standard in a study of an information resource supporting medical diagnosis.[10] Although it is known that a discharge diagnosis sometimes proves later to have been incorrect, it is the best measure available, and so it is accepted. The alternative to accepting a less-than-perfect standard would be not to do the study. An error-free appraisal of the patient's diagnosis may not be available until the patient's death—and may never be available if the patient fully recovers from his or her illness. Consistent with this view, the investigators obligation in objectivist studies is to develop the best possible way of measuring a standard suited to the context of the research, conduct measurement studies to estimate the error associated with measurement of the standard, and then, in demonstration studies, incorporate this error estimate appropriately into statistical analyses and interpretation of the results. Human experts often are employed in informatics studies to generate a less-than-perfect performance standard.[11] This topic will be returned to, in detail, in Chapter 6.

Each domain of biomedical practice creates its own challenges for evaluators, who inevitably find themselves in the roles of both developer and measurer of standards. Some domains make this task more challenging than do others. The "carat level" of a standard can be spoken of somewhat loosely as a heuristic estimate of the level of error with which it can be measured: the accuracy and precision with which the standard's true value can be known. Table 4.2 lists some of the domains that are addressed in biomedical informatics studies, as well as a heuristic "carat level" reflecting the intrinsic difficulty of making precise measurements in that domain. (Table 4.2 is offered for illustrative purposes only, and no specific interpretation should be attached to the numbers provided.)

According to Table 4.2, there is no absolute 24-carat gold standard for any problem in biomedicine. Even a pathological process identified on autopsy might be erroneously identified, or might be unrelated to the patient's symptoms. As seen later in our theory of error, the carat level of a standard can be estimated, but it cannot be determined precisely. For each member of a class of objects, precise determination would require knowledge of the true value of an attribute against which the purported standard can be compared; if the true value were known, it would by definition become the 24-carat standard. In addition, there are some clinical situations where an almost-perfect standard can be known, but only through studies too expensive or dangerous to conduct. In such cases, the more approximate, lower carat standard is accepted. For example, myocardial perfusion scintigraphy is a currently accepted protocol for evaluating coronary artery disease because an arteriogram involves too much risk in patients with minimal symptoms.

TABLE 4.2. Prototypical "carat scale" of gold standards.

Carats	Criteria
23+	Diagnosis of a patient who underwent a definitive test
20	Diagnosis of a patient about whom a great deal is known but for whom there is no definitive diagnosis
18	Appropriateness of a therapy plan for a patient with a specific diagnosis
15	Correctness of a critique issued by an advisory system
13	Adequacy of a diagnostic workup plan
10	Quality of a substance-abuse screening interview

The Structure of Demonstration Studies

We now move from a discussion of measurement to a discussion of demonstration. Demonstration studies differ from measurement studies in several respects. First, they aim to say something meaningful about a biomedical information resource or answer some other question of substantive interest in informatics. With measurement studies, the concern is with the error inherent in assigning a value of an attribute to each individual object, whereas with demonstration studies, the concern is redirected. Demonstration studies are concerned with determining the actual magnitude of that attribute in a group of objects, or determining if groups of objects differ in the magnitude of that attribute. For example, in a study of an information resource to support management of patients in the intensive care unit, a measurement study would be concerned with how accurately and precisely the "optimal care" (attribute) for a patient (object) can be determined. The demonstration study might explore whether care providers supported by the resource deliver care more closely approximating optimal care. In the study of an information resource to support students learning to interpret histological specimens, a measurement study may focus on how well the accuracy of students' diagnoses can be measured. The subsequent demonstration study would compare supported and unsupported students' performances on this test.

The terminology of demonstration studies also changes from that used for measurement studies. Most notable are the following points:

- The *object* of measurement in a measurement study is typically referred to as a *subject or participant* in a demonstration study.
- An *attribute* in a measurement study is typically referred to as a *variable* in a demonstration study.

In theory, these terminology differences are disconcerting, but in practice, they seldom cause confusion.

When designing objectivist studies, variables are divided into two categories: dependent and independent. The *dependent variables* are a subset of the variables in the study that capture outcomes of interest to the investigator. For this reason, dependent variables are also called "outcome variables." The *independent variables* are those included in a study to explain the measured values of the dependent variables.

Demonstration Study Designs

The intent, and thus the design, of demonstration studies can be descriptive, comparative, or correlational—as described in the following text and illustrated in Figure 4.3.

(A)

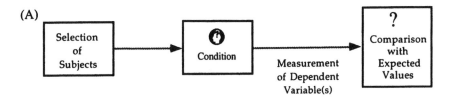

(B)

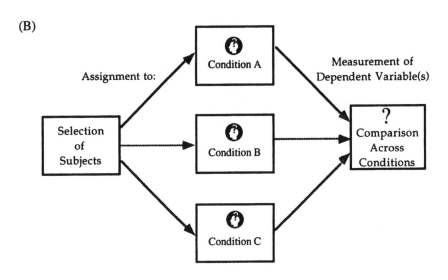

(C)

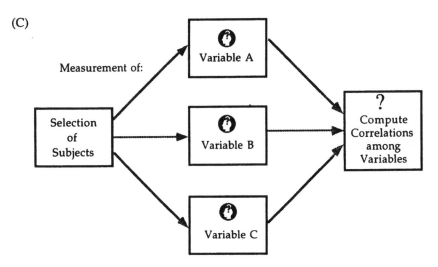

FIGURE 4.3. (A) Descriptive study design; (B) comparative study design; (C) correlational study design.

Descriptive Studies

A *descriptive* design seeks only to estimate the value of a dependent variable or set of dependent variables in a selected sample of subjects. Descriptive designs have no independent variable. If a group of nurses were given a rating form (previously validated through a measurement study) to ascertain the "ease of use" of a nursing information system, the mean value of this variable would be the key result of a descriptive study. If this value were found to be toward the low end of the scale, the researchers might conclude from this descriptive study that the system was in need of substantial revision. Although they seem deceptively simple, descriptive studies can be highly informative. Teach and Shortliffe's[12] examination of physicians' attitudes toward medical decision support is an example of a descriptive study that has had substantial impact "simply" by asserting that physicians, as a group, appear to share certain beliefs. Studies of the quality of health information on the Internet also illustrate the importance of well-conducted descriptive studies.[13] Descriptive studies also can be tied to the "objectives-based" approach to evaluation described in Chapter 2. When an investigator seeks to determine whether a resource has met a predetermined set of performance objectives, the logic and design of the resulting demonstration study may be seen as descriptive.

Comparative Studies

In a *comparative* study, the investigator typically creates a contrasting set of conditions. After identifying a sample of subjects for the study, the researcher either assigns each subject to one of these conditions or classifies them into one of the conditions based on some predetermined characteristic. Some variable of interest is then measured for each subject, and the measured values of this variable are compared across the conditions. The contrasting conditions comprise the independent variable(s) for the study, and the "variable of interest" is the dependent variable. The study by MacDonald and colleagues[14] of the effects of reminder systems is a classic example of a comparative study applied to informatics. In this study, groups of clinicians (subjects) either received or did not receive computer-generated reminders (conditions comprising the independent variable), and the investigators measured the extent to which clinicians took clinical actions consistent with the reminders (dependent variable). Comparative studies are aligned with the "comparison-based" approach to evaluation introduced in Chapter 2.

When the experimental conditions are created prospectively by the investigator and all other differences are eliminated by random assignment of subjects, it is possible to isolate and explore the effect due solely to the difference between the conditions. Under this design, the investigator also may assert that these effects are causal rather than merely coincidental. The randomized clinical trial, as described in the literature of clinical epidemiology,[15] is the consummate demonstration study.

It is not always possible, however, to manipulate the environment to the extent required to conduct such a pure experiment. In some study settings, the investigator may be compelled to forego random assignment of subjects to groups, and thus conduct what is called a "quasi-experiment." For example, health professionals who work in unionized organizations may refuse to be randomized into studies, insisting instead that they be able to choose the alternative that they believe in advance is best suited for them. Even when the results of a quasi-experiment reveal a difference between groups of subjects on the dependent measure, the source of the effect cannot be isolated as the independent variable. If the subjects selected themselves into groups instead of being randomly assigned, some unknown difference between the groups' members may be the causal factor.

Correlational Studies

In other cases, investigators conduct *correlational* studies that explore the hypothesized relationships among a set of variables the researcher measures but does not manipulate in any way. Correlational studies are guided by the researcher's hypotheses, which direct the choice of variables included in the study. The independent variables are the hypothesized predictors of an outcome of interest, which is the dependent variable. Correlational studies are linked most closely to the "comparison-based" and "decision-facilitation" approaches to evaluation discussed in Chapter 2. Correlational studies are also called observational, retrospective, or ex post facto studies. So-called data-mining studies that seek to extract interesting relationships from existing datasets are a form of correlational study. Data-mining studies are becoming increasingly common in both clinical and biological application domains.[16,17] Outcomes research and case-control studies in epidemiology can be seen to fall into this category as well.

In informatics, an example of a correlational study is one in which the researcher analyzes the extent of use of an information resource (the dependent variable) as a function of the clinical workload and the seniority (two independent variables) of each care provider (the subjects) in a hospital. In this study, the values of all the variables are properties of the subjects that cannot be manipulated and are studied retrospectively. As another example of a correlational study, the proportion of physicians in a hospital who enter their own medication orders may be followed over time. If an increase in this proportion is observed soon after a new user interface is implemented, the investigator might argue that the change in user interface was the cause of the increase. Although such an uncontrolled study cannot be the basis of a strong inference of cause and effect, correlational studies can be highly persuasive when carefully conceived and conducted.

As a general rule, and using the definitions introduced in Chapter 3, laboratory studies of information resources at an early stage of development will be descriptive in nature. These studies will focus on the performance of the resource in relation to design specifications only. Laboratory studies of more mature information resources will tend to be comparative in nature because laboratory settings allow for careful and planned manipulation by the experimenter. Field studies can be descriptive, comparative, or correlational in nature. Although it is possible, with great effort and at substantial expense, to conduct a carefully controlled comparative study in the field, it is difficult in some settings—and sometimes even unethical—to manipulate variables and impose experimental controls where ongoing health care is being delivered. Such a dilemma may arise, for example, with an alerting system that warns clinicians of drug interactions. If laboratory studies that have already been conducted suggest that the advice of this resource is accurate, a human-subjects review committee (also known as an Institutional Review Board, or IRB) might disallow a randomized trial of the resource because it is considered unethical to withhold this advice from the care of any patient. To cite one example, a clinical trial of the MEDIPHOR system at Stanford University was disallowed on these grounds (S.N. Cohen, personal communication, 1996). Such ethical issues are explored in more detail in Chapter 12.

Shared Features of Objectivist Studies

By comparing Figures 4.3 (A–C), it can be seen that these different study designs share several features. They all entail a deliberate selection of subjects, an explicit identification of variables, and a measurement process yielding data for analysis. They differ, as discussed above, in their general aims, the degree of imposed control or manipulation, and the logic of data analysis.

It is important, as a prerequisite to undertaking the design of studies, to understand the distinctions offered in this section. The distinction between independent and dependent variables is central.

Self-Test 4.4

Classify each of the following demonstration study designs as descriptive, comparative, or correlational. In each study, who or what are the subjects? Identify the independent and dependent variables.

1. In Chapter 2, the T-HELPER system was discussed. One of this resource's goals is to identify patients who are eligible for specific clinical protocols. A demonstration study of T-HELPER is implemented to examine protocol enrollment rates at sites where T-HELPER was and was not installed.

2. A new clinical workstation is introduced into a network of medical offices. Logs of one week of resource use by nurses are studied. The report enumerates sessions on the workstation, broken down into logical categories.

3. A number of computer-based information resources have been installed to support care on an inpatient service. The information resources log the identity of the patients about whom inquiries are made. By chart audit, the investigators identify a number of clinical characteristics of each patient's clinical problems. The investigators then study which characteristics of patients are predictive of the use of resources to obtain further information about that patient.

4. A researcher compiles a database of single nucleotide polymorphisms (SNPs), which are variations in an individual's genomic sequences. The researcher then examines these SNPs in relation to diseases that these individuals develop, as reflected in a clinical data repository.

5. Students are given access to a database to help them solve problems in a biomedical domain. By random assignment, half of the students use a version of the database emphasizing hypertext browsing capabilities; half use a version emphasizing Boolean queries for information. The proficiency of these students at solving problems is assessed at the beginning and end of the second year of medical school.

Meshing Aims, Approaches, and Designs in Demonstration Studies

This chapter closes with a description of the steps required to develop a demonstration study. This discussion is a preview of the much more complete exploration of designs for demonstration studies in Chapters 7 and 8. It is included to alert the reader to the complexities of demonstration studies, particularly those carried out in ongoing patient care, research, or educational settings. In Chapter 12, we will return to issues of study planning, as well as how study plans are formally expressed in proposals and evaluation contracts.

Planning a demonstration study can be seen as a three-stage process, as shown in Figure 4.4. First, one must carefully define the problem the study is intended to address. This step requires eliciting the aim of the study and the main questions to be answered. It is then useful to classify the study, based on its aims and the setting in which it will be conducted, using the distinctions offered in Chapter 3. A study may emphasize structure, function, or impact, and it may be seen as occurring primarily in a laboratory or field setting. From this information, a general design for the study—descriptive, comparative, correlational—can be selected. The needs of studies that address resource structure and function often are satisfied by an objectives-based approach (Is the resource performing up to the level

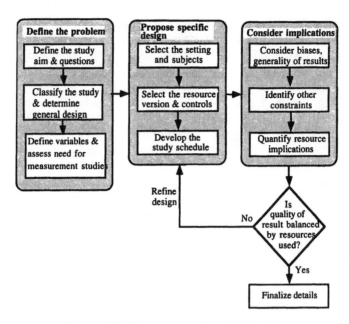

FIGURE 4.4. Three stages of study planning.

the designers expected?), which would recommend a descriptive study design. If a study addresses impact (Does the resource make a difference in research or health care?), a comparative or correlational design must be employed depending on the amount of control that can be imposed on the study setting. Comparative designs also are employed in studies seeking to show that the information resource is an improvement over what it replaced. Once the general design has been determined, evaluators can proceed to define the dependent and independent variables and consider how these factors might be measured. If the measurement instruments and procedures proposed for use do not have a "track record" (see Figure 4.2), it is usually necessary to undertake measurement studies before the demonstration study itself can be completed.

The second stage of planning a study is to propose a more-specific design. As suggested in Figure 4.4, a study design consists of three parts. There must be a statement of the setting in which the study will be conducted and of the source, kind, and number of subjects. The conditions of the study must be established if the study is comparative in nature. The version of the resource and any "control" resource to be tested must be selected. The final part is to outline the study schedule. In the case of evaluations of resource function, the schedule may be simple; but in studies concerned with the impact of the resource on its users or on health care, the schedule may be complex because the study must be embedded in an organized routine that usually cannot be altered substantially to suit the needs of the study. The schedule must clarify which subjects have access to which version of the resource at each phase of the study.

The third stage of planning an evaluation is to consider the issues arising from the proposed study design. The most important of these issues are biases that threaten the objectivist study's scientific validity. Specific biases to consider are discussed in detail in Chapter 7. Even if there are no significant biases, there may be limits to the generalizability of the study results or other constraints (related to ethics, time, or other factors) that make certain study plans not feasible. Each plan also has staffing and budget implications that may require careful examination.

Once the implications of the proposed plan have been listed, evaluators can balance the probable quality of the intended results with the time, energy, and financial resources necessary to obtain them. If this balance proves initially to be unsatisfactory, it becomes necessary to refine the proposed plan and reconsider its implications several times before an acceptable plan emerges. Finally, investigators must clarify the details of the study plan, and express it in a study contract before the study is started, to ensure that as many problems as possible are anticipated and defused. Every investigator designing a study must do so with the realization that, even after the central questions have been identified, every study is in some significant way a compromise. The investigator must balance the desire to assess many variables with many subjects under the most ideal conditions against the realities of limited funding and what is permissible in the environment. There are no formulae guiding this balancing act. This is one of many places where the "art" of evaluation becomes as important as its underlying science.

Answers to Self-Tests

Self-Test 4.1

1. The attribute is "appropriateness" of each alert. "Alerts" comprise the object class. (Note that cases are *not* the object class here because each alert is what is directly rated—the attribute of "appropriateness" is a characteristic of each alert—and because each case may have generated multiple alerts related to different clinical aspects of the case.) The instrument is the rating form as completed by a human judge. Each individual judge's rating of the appropriateness of an alert constitutes an independent observation.

2. The attribute is "knowledge of the clinical information system." Physicians comprise the object class. The instrument is the written test. Each question on the test constitutes an independent observation.

3. The attribute is "correctness" of the indexing. "Cases" comprise the object class.

4. A DNA chip is measuring multiple attributes at one time. Each attribute is the extent of fluorescence at a particular location on the chip, which corresponds to the extent of genetic sequence match between the sample and the DNA strands at that location. The object class is the biological sample with unknown sequence. Multiple observations are employed because each site on the chip has multiple, presumably identical, DNA "test strands."

Self-Test 4.2

1. Ratio
2. Ordinal
3. Ratio
4. Ordinal
5. Nominal
6. Nominal
7. Interval (the average score, which corresponds to the zero point in this case, is completely arbitrary)

Self-Test 4.3

The attribute is "adequacy of management"; cases (trauma patients) comprise the object class; the instrumentation includes the judges and the form used to record their ratings.

The measurement study could elucidate (1) whether there is a difference between local and national judges, which may be embodied in practice norms that are part of the institutional culture; (2) how many judges are needed to rate each case with an acceptable error rate; (3) if the training for the task and forms used for the task need improvement; and (4) if the test cases show sufficient difficulty as a set to be useful in demonstration studies. If all cases are managed perfectly by both TraumAID and the care providers, they are not challenging enough to be used in the demonstration study.

Self-Test 4.4

1. It is a comparative study because the investigators presumably had some control over where the resource was or was not installed. The site is the "subject" for this study. (Note that this point is a bit ambiguous. Patients could possibly be seen as the subjects in the study; however, as the question is phrased, the enrollment rates at the sites are going to the basis of comparison. Because the enrollment rate must be computed for a *site*, then site must be the "subject.") It follows that the dependent variable is the protocol enrollment rates; the independent variable is the presence or absence of T-HELPER.

2. It is a descriptive study. Sessions on the workstation are the "subjects." There is no independent variable. Dependent variables are the extent of workstation use in each category.

3. It is a correlational study. The patients on the service are the subjects. The independent variables are the clinical characteristics of the patients; the dependent variable is the extent of use of information resources.

4. This is also a correlational study. Patients are the subjects. The independent variable is the genetic information; the dependent variable is the diseases they develop. There is, however, no manipulation or experimental control.

5. Comparative study. Students are the subjects. Independent variable(s) are the version of the database and time of assessment. The dependent variable is the score on the problem-solving assessment.

References

1. Feinstein AR. *Clinimetrics*. New Haven: Yale University Press; 1987:viii.
2. Cork RD, Detmer WM, Friedman CP. Development and initial validation of an instrument to measure physicians' use of, knowledge about, and attitudes toward computers. J Am Med Inform Assoc 1998;5:164–176.
3. Friedman CP, Abbas UL. Is medical informatics a mature science? A review of measurement practice in outcome studies of clinical systems. Int J Med Inf 2003;69:261–272.
4. Michaelis J, Wellek S, Willems JL. Reference standards for software evaluation. Methods Inf Med 1990;29:289–297.
5. Clarke JR, Webber BL, Gertner A, Rymon KJ. On-line decision support for emergency trauma management. Proc Symp Comput Applications Med Care 1994;18:1028.
6. Shortliffe E. Computer programs to support medical decisions. JAMA 1987;258: 61–66.
7. Quaglini S, Stefanelli M, Barosi G, Berzuini A. A performance evaluation of the expert system ANAEMIA. Comp Biomed Res 1987;21:307–323.
8. Walter SD, Irwig LM. Estimation of test error rates, disease prevalence and relative risk from misclassified data: a review. J Clin Epidemiol 1988;41:923–937.
9. Phelps CD, Hutson A. Estimating diagnostic test accuracy using a "fuzzy gold standard." Med Decis Making 1995;15:44–57.
10. Bankowitz RA, McNeil MA, Challinor SM, Parker RC, Kapoor WN, Miller RA. A computer-assisted medical diagnostic consultation service: implementation and prospective evaluation of a prototype. Ann Intern Med 1989;110:824–832.
11. Hripcsak G, Wilcox A. Reference standards, judges, and comparison subjects: Roles for experts in evaluating system performance. J Am Med Inform Assoc 2002;9:1–15.
12. Teach RL, Shortliffe EH. An analysis of physician attitudes regarding computer-based clinical consultation systems. Comput Biomed Res 1981;14:542–558.
13. Impiccatore P, Pandolfini, Casella N, Bonati M. Reliabilty of health information for the public on the world wide web: systematic survey of advice on managing fever in children at home. BMJ 1997;314:1875–1879.

14. McDonald CJ, Hui SL, Smith DM, et al. Reminders to physicians from an intro-spective computer medical record: a two-year randomized trial. Ann Intern Med 1984;100:130–138.
15. Sackett DL, Haynes RB, Guyatt GH, Tugwell P. *Clinical Epidemiology: A Basic Science for Clinical Medicine*. Boston: Little Brown; 1991.
16. Winslow RL, Boguski MS. Genome informatics: Current status and future prospects. Circ Res 2003;92:953–961.
17. Hripcsak G, Bakken S, Stetson PD, Patel VL. Mining complex clinical data for patient safety research: a framework for event discovery. J Biomed Inform 2003;36:120–130.

5
Measurement Fundamentals

There is growing understanding that all measuring instruments must be critically and empirically examined for their reliability and validity. The day of tolerance of inadequate measurement has ended.[1]

This quotation from 1986 remains true to this day, and motivates the attention to measurement in this volume. In Chapter 4 we established a clear distinction between *measurement studies* that determine how well (with how much error) we can measure an attribute of interest, and *demonstration studies* that use these measures to make descriptive or comparative assertions. We might conclude from a measurement study that a certain process makes it possible to measure the "speed" of a resource in executing a certain family of tasks to a precision of ±10%. By contrast, we would conclude from a demonstration study that a hospital where Resource A is deployed completes this task with greater speed than a hospital using Resource B. Demonstration studies are the foci of Chapters 7 and 8; measurement and measurement studies are the foci of this chapter and the next.

Recall from Chapter 4 that measurement studies are, ideally, conducted before any related demonstration studies. All measurement studies have a common general structure and employ an established family of analytical techniques, which are introduced in this chapter. In measurement studies, the measurement of interest is undertaken with a sample of objects under conditions similar to those expected in the demonstration study, to the extent that those conditions can be created or simulated. The data generated by a measurement study are analyzed to estimate the error inherent in the measurement process. The estimated error—which is indeed an estimate because it derives from a *sample* of objects and perhaps also from a sample of circumstances under which the measurement will be made—is the primary result. In general, the greater the sample size used in a measurement study, the greater the confidence the investigator can place in the estimate of the size of the measurement error. Sometimes the results of a measurement study suggest that measurement methods must be further refined before the demonstration study can be undertaken with confidence, and the results often also suggest the specific refinements that are needed. After refinements are made, the investigator may wish to repeat the measurement study to verify that the expected reduction in error has occurred.

A demonstration study usually yields, as a by-product, data that can be analyzed to estimate some kinds of measurement error. For example, the patterns of responses to a questionnaire by subjects in a demonstration study can be analyzed to estimate the reliability of the questionnaire in that specific sample of subjects. It is often useful to carry out these analyses to confirm that measurement errors are in accord with expected levels; however, this does not substitute for orthodox measurement studies conducted fully in advance. Estimates derived from demonstration study data may reveal unacceptable levels of measurement error, invalidating the demonstration study and the time and effort that went into it.

In the presence of published results of measurement studies they can cite, investigators can proceed with confidence to conduct their demonstration studies, so long as they are using the measurement instruments under circumstances similar to those described in the published measurement studies. For this reason, carefully designed and conducted measurement studies are themselves important contributions to the literature. These publications are a service to the entire field of informatics, enabling the full community of investigators to choose measurement methods with greater confidence and often without having to conduct measurement studies of their own.

Error: Reliability and Validity of Measurement

Nothing is perfect. All measurements have errors. Much of the work in measurement is devoted to (1) estimating the magnitude of the error and (2) minimizing the error. We initially develop the notion of error according to a classical theory of measurement, within which the two central concepts are reliability and validity.[1,2]

In classical theory, reliability is the degree to which measurement is consistent or reproducible. A measurement that is reasonably reliable is measuring *something*. Validity is the degree to which that *something* is what the investigator wants to measure. Reliability is a logical and pragmatic precursor to validity. We cannot even discuss the validity of a measurement process until we demonstrate it to be reasonably reliable. Note that reliability and validity are not properties solely of the measurement instrument but, rather, of the total measurement process. Changing any aspect of the total measurement process may introduce error or change the nature of the error. For example, a questionnaire written using technical computer language and shown to be reliable when administered to a sophisticated group of computer users may be much less reliable when administered to persons untrained in technology. When answering the questions, these untrained persons will make misinterpretations that are unpredictable in nature. Another example is an altimeter, which retains its reliability but becomes invalid if the barometric pressure changes due to changes in the weather. (We will expand on this example below.)

Classical theory makes the assumption that an observed score for any object can be represented as the sum of the unknowable result of a perfectly reproducible measurement (the "true" score) and measurement error. This point is illustrated in Figure 5.1. The "true" score, in addition to being unknowable, is something of a misnomer because it still may not be fully accurate. Although perfectly reproducible for each object and therefore totally reliable, the true score may actually be revealing a composite of the attribute of interest and some other attributes. The true score thus has two components: a valid component, capturing the extent to which it reflects the intended attribute; and an invalid component, reflecting the extent to which the measured value also reflects some other attribute(s). The highly reliable reading on a simple altimeter, for example, reflects in part the attribute of interest (an airplane's elevation above sea level) and in part something extraneous that is related to the local weather conditions.

In classical theory, the errors that contribute to unreliability are unsystematic. They are assumed to be normally distributed about a mean of zero and uncorrelated with true scores and any other sources of error. In effect, these errors introduce noise into the result of a set of measurements. They affect the results of measurements in ways that are estimable in magnitude, over a set of observations, but unpredictable in detail as they affect the results of measurements on individual objects. There is no way to correct or adjust for unreliability in the results of measurements on individual objects. By contrast, the errors that contribute to invalidity tend to affect measurement results in ways that can potentially be explained and even adjusted for. For example, measurement of a patient's blood pressure is usually highly reliable over short time periods, because measurements

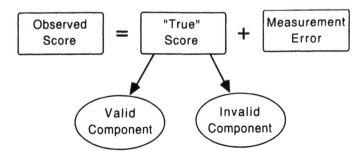

FIGURE 5.1. Components of an observed (measured) score in classical theory. (Note that the "true score" is not all that its name implies!)

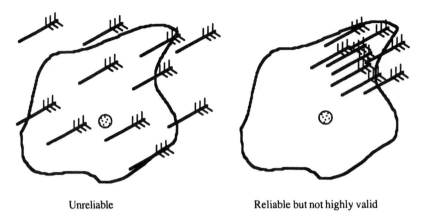

Unreliable   Reliable but not highly valid

FIGURE 5.2. Measurement as archery.

taken a few minutes apart will yield results with little variation. However, measurements taken in a physician's office are usually elevated due to the patient's anxiety. So a patient's "true score" for blood pressure is invalid to the extent that it also reflects the extraneous attribute of anxiety.*

The analogy to an archer shooting at a set of irregularly shaped targets, as shown in Figure 5.2, may be instructive. Each target corresponds to an object with a hidden "bull's-eye" corresponding to an (unknowable) exact value of the attribute for the object, and thus a completely exact result of the measurement. Each arrow corresponds to a single observation, the result of one act of measurement. The irregular shape of the target suggests to the archer the location of its hidden bull's-eye, but does not reveal it. The differing shapes of the targets correspond to differing values of the attribute for each object. So for each target, the archer aims at where he *thinks* the bull's-eye is. If there is enough consistency to the archer's shooting to speak meaningfully of a central point on the target around which the arrows cluster, the archer has enough reliability to prompt a meaningful discussion of validity. The reliability is inversely related to the amount of scatter of the arrows around the central point. The central point, even if no arrows strike it exactly, estimates the result for which the archer was aiming. If the archer shoots an infinite number of arrows at each target, the central point about which these arrows cluster would be exactly equal to the point the archer was aiming for. This central point is analogous to the true score. The smaller the distance between this central point—the point for which the archer was aiming—and the actual location of the hidden bull's-eye on each target, the greater the archer's validity. We can estimate the reliability of a measure-

* Validity must also be considered in terms of the definition of, and thus the name given to, the attribute. If we defined and name the attribute "blood pressure in the office" when we measure blood pressure in the office, the measurement process becomes much more valid.

ment process through the relatively easy task of measuring the scatter of the arrows over a series of targets. Determining the validity of the measurement entails a much more complicated and uncertain process of trying to determine the actual location of the bull's-eyes in relation to where the archer believed them to be.

In other disciplines, terms very closely related to reliability and validity are used to describe and quantify measurement error. Clinical epidemiologists typically use *precision* as a term corresponding to reliability and *accuracy* as a term corresponding to validity.[3] Feinstein[4] suggested that "consistency" may be a preferable substitute for both reliability and precision.

Methods to Estimate Reliability

In general, the reliability of a measurement can be improved by increasing the number of independent observations for each object and averaging the results. In this way, the observed score for each object more closely approximates the true score. Returning to the archery metaphor, the more arrows the archer shoots, the more precisely the results estimate the point at which the archer is aiming.

Moving from the world of archers, how do we undertake multiple measurements in our world? One logical, and often useful, way is to repeat them over time. This method provides an estimate of what is known as *test-retest reliability*. This approach is conceptually elegant and works well in a laboratory where the objects of study are usually inanimate and relatively stable over time, such as with measurements of machine performance. However, the repeated measurements (test-retest) technique often does not work well when studying the attributes of humans or of humans in interaction with machines, as is often the case in biomedical informatics. When humans are involved in test-retest studies, it is necessary to bring them back for the repeat study at just the right time and to re-create exactly the circumstances of the initial measurement. The timing is critical. If too little time has elapsed, perhaps only 1 day, humans remember what they did the last time and just do it again, which tends to overestimate the reliability of the measurement. If too much time has elapsed, perhaps as little as 1 month, the values of the attribute may have shifted, owing to events in the world affecting these persons, which then tends to underestimate the reliability of the measurement. The test-retest approach to reliability, with persons as the objects of measurement, may thus be problematic for two very practical reasons: first, because it is difficult to convince people to do anything again, and second, because it can be even more difficult to get them to return at precisely the correct interval for the particular measurement under study.

An alternative approach, often necessary for studies of persons as objects, employs multiple observations conducted on the *same occasion*. These multiple co-occurring observations cannot be carried out identically, of course. In that case, persons would respond identically to each one. *The observations can be crafted in ways that are different enough for each observation to create a unique challenge for the object yet similar enough that they all measure essentially the same attribute.* The agreement between the results of these multiple observations provides an estimate of *internal consistency reliability.* Using the archery metaphor, the method of co-occurring observations is roughly analogous to having a set of archers, each placed at a slightly different angle so each has a slightly different view of the target. On command, each archer shoots one arrow simultaneously with the other archers (Figure 5.3). Each archer aims at where he thinks the bull's-eye is, taking cues from the shape of the target. The assumption is made that each archer interprets these cues in the same way. We will return to this assumption later in this chapter.

To see the contrast between the approaches, reconsider the TraumAID system, originally introduced in the previous chapter, to advise on the care of patients with penetrating injuries of the chest and abdomen.[5] This information resource might be studied by asking expert judges to rate the appropriateness of the medical procedures suggested by the system over a series of trauma cases. Thus the objects are the cases (and more specifically the set of procedures recommended for each case), the judges' ratings comprise the observations, and the attribute is the "appropriateness" of the recommended care for each case. If one or more judges rated each case and then, 3 months later, rated the same set of cases again, the agreement of each judge with him/herself from one occasion to the next would assess test-retest reliability. If all judges rated each case on only one occasion, the agreement among the different judges would be a measure of internal consistency reliability. The appeal of the test-retest approach is limited because the judges may recall the cases, and their ratings of them, even after an

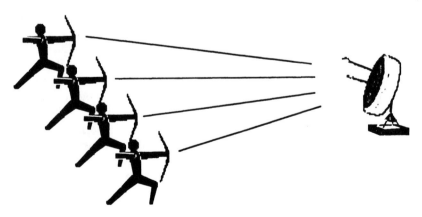

FIGURE 5.3. Archery and the method of multiple simultaneous observations.

interval as long as 3 months, or they may be unwilling to carry out the ratings twice. Lengthening the time interval between ratings increases the risk that changes in the prevailing standard of care against which TraumAID's advice is judged, or personal experiences of the judges that alter their perceptions of what constitutes good care, might change the context in which these judgments are made. Under these circumstances disagreements between test and retest judgments could be attributed to sources other than measurement error.

A set of somewhat differing observations taken at approximately the same time, each purporting to measure the same attribute, may be called a *scale* or an *index*.* Examples include sets of items on a written test or questionnaire, a set of human judges or observers, or a set of performance indicators that occur naturally in the world. The Dow Jones index is computed from the market values of a selected set of stocks, and is accepted as an indicator of the more abstract attribute of the performance of the New York Stock Exchange. Thinking of measurement problems in terms of multiple observations, forming a scale or index to assess a single attribute, is useful for several reasons. First, without these multiple observations we may have no way of estimating the reliability of a measurement process, because the test-retest approach is often impractical. Second, a one-observation measurement rarely is sufficiently reliable or valid for use in objectivist studies. (How can we possibly determine, based on one arrow, at what point an archer was aiming? Including only one company in the Dow Jones index could not possibly reflect the performance of the market as a whole.) Hence multiple observations are usually necessary to produce a functioning instrument. One shortcoming of the multiple observations approach is that the observations we believe to be assessing a common attribute, and thus to comprise a valid scale, may not behave as intended. (The archers who shoot simultaneously may have different interpretations of where the bull's-eye is.) To address this problem, there is a well-codified methodology for constructing scales, to be discussed in Chapter 6.

Whether we use the test-retest method or the internal consistency approach with co-occurring observations, the best estimate of the true value of the attribute for each object is the average of the independent observations. To compute the result of a measurement, we typically sum or average the scores on the items comprising a scale or index. If we know the reliability of a measurement process, we can then estimate the error due to

---

* Technically, there is a difference between a *scale* and an *index*,[6] but for purposes of this discussion the terms can be used interchangeably. Also note that the term *scale* has two uses in measurement. In addition to the definition given above, *scale* can also refer to the set of response options from which one chooses when completing a rating form or questionnaire. In popular parlance, one might say "respond on a scale of 1 to 10" of how satisfied you are with this information resource. We often move freely, and without too much confusion, between these two uses of the term *scale*.

random or unsystematic sources in any individual object's score. This error estimate is known as the standard error of measurement and is defined more precisely in the next section. Also, knowledge of the reliability of a measurement process can help us understand to what degree errors of measurement are contributing to a possible underestimate of group differences in demonstration studies.

Quantifying Reliability and Measurement Errors

One important goal of a measurement study is to quantify the reliability of a measurement process. We have seen that quantification can be accomplished by two general methods. Using a representative sample of objects we can employ a measurement process using multiple co-occurring observations to estimate internal consistency reliability; or we can repeat a measurement process on separate occasions, which enables estimation of test-retest reliability. A key aspect of reliability, from a measurement perspective, is that *any measurement process consisting of multiple observations can reveal the magnitude of its own reliability.* This contrasts with estimation of validity, that, as we will see later, requires collection of additional data.

For either the test-retest or internal consistency approach, we can compute a reliability coefficient with a maximum value of 1.0. The reliability coefficient (ρ) is defined, somewhat abstractly, as the fraction of the total variability in the scores of all objects that is attributable to differences in the true scores of the objects themselves. That is,

$$\rho = \frac{V_\infty}{V_{total}}$$

where V_∞ = variability due to true score differences
V_{total} = total variability in the measurements

This formula, as it stands, is not helpful. The true score variability cannot be observed directly from the results of a measurement process because the true scores themselves are unknown. However, by using measurement theory and performing some algebra not shown here, we can put this formula in a more useful form. Using the assumption that the errors reducing reliability of measurement are random and thus uncorrelated with true scores, we can conclude that the true score variability is equal to the total variability minus the variability due to measurement error. We may thus write:

$$\rho = \frac{V_{total} - V_{error}}{V_{total}}$$

This is more helpful because both quantities on the right side of the formula can be computed directly from the data generated by a measurement study.

TABLE 5.1. Perfectly reliable measurement.

Object	Observations					Object score
	1	2	3	4	5	
A	3	3	3	3	3	3
B	4	4	4	4	4	4
C	2	2	2	2	2	2
D	5	5	5	5	5	5

The total variability is the statistical variance of all observations over all objects used in the measurement study, and the variability due to error can be estimated as the extent to which the results of individual observations vary within each object. Returning to the archery metaphor, V_{error} can be likened to the directly observable scatter of the arrows the archer(s) fire at each target. The greater the scatter, the lower the reliability.

As a first example, consider the following result of a measurement study (Table 5.1), a result rarely seen in nature. Each object displays an identical result for all five observations thought to comprise a scale. The objects in this example could be clinical cases, and the observations could be the ratings by expert judges of the quality of care provided in each case. Alternatively, the objects could be people, and the observations could be their responses on a questionnaire to a set of questions that address a specific attribute. Table 5.1 is the first example of an objects-by-observations matrix, which is the way results of measurement studies are typically portrayed. Because scores for each object are identical across observations, the best estimate of the error is 0 and the best estimate of the reliability, denoted as ρ, is 1.0. (In this situation, each arrow always lands in the same place on each target!) Because the average of the observations is the result of the measurement, Object A's score would be 3, Object B's score would be 4, and so forth. There is no scatter or variability in the results from the individual observations, so we place high confidence in these results as a measurement of *something*. (A separate issue is whether this *something* is in fact what the investigator thinks it is. This is the issue of validity, discussed later.) If the matrix in Table 5.1 were the result of a measurement study, this estimate of perfect reliability would generalize only to the real or hypothetical population of objects from which the specific objects employed in the study were sampled. Because the number of objects in this particular example is small, we should place low credence in a belief that the measurement process has perfect reliability. If just one additional object were added to the sample in the measurement study, and for that object the results of all five observations were not identical, this modification in the measurement study results would substantially lower the estimated reliability.

In a more typical example (Table 5.2), the results of the observations vary within each object. Each object's score is now the average of observations whose results are not identical. The total variability has a component due to error, the magnitude of which can be estimated from the amount of disagreement among the observations for each object. The reliability coefficient (ρ) in this particular case is 0.81. We still place high credence in the results as a measurement of *something*, but the measurement is now associated with an error whose magnitude we can estimate. How much reliability is "enough" will be discussed later in this chapter.

The details of computing the reliability coefficient are beyond this discussion. A variety of statistical packages perform this reliability calculation, or it can be readily programmed on a spreadsheet using formulae provided in Appendix A. The reliability coefficient generated by these methods is known as Cronbach's alpha (α).[7] Other reliability coefficients exist, but α is commonly used and is applicable to a wide range of situations.

To the extent that a measurement lacks reliability, we associate random or unsystematic error with the results of the measurement process. We cannot specify the magnitude or direction of the error for each object—if we could, we could correct the result—but, using the classical theory of measurement, we can estimate the *standard error of measurement* (SE) as

$$SE_{meas} = SD\sqrt{1-\rho}$$

where ρ is the relevant coefficient of reliability and SD is the standard deviation of all measurement results: the standard deviation of the "object scores" in Table 5.2.

The standard error of measurement allows us to place an error bracket around the result of a measurement for each object. The standard error of measurement is the estimated value of the standard deviation for a set of independent observations made on the same object. The mean of the measurements estimates the "true score." Recall that measurement errors are assumed to be normally distributed and that, for a normally distributed variable, 68% of the observations fall within one standard deviation of the mean. It follows that 68% of the observations of an object fall within one standard error of measurement on either side of the true score, as illustrated in Figure 5.4. In Table 5.1, the standard deviation of the scores for the four objects is 1.29, but because the reliability is perfect ($\rho = 1$), the standard

TABLE 5.2. More typical measurement result.

Object	\multicolumn{5}{c}{Observations}	Object score
	1	2	3	4	5	
A	4	5	3	5	5	4.4
B	3	5	5	3	4	4.0
C	4	4	4	4	5	4.2
D	3	2	3	2	3	2.6

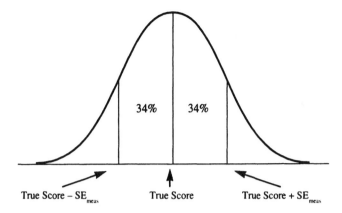

FIGURE 5.4. Distribution of measurement results illustrating the standard error of measurement.

error of measurement for any single object is 0. In the more realistic example of Table 5.2, the standard deviation of the results is 0.82, and the standard error of measurement (applying the above formula) is 0.36. For object 1, then, the measured score of 4.4 should be roughly interpreted as 4.4 ± 0.4.*

This classical approach to measurement is limited in that only one source of measurement error, which we have generically labeled "error due to observations," can be considered at a time. Using a more sophisticated approach, known as generalizability theory, it is possible to compute a reliability estimate that takes multiple sources of error into account. Despite its limitations, the classical approach has substantial applicability because measurement problems with one important source of error arise frequently in informatics. Hripcsak and colleagues[8] present an excellent discussion of the bounds of classical measurement theory in informatics and offer an example of how generalizability theory can be applied when it needs to be.

Self-Test 5.1

1. What are the effects on the standard error of measurement of (a) adding a constant to each measurement result and (b) multiplying each measurement result by a constant?
2. The measurement result given below has a reliability of 0.88.

---

* Those familiar with the concept of confidence intervals might think of the standard error of measurement as approximately equal to the "68% confidence interval" for the true score.

Object	Observations			
	1	2	3	4
1	2	4	4	3
2	3	3	3	4
3	2	3	3	2
4	4	3	4	4
5	1	2	1	2
6	2	2	2	2

a. Compute the score for each object and the standard deviation of these scores. (Standard deviations can be computed by most spreadsheet programs. The formula can be found in any basic statistics text.)
b. Compute the standard error of measurement.
c. Would changing the result of Observation 1 on Object 1 from 2 to 4 increase or decrease the reliability?

Reliability and Measurement Studies

Let us assume that the data in Table 5.2 are the results of a measurement study, conducted with four objects and five observations, to estimate the error when measuring some attribute. The first aspect of these results to note is that the reliability estimate must be interpreted much like the results of any study. The study results can be generalized only with great care. If the objects were sampled in some representative way from a larger population of objects, the result can be generalized only to that population. The estimate of measurement error might be different if objects were sampled from a different group. For example, assume that Table 5.2 gives the results of a measurement study where the attribute to be measured was speed of information retrieval (in tenths of a second), the objects were database search engines, and the observations were execution times for a selected set of information retrieval tasks. The measurement study results, with $\rho = 0.81$, suggest that the tasks are measuring with reasonably high reliability the attribute of speed. However, it cannot be assumed that these same tasks, when applied to a new generation of information systems designed on different software principles, will yield the same reliability when the speed of these new systems is assessed using the same set of tasks. (Note that the measurement issue here is the consistency of the observations across tasks. Whether the new generation of software is actually faster in executing this "battery" of tasks is a demonstration issue.)

As illustrated in Tables 5.1 and 5.2, the results of a measurement study take the form of an objects-by-observations matrix. We now discuss the effects of changing the dimensions of this matrix, beginning with the horizontal (observations) dimension.

Effects on Reliability of Changing the Number of Observations

Increasing the number of observations typically increases the magnitude of the estimated reliability. We offer this result without proof, but it can be seen intuitively by returning to the archery metaphor. If, for each target, the archer is aiming at a particular point, the greater the number of arrows he shoots, the more accurately the central point of where the arrows land estimates the location of the point of aim. More rigorously, the Spearman-Brown prophecy formula provides a way to estimate the effect on reliability of adding observations to or deleting observations from a measurement process. If one knows the reliability ρ_k of a measurement process with k observations, an estimate of its reliability ρ_n with n observations is given by

$$\rho_n = \frac{q\rho_k}{1+(q-1)\rho_k}$$

where $q = n/k$.

This formula assumes that the added observations perform equivalently to the observations already in the measurement process. (Or, by our running analogy, that the new archers had the same kinds of bows and arrows as the ones already employed.) So the prophecy formula is just what its name implies. One never knows, in advance of the experience, what the effect of changing the number of observations will be. This is a huge assumption, often ignored as such in research practice. To illustrate the prophecy formula's estimated effect of changing the number of observations, consider a hypothetical situation where four judges are asked to independently assess the quality of care for each of a set of 30 clinical cases. In this situation, judges are the observations, cases are the objects, and quality of care is the attribute. If the reliability of the four judges is calculated to be 0.65, Table 5.3 shows the prophesied effects, using the above formula, of adding or deleting judges who perform equivalently to those already in the study. The result in boldface is the result of the measurement study as actually conducted. All other values were derived by the prophecy formula.

Table 5.3 suggests that the reliability of a measurement process is at least partially in the hands of the investigator. Measurement can often be engineered to meet a predetermined reliability goal or expectation. This in turn

TABLE 5.3. Application of the prophecy formula.

	Number of judges							
	1	2	**4**	6	8	10	20	100
Adjustment factor	0.25	0.5	**1.0**	1.5	2.0	2.5	5.0	25.0
Reliability	0.317	0.481	**0.650**	0.736	0.788	0.823	0.903	0.979

raises the question of how much reliability is "good enough." There is not a cut-and-dried answer to this question. How much reliability is necessary depends primarily on how the results of the measurement are to be used. If the measurement results are to be used for demonstration studies where the focus is comparisons of groups of objects, a reliability coefficient of 0.7 or above is usually adequate, although higher reliability is always desirable when allowed by available resources. By contrast, a reliability coefficient of 0.9 or above is often necessary when the concern is assignment of scores to individual objects with a high degree of precision—for example, when a decision has to be made as to whether a particular information resource has achieved a prestated performance specification, or whether a clinician has attained a level of proficiency necessary to safely perform a procedure. In these situations, investigators often set a target level of the standard error of measurement and seek to attain a reliability that allows them to reach their target. The question of how much reliability is enough is often answered with: "enough to make the standard error of measurement as small as we need it to be to draw the conclusions we need to draw." Measurements with reliabilities of 0.5 or less are rarely adequate for anything but very preliminary studies. *As a general rule, the reliability of measures used in any study should be estimated and reported by the investigators.*

With reference to Table 5.3, if our concern is a demonstration study where we compare the quality of care for groups of cases, the collective opinions of at least six judges would be adequate in this hypothetical example to achieve a reliability of more than 0.7. However, if our concern is to assign a very precise "quality of care" score to each case, more than 20 judges would be needed to reach a reliability of 0.9. The reliability of one or two judges, for this hypothetical study, would therefore be less than acceptable.

Effects of Changing the Number of Objects

Increasing the number of objects typically increases confidence in the estimate of the reliability. The result of a measurement study provides an *estimate* of the reliability of the measurement process. In general, the greater the number of objects in the measurement study, the greater over confidence in this estimate. We can see intuitively from Tables 5.1 and 5.2, which portray measurement studies with four objects each, that addition of a fifth object for which the observations were highly discrepant would have a dramatic effect on the reliability estimate. However, if the measurement study included 25 objects, the incremental effect of a discrepant 26th object would be less profound. Reliability estimates based on large numbers of objects are thus more stable.

For measurement study design where an almost unlimited number of objects is available, at least 100 objects should be employed for stable estimates of reliability. For example, in a measurement study of an attitude questionnaire to be completed by registered nurses, the number of available "objects" (nurses in this case) is large and a minimum sample of 100 should be employed. In situations where the number of available objects is limited, the designer of a measurement process faces a difficult challenge, since it is not desirable to include the same persons in measurement and demonstration studies. So, for example, if patients with a rare disease were the objects of measurement and 500 cases are all that exist, a measurement study using 50 of these persons would be a pragmatic choice while still providing a reasonably stable estimate of reliability. It is important to emphasize that the examples in Tables 5.1 and 5.2 were purposely flawed to enable concise presentation. Both examples contain too few objects for confident estimation of reliability.

Self-Test 5.2

1. For the data in question 2 of Self-Test 5.1, what is the predicted reliability if the number of observations were (a) increased to 10 or (b) decreased to 1.

2. The Critical Assessment of Techniques for Protein Structure Assessment (CASP) is an annual competition that tests methods for predicting the structure of proteins. Alternative prediction methods are challenged by sets of test amino acid sequences. Each sequence corresponds to a three-dimensional protein structure that is unknown to the competitors but has been determined experimentally. Quality of the prediction methods is based on the percentage of carbon atoms in the predicted structure that are within some specified distance of their actual location in the protein structure, as determined experimentally. In the CASP4 competition conducted in 2001,[9] 14 test sequences were used with 123 prediction methods. Assume, although this was not the case, that in the competition all methods were applied against all test sequences.

    a. Frame this as a measurement problem. Name the attribute, observations, and objects.

    b. What would be the dimensionality of the objects by observations matrix for CASP4?

    c. In order to designate one method as the winner, by classical theory what level of reliability would the organizers of CASP likely wish to achieve?

Measurement Error and Demonstration Studies

Up to this point, we have discussed the effect of measurement error (random errors that erode reliability) on the result of a measurement for each individual object. What about the effects of such errors on the estimated mean of some attribute for a *group* of objects, which is the main concern of a demonstration study? For any sample of size N, the mean of a variable is associated with a standard error of the mean computed as:

$$SE_{mean} = \frac{SD}{\sqrt{N}}$$

As a general rule, random measurement error adds variability to the results of a measurement process. The greater the error, the greater the standard deviation (SD) of the scores for each object, and as the standard deviation increases, so does the standard error of the mean. Thus, measurement error contributes to the uncertainty with which we can know the mean value of some attribute in a sample. Random errors do not bias the estimates of the means of a group; they affect only the scatter or variability of measured values around the mean.

In comparative demonstration studies we are often interested in whether the mean of some attribute differs among specified groups or samples of objects. Because measurement error adds imprecision to the estimates of the means for each group, the lack of reliability decreases the probability that a true difference between the mean values in the groups, if such a difference exists, will be detected by the study.* So measurement error reduces the statistical "power" of demonstration studies. For example, we might compare the costs of managing hypertensive patients with and without support from a clinical decision support tool. With samples of 100 patients in each group, the observed mean ($\pm SE_{mean}$) of these costs might be $595 ($\pm$2) per patient per year with the tool and $600 ($\pm$2) without it. This difference is not statistically significant. Suppose, however, it was found that the measurement methods used to determine these costs were so unreliable that measurement error was contributing a substantial part of the variability reflected in the standard error of the mean. Through use of improved measurement methods, it may be possible to reduce the standard error of the mean by 25%. If this were done, the most likely results of a hypothetical replication of the study would then be $595 ($\pm$1.60) for the advisor group and $600 ($\pm$1.60) for the control group. This difference *is* statistically significant.**

In correlational demonstration studies, we are not interested in the values of the means across various groups, but rather in the correlations between two attributes in a single sample. For example, we might want to compare,

---

* The concept of statistical power is formally introduced in Chapters 7 and 8. Also in these later chapters, we will see that the standard error of the mean is closely related to the concept of the 95% confidence interval, to be introduced there.
** For those experienced in inferential statistics, a t-test performed on the case with the larger standard errors reveals $t = 1.77$, $df = 198$, $p = .08$. With the reduced standard errors, $t = 2.21$, $df = 198$, $p = .03$.

for a sample of health care providers, the extent of use of a clinical work-station with each provider's score on a knowledge test administered at the end of a training session. In this type of study, the effect of measurement error is to reduce the observed magnitude of the correlation. The "true" level of correlation between the extent of use and test score is higher than that suggested by the results of the study. This effect of measurement error on correlation is known as *attenuation*. An approximate correction for attenuation can be used if the reliabilities of the measures are known:

$$r_{corrected} = \frac{r_{observed}}{\sqrt{\rho_1 \rho_2}}$$

where $r_{corrected}$ = correlation corrected for measurement error (attenuation)
$\quad r_{observed}$ = observed or actually measured correlation
$\quad \rho_1$ = reliability of measure 1
$\quad \rho_2$ = reliability of measure 2.

Because the reliability of any measure cannot exceed unity, the absolute magnitude of the corrected correlation is either equal to or exceeds the absolute magnitude of the observed value. This correction must be applied with caution because it makes the standard assumptions of classical measurement theory—that all measurement errors are random and thus not correlated with anything else. If this assumption is violated, it is possible to obtain corrected correlations that are overinflated.[10] Nonetheless, the attenuation phenomenon is important in biomedical informatics. An example is discussed in detail later in the chapter.

To see why this attenuation happens, first consider two variables (Y_{true} and X_{true}), each measured with perfect reliability ($\rho = 1$) and between which the correlation is high. The relation between Y_{true} and X_{true} is shown in the upper part of Figure 5.5. The values of Y_{true} and X_{true} fall nearly on a straight line and the correlation coefficient is 0.95. By applying a small, normally distributed error function to Y_{true} and X_{true}, we generate representative values of these variables as they might be measured with less than perfect reliability: Y_{error} and X_{error}. The plot of Y_{error} versus X_{error} in the lower part of Figure 5.5 shows the degradation of the relationship and the corresponding attenuation of the correlation coefficient in this case from 0.95 to 0.68.

Self Test 5.3

Assume that the assumptions underlying the correction for attenuation hold. Use the correction formula to show that $r_{observed} \leq \sqrt{\rho_1 \rho_2}$. (*Hint:* Use the fact that the corrected correlation must be ≤1.0.) This equation is important because it points out that the reliability of a measure sets an upper

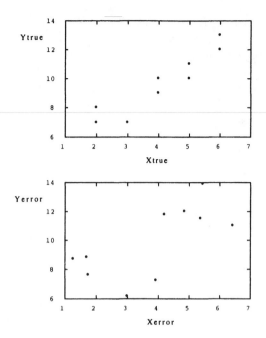

FIGURE 5.5. Effect of measurement error on the correlation between two variables.

bound on the correlation that can be measured between it and other measures.

Validity and Its Estimation

Reliability estimates indicate the degree of random, unsystematic "noise" in a measurement. The other important aspect of a measurement process is its validity, which indicates the degree of "misdirection" in the measurement. To the extent that a measurement is reliable, the results have meaning. To the extent that a measurement process is valid, the results mean what the investigator believes them to mean. More rigorously, the validity of a measurement process is the fraction of the perfectly reliable true scores that reflects the attribute of interest (see Figure 5.1). Returning to the archery metaphor, the validity is the extent of concordance, over a series of targets, between the point at which the archer was aiming on each target and the unknown location of each target's bull's-eye.

We previously saw that a measurement process, if conducted appropriately so it includes multiple observations, can reveal its own reliability through analysis of the consistency of the results of the observations. Estimation of validity is a different process requiring the collection of additional information. Whereas the reliability of our archers can be determined from the scatter of the arrows on each target, we need to collect additional information if we want to estimate how close to the invisible bull's-eyes the archers' points of aim really were. One way to do this is to ask each archer to verbalize how she decided where to aim and then ask some knowledgeable judges whether this reasoning made sense. This procedure, while providing some useful information about validity, is not likely to be definitive. This analogy illustrates the fundamental challenge of estimating validity. Although we can collect collateral information to establish validity, no single source of such information is completely credible, and often multiple different sources must be used. To take an example from the real world, the reliability of traffic reports on the radio can be estimated by monitoring several radio stations that base their traffic reports on informants in curse. To the extent that they report the same traffic conditions at a point in time, the reports can be considered reliable. However, if these reports are valid, there must *really* be a traffic jam where and when the stations report it. Validation requires collateral information, perhaps best obtained in this case by dispatching a helicopter to the site of the reported problem. Still, the conditions may have changed in the time it takes the helicopter to arrive.

Complete measurement studies seek to establish the validity of a measurement process as well as its reliability. In real measurement activities, we can estimate validity by asking people to examine the instruments used and opine as to what attribute the process appears to be addressing, or we can estimate validity by conducting more formal statistical studies that require the collection of additional data. Such studies might examine the relationship between the results of the measurement process under study and, for the same objects, the results of related measurements whose validity has been previously established. These relationships are typically expressed as correlations between the measurement process under study and the additional processes selected as comparisons. If the results of such studies are in accord with expectations, a case can be made for the validity of the new measurement process.

There are many more ways to study validity than there are to study reliability. Often multiple approaches are used, and the strongest case for the validity of a measurement process is made by accumulating evidence across a series of studies. More rigorously, studies of validity are of three general types: content, criterion-related, and construct.[11] These are summarized in Table 5.4.

Content Validity

This is the most basic notion of validity, known more loosely as "face" validity. Estimation of content validity addresses questions such as: By inspection of the instruments, do the observations appear to address the attribute that is the measurement target? Does the measurement process make sense?

TABLE 5.4. Approaches to validation.

Approach	Other/related names	Driving question	Strengths	Weaknesses
Content validation	Face validation	Does it look valid?	Relatively easy to study	Makes a weak (subjective) case for validity
Criterion-related validation	Predictive validation Concurrent validation	Does it correlate with an external standard?	Can be compelling, when a standard exists	Standards may not exist or may be controversial
Construct validation	Convergent validation Divergent or discriminant validation	Does it reproduce a hypothesized pattern of correlations with other measures?	Makes the strongest case for validity	Requires much additional data collection

Assessment of content validity requires the instrument and procedures to be inspected rather than administered. Content validity often is estimated by seeking opinions from informed individuals, for example by asking panels to review the observations purported to constitute a scale. In this case, the opinions of the informed individuals comprise the additional data that are always required in validation studies. (Our earlier example of asking archers to verbalize how they determined their point of aim, and then asking external judges to review these statements, can be seen as a process of ascertaining content validity.)

Although it should be expected that most measurement processes have at least adequate content validity, the issues involved in verifying this can become subtle. For example, an investigator may be constructing a checklist to measure an information resource's "ease of use." Using the method of multiple simultaneous observations, the checklist would contain several observations hypothesized to comprise a scale, each item purporting to measure "ease of use" from a slightly different perspective. In a content validity study, a group of judges may be asked: Which of the following items belong on the "ease of use" scale?

- Accessibility of help
- System response time
- Format of displayed information
- Clarity of user interface

There might be little disagreement about the validity of the items addressing user interface and information displays, but some judges might argue that the "system response time" item addresses the resource's performance rather than its ease of use, and that "accessibility of help" is not a characteristic of the resource itself but rather of the environment in which the resource is installed. As shown in Table 5.4, content validity is relatively easy to assess, but it provides a relatively weak argument, grounded in subjective judgment, for the validity of a measurement process. Nonetheless, the content validity of a measurement process cannot be assumed and must be verified through appropriately designed explorations.

Criterion-Related Validity

For criterion-related validity the central question is different: Do the results of a measurement process correlate with some external standard or predict an outcome of particular interest? For example, do those who score highly on a scale purported to measure computer literacy also learn more quickly to navigate an unfamiliar piece of software? Does a scale that rates the quality of radiotherapy treatment plans identify treatment plans associated with longer patient survival? Determination of criterion-related validity depends on the identification of specific criteria that will be accepted as reasonably definitive standards and for which reliable and valid measurement methods already exist. If the measurement process under study is to be considered valid, the correlation with a criterion measure would be expected to be moderately high, with coefficients of at least 0.5, and preferably higher.

Unlike content validity, which can be assessed through inspection of the measurement instruments and processes themselves, determination of criterion-related validity requires a study where measurements are made, on a representative sample of objects, using the instrument being validated as well as the instruments needed to assess the criterion. Using our previous example, estimating the criterion-related validity of a computer literacy scale in a formal measurement study requires that the scale be completed by a sample of health professionals who also try their hand at using an unfamiliar piece (or pieces) of software. Their scores on the literacy scale would then be analyzed in relation to the time taken to master the unfamiliar software. The greater the statistical correlation between literacy scores and mastery time, the greater the criterion-related validity of the scale. Note that in this case, the polarity of the relationship would be expected to be negative: lower mastery times associated with increased literacy scores.

When the criterion is an attribute that can only be known in the future, criterion-related validity is often referred to as "predictive" validity. It is often possible to identify predictive standards for validation of new measurement methods, but predictive validation studies can take months or years to complete. Using survival rates of patients as a criterion to validate methods for rating the quality of radiotherapy treatment plans is an example of a predictive validity study. When the criterion is an attribute that can be measured at the same time as the measurement process under study, this is often termed a "concurrent" validation. The above example of a computer literacy scale is illustrative of concurrent validation.

Construct Validity

Construct validity resembles criterion-related validity, but the approach is more sophisticated. When exploring construct validity, we ask: Does the measurement of the attribute under study correlate with several measurements of other attributes (also known as constructs) in ways that would be expected theoretically? This method is the most complex, but in many ways the most compelling, way to estimate validity. Assessment of construct validity in a measurement study involves multiple additional attributes, unlike assessment of criterion-related validity where the emphasis is on a single standard. The focus in construct validity is on verifying a set of relationships that have been hypothesized in advance. Some of the relationships between the attribute under study and the additional attributes included in the measurement study will be hypothesized to be high; others will be hypothesized to be small or zero. Again in contrast to criterion-related validation, where the desirable result is always high correlation, for construct validity the desirable result is the replication of a hypothesized pattern of correlations, whatever that pattern happens to be. In some scientific circles, the correlations that are hypothesized to be high are referred to as indicators of convergent validity; the correlations that are hypothesized to be low are referred to indicators of divergent or discriminant validity.

Consider as an example the development of an instrument to assess the attribute of "ease of use" for a biomedical information resource (Figure 5.6). The attribute of "ease of use" might be expected to correlate highly, but not perfectly, with other attributes, such as "maturity of the resource" and the "extent of the training" the users had received. Ease of use would *not* be expected to correlate highly with the ages of the resource users, and only a low correlation might be expected with the speed of the hardware on which the software runs. To assess construct validity, data on all four additional attributes shown in Figure 5.6 would be collected, using previously validated procedures, along with the ease-of-use data collected via the measurement process to be validated. Correlation coefficients between these measures, as computed from the measurement data on all five attributes, would be computed and the results compared with those hypothesized. If the expected pattern is reproduced, the investigator can make a strong case for the validity of the new measure. When the hypothesized pattern of correlations is not reproduced, the deviations often can cue the investigators to which unwanted attributes are being tapped by the new instrument—and thus point the way to modifications that will increase its validity.

In sum, concern about validity of measurement extends throughout all of science. When astrophysicists detect a signal (some nonrandom pattern

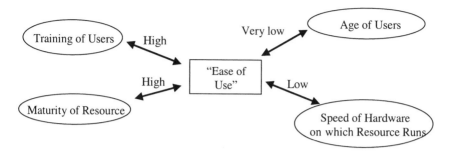

FIGURE 5.6. Construct validity study.

of waveforms) in their radiotelescopes and try to determine what it means, their concern is with validity. In general, concern with validity increases when the attributes are more abstract and only indirectly observable, but this concern never vanishes. For example, the notion of computer speed is relatively concrete, and there exists a relatively robust consensus about what the concept of speed means. Yet if a study is undertaken whereby a computer is put through a series of tasks, how can the investigator be sure that the result of the measurement solely reflects speed, uncorrupted by some other characteristic of the machine? The picture becomes more complex as one moves into the realm of human behavior and its associated attributes. When attitudes and other states of mind, such as "satisfaction," become the focus of measurement, the need for formal measurement studies that address validity becomes self-evident.

Self-Test 5.4

Is each of the following studies primarily concerned with content, criterion-related, or construct validity?

1. An investigator develops a rating form to ascertain the "quality" of a differential diagnosis for patients with illnesses of unknown cause. The ratings for a set of test cases are studied in relation to the time until a definitive diagnosis is established.

2. An investigator developing a computer literacy questionnaire convenes a panel of experts to identify the core competencies defining computer literacy.

3. An investigator develops a measure of the speed of a medical software program using a set of benchmark information processing tasks. For a set of information systems, the results of the new measure are studied in relationship to (a) the overall satisfaction with each system, as judged by samples of users in settings where the program has been installed, and (b) the manufacturer of the hardware on which the software runs.

Demonstration Study Results and Measurement Error: An Example

In demonstration studies, failing to take measurement error properly into account can have several detrimental effects. We have argued that investigators should carry out measurement studies, preferably in advance of demonstration studies, to estimate the nature and degree of measurement error. If the nature and extent of measurement errors are not known, investigators are at their mercy. The investigators must act as if the measurements are without error but knowing this is not the case.

Consider a demonstration study where the performance of a resource is compared to a standard whose carat level is taken to be a perfect "24" but in fact is less. Unconsidered measurement error in the standard will lead the investigator to underestimate the true value of the correlation between the resource and the standard. To see how this phenomenon works in practice, we examine the work of van der Lei and colleagues,[12] who studied the performance of Hypercritic, a knowledge-based system that offers critiques of the treatment of hypertensive patients through computational examination of the electronic records of these patients.* For illustrative purposes, we present a somewhat simplified version of the original study as well as a different approach to analysis of the data. The reader is encouraged to read the original paper.

In the simplified version, we assume that Hypercritic and each member of a panel of eight physicians have independently examined the records of a set of hypertensive patients for the purpose of generating comments about the care of each patient. As a result of this initial review, a set of 298 comments was generated, and we make the assumption that only one comment was generated from the record of each patient. Each comment in the set could have been generated by Hypercritic and/or by one or more of the physician panelists. Subsequently, each physician independently reviewed all 298 comments and judged each to be either correct or incorrect. If Hypercritic generated a comment as it scanned the patient records during the initial review, we assume that Hypercritic considered the comment to be correct. The structure of the study is illustrated in Figure 5.7.

The results of the study can be portrayed in a table, with each comment comprising a row, one column reflecting the ratings of that comment by each judge, and a separate column indicating whether each comment was generated by Hypercritic during the initial record review. Table 5.5 presents the study results for a subset of 12 comments. The judges are labeled A through H, and judges' ratings of comments are coded as 1 for correct and 0 for incorrect. With reference to Table 5.5, it is evident that Hypercritic and the

---

* The authors are grateful to Johan van der Lei and his colleagues for sharing the original data from their study and allowing us to develop this example.

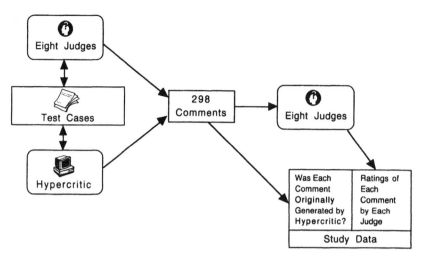

FIGURE 5.7. Hypercritic study.

judges did not always agree, and that the judges did not always agree among themselves. Comment 1 was generated by Hypercritic—and perhaps by one or more judges as well—on the initial review of the patient's record and was subsequently rated as correct by judges A, B, and D. Comment 2 was not generated by Hypercritic. On the initial review it was generated by one or more of the judges, and it was subsequently endorsed by judges B, C, D, and G. A demonstration study exploring the accuracy of Hypercritic's advice would seek to correlate the level of judges' endorsement of these comments on the second review with Hypercritic's "endorsement," as inferred from whether Hypercritic generated the comment on the initial review. We can consider the pooled ratings of the judges to be a less-than-

TABLE 5.5. Results from a subset of 12 comments in the Hypercritic study.

Comment no.	Generated by Hypercritic?	Ratings by each judge								Judges' "correctness" score
		A	B	C	D	E	F	G	H	
1	Yes	1	1	0	1	0	0	0	0	3
2	No	0	1	1	1	0	0	1	0	4
3	No	1	1	1	1	0	0	1	0	5
4	Yes	1	1	0	1	0	0	1	1	5
5	No	1	1	1	1	1	0	0	1	6
6	No	0	1	1	1	0	0	1	1	5
7	No	1	1	1	1	0	0	1	1	6
8	No	1	1	1	1	0	0	1	1	6
9	Yes	1	1	0	1	1	1	1	1	7
10	Yes	1	1	1	1	1	0	1	1	7
11	No	1	1	1	1	1	1	0	1	7
12	Yes	1	1	0	1	1	1	1	1	7

perfect standard against which Hypercritic may be tested. The extent of disagreement among the judges can provide an estimate of measurement error in this standard. Because the authors of the original work did not perform a measurement study in advance with data different from that used in their demonstration study, we will estimate the measurement error from their demonstration study data.

Measurement Error Estimate

The "measurement study" is concerned only with the ratings of the judges (A through H in Table 5.5). Hypercritic's performance is irrelevant at this point, because that is a demonstration study issue. Casting the judges' ratings more precisely in terms of our measurement theory, the objects of measurement are the comments, and the attribute of primary interest may be seen as the correctness of these comments. We may consider each judge's rating to be an assessment of the correctness attribute for each comment. Each rating by a judge is thus an independent observation. Classical measurement theory then directs us to sum or average these independent judgments to obtain the best estimate of the correctness of each comment. (*Note:* If you do not follow this conceptualization, you should review the earlier section, "Quantifying Reliability and Measurement Errors," before proceeding further.)

Applying this approach generates for each comment a correctness score equal to the number of judges who considered that comment to be correct. The correctness score is shown in the rightmost column of Table 5.5. From Table 5.5, Comment 1 would have a correctness score of 3 and Comment 11 a correctness score of 7. For the complete data in this study, we can estimate the reliability of these correctness scores by using the matrix of judges' ratings across all 298 comments. The full set of 298 correctness scores has a mean of 5.2 and a standard deviation of 2.0. The reliability coefficient, when computed for all 298 cases, is 0.65. The standard error of measurement of each correctness score is 1.2.*

The results of this measurement study allow us to conclude that the ratings by the judges have sufficient reliability to be measuring something meaningful. A somewhat higher reliability, obtainable using more judges or other methods discussed in the next chapter, would be desirable. To complete the measurement study, we would also need to consider the validity of these ratings: to what extent the ratings actually represent the attribute of correctness versus some other attribute(s). Content or face validity of the ratings might be explored by examining the credentials of the judges,

---

* Readers familiar with theories of reliability might observe that coefficient alpha, which does not take into account rater stringency or leniency as a source of error, might overestimate the reliability in this example. In this case, however, use of an alternate reliability coefficient[13] has a negligible effect.

verifying that they had adequate qualifications for and experience in managing hypertension. A measure of criterion-related validity might be obtained by examining the incidence of hypertension-related complications for the patients included in the study in relation to the correctness scores of the comments about their care, for cases where the corrective action recommended by the comment was *not* taken. A positive correlation between complication rates and correctness scores would be an indication of criterion-related validity in the predictive sense. Criterion-related validity of the correctness attribute, in the concurrent sense, might be assessed by comparing comments with published clinical guidelines. Construct validity might be explored by collecting additional data needed to consider a number of hypotheses, for example, that the correctness of comments would be moderately (and inversely) related to each patient's comorbidity. The greater the number of other diseases a patient had, the less likely it would be for comments about his/her hypertension management to be correct.

Demonstration Study

Having computed the reliability of the correctness scores, we are in a stronger position to undertake a demonstration study to estimate the clinical value of the comments generated by Hypercritic itself.* One measure of the accuracy of Hypercritic is the correlation between Hypercritic's assessment of each comment—determined by whether Hypercritic generated the comment on its review of the patients' charts—and the correctness score obtained by pooling the eight judges' comments. The correlation coefficient based on all 298 comments is 0.50, which signals a moderate and statistically significant relationship. We might also suspect that this observed correlation underestimates the magnitude of the relation between Hypercritic's output and the correctness scores because the observed correlation has been attenuated by measurement error in these correctness scores. To estimate the effects of error on the observed correlation, we might apply the correction for attenuation (see page 129) and obtain a corrected correlation coefficient of 0.62. By comparing the estimated corrected correlation of 0.62 with the observed correlation of 0.50, we may conclude that failure to consider measurement error will lead to underestimation of Hypercritic's accuracy by approximately 24%.

As we will discover in Chapter 8 when demonstration studies are discussed in detail, the correlation coefficient is a measure of system accuracy that has useful statistical meaning but says little about the nature of the disagreement between Hypercritic and the pooled ratings of the judges. For the purpose of a comprehensive evaluation of a system such as Hypercritic,

---

* Since we have no actual data to estimate the validity of the correctness scores, we will assume that the validity is perfect and consider unreliability to be the only aspect contributing to less-than-perfect measurement.

TABLE 5.6. Hypercritic demonstration study results in contingency table format.

| Hypercritic | Pooled rating by judges | | |
	Comment valid ($\geq$5 judges)	Comment not valid (<5 judges)	Total
Comment generated	145	24	169
Comment not generated	55	74	129
Total	200	98	298

additional analyses therefore would be performed. Contingency table methods, discussed in detail in Chapter 8, might be used to look at the number and nature of the disagreements between the resource and the judges. Such an analysis would require the investigators to choose a threshold level corresponding to the number of judges' endorsements a comment would require in order to be considered correct. Doing this reduces interval to ordinal the level of measurement of correctness; and, as such, results in some loss of information. (All comments coded as "correct" are considered to be equally correct, and all comments coded as "incorrect" are considered to be equally incorrect.) The original authors of the study used endorsement of a comment by five or more judges as a criterion for overall correctness. Using this same criterion, the data may be mapped into a contingency table as shown in Table 5.6.

The contingency table analysis illustrated in Table 5.6 is useful because it shows that two different kinds of errors occur in roughly equal proportion, if endorsement by five or more judges is taken as the threshold for considering a comment to be correct. Hypercritic failed to generate 55 of the 200 comments (28%) that were endorsed by five or more judges. Hypercritic did generate 24 of the 98 comments (24%) rated incorrect by the judges, because fewer than five judges endorsed them. Note that these error rates depend on the investigator's choice of a threshold.

Self-Test 5.5

Assume that the data in Table 5.5, based only on 12 comments, constitute a complete pilot study. The reliability of these data, based on 12 comments (objects) and eight judges (observations) is 0.29. (Note that this illustrates the danger of conducting measurement studies with small samples of objects, as the reliability estimated from this small sample is different from that obtained with the full sample of 298 comments). For this pilot study:

1. What is the standard error of measurement of the "correctness of a comment" as determined by these eight judges?
2. If there were four judges instead of eight, what would be the estimated reliability of the measurement? What if there were 10 judges?

3. Using the pooled ratings of all eight judges as the standard for accuracy, express the accuracy of Hypercritic's relevance judgments as a contingency table using endorsement by six or more judges as the threshold for assuming a comment to be correct.
4. For these data, the correlation between Hypercritic's judgments and the pooled ratings is 0.09. What effect does the correction for attenuation have on this correlation?
5. Optional: Using the formulae in Appendix A, verify that the reliability is 0.29 and compute the various sums of squares that are part of the computation.

References

1. Kerlinger F. Foundations of Behavioral Research. New York: Holt, Rinehart and Winston, 1986.
2. Thorndike RL, Hagen E. Measurement and Evaluation in Psychology and Education. New York: Wiley, 1977.
3. Weinstein MC, Fineberg HV, Elstein AS, et al. Clinical Decision Analysis. Philadelphia: Saunders, 1980.
4. Feinstein AR. Clinimetrics. New Haven, CT: Yale University Press, 1987.
5. Clarke JR, Cebula, DP, Webber BL. Artificial intelligence: a computerized decision aid for trauma. J Trauma 1988;28:1250–1254.
6. Babbie ER. The Practice of Social Research. Belmont, CA: Wadsworth, 1992.
7. Cronbach L. Coefficient alpha and the internal structure of tests. Psychometrika 1951;16:297–334.
8. Hripcsak G, Heitjan DF. Measuring agreement in informatics reliability studies. J Biomed Inform 2002;35:99–110.
9. Marti-Renom MA, Madhusudhan MS, Fiser A, Rost B, Sali A. Reliability of assessment of protein structure prediction methods. Structure 2002;10:435–440.
10. Phelps CD, Hutson A. Estimating diagnostic test accuracy using a "fuzzy gold standard." Med Decis Making 1995;15:44–57.
11. American Psychological Association. Standards for Educational and Psychological Tests. Washington, DC: APA, 1974.
12. Van der Lei J, Musen MA, van der Does E, Man in`t Veld AJ, van Bemmel JH. Comparison of computer-aided and human review of general practitioners' management of hypertension. Lancet 1991;338:1504–1508.
13. Shrout PE, Fleiss JL. Intraclass correlations: uses in assessing rater reliability. Psychol Bull 1979;86:420–428.

Answers to Self-Tests

Self-Test 5.1

1. a. Adding a constant has no effect on the standard error of measurement, as it affects neither the standard deviation nor the reliability.
   b. Multiplication by a constant increases the standard error by that same constant.

2. a. The scores are 13, 13, 10, 15, 6, 8 for objects 1–6. The standard deviation of the six scores is 3.43.
   b. 1.19.
   c. The reliability would increase because the scores for object 1, across
observations, become more consistent. The reliability in fact increases
to 0.92.

Self-Test 5.2

1. a. 0.95.
   b. 0.65.
2. a. The attribute is, for a given method and test sequence, the percentage of carbon atoms within the threshold distance. The observations
are the test sequences. The objects are the prediction methods.
   b. The matrix would have 14 columns corresponding to the test
sequences as observations and 123 rows corresponding to prediction
methods as objects.
   c. A very high reliability, on the order of .9 would be sought. The demonstration study seeks to rank order the objects themselves, as opposed
to comparing groups of objects. This suggests the use of a large
number of test sequences.

Self-Test 5.3

The answer may be obtained by substituting $r_{corrected} \leq 1$ into the formula:

$$r_{corrected} = \frac{r_{observed}}{\sqrt{\rho_1 \rho_2}}$$

to obtain the inequality:

$$1 \geq \frac{r_{observed}}{\sqrt{\rho_1 \rho_2}}$$

Self-Test 5.4

1. Criterion-related validity. The time until a definitive diagnosis is established might be viewed as a universally accepted standard.
2. Content validity.
3. Construct validity. The relation between system speed and user satisfaction is complex, and the correlation would not be expected to be perfect.

Self-Test 5.5

1. SE_{meas} (eight judges) = 1.10.
2. Reliability (four judges) = 0.17; reliability (10 judges) = 0.34.

3.

| | Judges | |
Hypercritic	Valid	Not valid
Generated	3	2
Not generated	4	3

4. Corrected correlation is 0.17.
5. Total sum of squares (SS) = 19.84; judges (observations) SS = 5.84; comments (objects) SS = 2.33; error SS = 11.67.

Appendix A: Computing Reliability Coefficients

The computation of reliability coefficients is based on a matrix of objects by observations as shown in Table 5.7. This calculation is presented without proof. It will be familiar to those experienced with the analysis of variance (ANOVA). We use standard matrix notation, so each observation is given by X_{ij} where i denotes the object and j denotes the observation. In the matrix in Table 5.7, X_{23} is the value of the third observation on object B, with a value of 5. The total number of objects is therefore n_i, and the total number of observations is n_j.

We begin by calculating three sums of squares: total sum of squares (SS_{total}), the sum of squares for objects ($SS_{objects}$), and the sum of squares for observations ($SS_{observations}$). The total sum of squares is given by

$$SS_{total} = \sum_{ij} X_{ij}^2 - \frac{\left(\sum_{ij} X_{ij}\right)^2}{n_i n_j}$$

Note that $\sum_{ij} X_{ij}$ equals the sum of all observations for all objects, and $\sum_{ij} X_{ij}^2$ equals the sum of the squared values of all observations for all objects.

The sum of squares for objects is given by:

TABLE 5.7. Sample data for reliability calculation.

Object	Data, by no. of observations					Object sums
	1	2	3	4	5	
A	4	5	3	5	5	22
B	3	5	5	3	4	20
C	4	4	4	4	5	21
D	3	2	3	2	3	13
Observation sums	14	16	15	14	17	

$$SS_{objects} = \frac{\sum\limits_{i=1}^{n_i}\left(\sum\limits_{j=1}^{n_j} X_{ij}\right)^2}{n_j} - \frac{\left(\sum\limits_{ij} X_{ij}\right)^2}{n_i n_j}$$

The sum of squares for observations is given by:

$$SS_{observations} = \frac{\sum\limits_{j=1}^{n_j}\left(\sum\limits_{i=1}^{n_i} X_{ij}\right)^2}{n_i} - \frac{\left(\sum\limits_{ij} X_{ij}\right)^2}{n_i n_j}$$

From these three quantities, we can compute the sum of squares for error as

$$SS_{error} = SS_{total} - SS_{objects} - SS_{observations}$$

Now the reliability coefficient (alpha) can be computed using the formula:

$$\rho = \left[\frac{1 - [SS_{error}/(n_i - 1)(n_j - 1)]}{[SS_{objects}/(n_i - 1)]}\right]$$

In the sample matrix in Table 5.7, using these formulas, we obtain:

Total sum of squares = 19.2
Sum of squares for objects = 10.0
Sum of squares for observations = 1.7
Error sum of squares = 7.5
Reliability = 0.81

6
Developing and Improving Measurement Methods

This chapter moves the theoretical emphasis of Chapter 5 to actual measurement practice. In Chapter 5 we introduced theories of measurement that were, in effect, theories of error. In this chapter we address specific procedures for estimating error and designing measurement methods to reduce error. We discuss the structure of measurement studies, the mechanics of conducting them, and how one uses the results of these studies to improve measurement techniques. We consider how to develop measurement methods that yield acceptably reliable and valid results. Recalling that the key to objectivist measurement is the use of equivalent independent observations, we organize much of this chapter around three different categories of independent observations that arise frequently in measurement problems in informatics: first, when the repeated observations in a measurement process are tasks completed by either persons or information resources; second, when the repeated observations are the opinions of judges about clinical cases or scientific problems; and third, when the repeated observations are items or questions on forms. Although the same general measurement concepts apply to all three categories, there are issues of implementation and technique specific to each.

Structure of Measurement Studies: Objects, Observations, and Scales

Recall from Chapter 5 that in measurement studies we typically make multiple independent observations on each of a set of objects. The data collected during a measurement study take the form of an objects-by-observation matrix (Figure 6.1). In the objectivist worldview, all independent observations of the same phenomenon should yield the same result. The closer the observations approach agreement for each object, the more reliable, and therefore objective and trustworthy, the measurement process can be considered to be. Disagreement reflects subjectivity on the part of

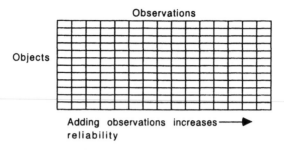

FIGURE 6.1. Objects-by-observations matrix.

the instruments, be they human, mechanical, electronic, or some combination thereof.

In Chapter 5, we developed quantitative methods for estimating errors of measurement, enabling the investigator to engineer the measurement process for optimal performance. We saw that the variability attributable to differences among objects contributes to true score variability, which should be maximized relative to variability from other sources. The variability due to all other sources contributes to measurement errors that should be minimized. In general, the reliability can be increased, and the standard error of measurement decreased, by increasing the number of independent observations. The methods introduced in Chapter 5 allow us to quantify the measurement errors that erode reliability directly from the objects-by-observations matrix using data generated by the measurement process itself.

We also saw in Chapter 5 that even reducing to zero the errors that are estimable from the measurement process itself, were that possible, does not guarantee a perfect measurement of the desired attribute. Even if the measurement is perfectly reliable, the results may be invalid. Human judges in near-perfect agreement about the accuracy of a decision support system's advice may still be incorrect if the judges share a fund of medical knowledge that is biased or obsolete. Separate validity studies, which typically require use of external standards, are needed to explore these additional issues. Because the conduct of a complete set of measurement studies, exploring both reliability and validity, is complex and time-consuming, it is vitally important that results of measurement studies be published so other informatics researchers can reuse the measurement methods developed and documented by their colleagues.

With this brief review as background, we now can describe the specific steps for conducting a measurement study:

1. Design the measurement process to be studied. Precisely define the attribute(s), object class, instrumentation, measurement procedures, and

what will constitute the multiple independent observations. Recall that the object class is an expression of who or what the measurements are made on.

2. Decide from which hypothetical population the objects in the measurement study will be sampled. It may also be necessary to decide from which population the observations will derive. (For example, if the observations are to be made by human judges, what real or hypothetical group do the selected judges represent?) This step is key because the results of the measurement study cannot be generalized beyond these populations.

3. Decide how many objects and how many independent observations will be included in the measurement study. This point determines the dimensionality of the objects-by-observations matrix for the data collected.

4. Collect data using the measurement procedures as designed and any additional data that may be used to explore validity. It is often useful to conduct a pilot study with a small number of objects before undertaking the complete measurement study.

5. Analyze the objects-by-observations matrix to estimate reliability. Cronbach's alpha can be computed using any of several computer programs for statistical analysis. Alternatively, the formulae in Appendix A of Chapter 5 can be used to create a spreadsheet that computes the reliability coefficient.

6. Conduct any content, criterion-related, or construct validity studies that are part of the measurement study. This will usually require collection of additional data.

7. If the reliability or validity proves to be too low, attempt to diagnose the problem. Recall that the Spearman-Brown formula can be used to estimate the effects on reliability of changing the number of independent observations.

8. Decide whether the results of the measurement study are sufficiently favorable to proceed directly to a demonstration study, or if a repeat of the measurement study, with revised measurement procedures, is needed.

Example

In a realistic but hypothetical situation, suppose that an investigator is interested in the performance of a decision support system and so seeks to assess the attribute "accuracy of advice" for each patient (case) evaluated by this information resource. Patients are the object class of measurement. Human judges, abstracts of each patient's history, a report of the system's advice, and the form used to elicit the ratings comprise the instrumentation. For the measurement study, the investigator elects to use 50 patients and six judges, each of whom will rate the accuracy of advice for each of the patients, to generate the multiple repeated observations. The dimensions of the matrix to be analyzed are 50 by 6. The choice of patients and judges is nontrivial because the results of the study cannot be generalized beyond the characteristics of populations from which these individuals are selected. To increase the generalizability, the investigator selects 50 patients from a citywide network of hospitals and six expert clinician judges from across the country. Conducting the study requires the resource to generate its advice for all 50 patients, and for each of the judges to review and rate the advice for all of the patients. The reliability of the ratings is estimated from the resulting objects-by-observations matrix to be 0.82. Using the Spearman-Brown formula, it is predicted that four judges will exhibit a reliability of 0.75. Given the time and effort required for the demonstration study to follow, the investigator decides to use only four judges in the demonstration study.

Steps to Improving Measurement

Two basic courses of action exist for an investigator if a measurement study reveals suboptimal reliability or validity: (1) modify the number of independent observations in the measurement process (typically affects reliability only); or (2) modify in more substantive ways the mechanics of the measurement (typically affects both reliability and validity). When a measurement study reveals a low reliability (typically a coefficient of less than 0.70), the investigator can improve it by increasing the number of independent observations drawn from the same population. Had the estimated reliability been too low in our example, the investigator could have added more judges chosen from the same national group, but it would have come at a cost. Increasing the number of observations increases the work involved in conducting each measurement, increasing the time and expense incurred when conducting the study—and often creating logistical challenges. In some other situations, as we saw above, a measurement study can yield higher-than-needed reliability, and the results of the measurement study can lead the investigator to streamline the study by reducing the number of independent observations per object. Increasing or decreasing the number of observations, *so long as they represent the same population*, can be assumed to affect reliability only.

Alternatively, the investigator can try to improve the mechanics or instrumentation of the measurement in pursuit of increasing the reliability. In our example, he or she might try better training of the judges, replacing a judge whose ratings seem unrelated to the ratings of his or her colleagues, or giving the judges an improved form on which to record the ratings. This approach, which addresses the substance of the measurement process, often has greater impact on reliability than merely increasing the number of observations. This approach also can increase reliability without increasing the resources required to conduct the measurement. It is important to understand, however, that such changes can affect *what* is being measured and thus can affect both reliability and validity. When an investigator responds to a measurement study result by changing the number of observations, it is typically not necessary to repeat the study because the impact of the change can be predicted from the Spearman-Brown formula. When the changes are more fundamental (e.g., a change in the format of a rating instrument or a change in the population from which judges are selected), it may be necessary to repeat the measurement study, possibly going through several iterations until the process reaches the required level of performance.

Self-Test 6.1

With reference to the example described earlier (see page 147):

1. What is the predicted reliability of this measurement process using one judge only? Would you consider this figure acceptable?
2. In the measurement study, the ratings were generated on a 1 to 4 response scale and had a mean of 2.3 with a standard deviation of 0.8. What was the magnitude of the standard error of measurement?
3. How might validity be explored in this hypothetical measurement study?

[Answers are found at the end of the chapter.]

Using Measurement Studies to Diagnose Measurement Problems

In this section we discuss how the investigator can decide, based on measurement study results, which specific strategies to pursue to improve measurement.

Analyzing the Objects-by-Observations Matrix

The diagnostic process entails some further analysis of the objects-by-observations matrix to determine which of the observations, if any, is eroding the reliability. Recall that each independent observation in the measurement process is hypothesized to assess the same attribute. If these observations do assess the same attribute, the results of each pair of observations across a sample of objects tend to be at least modestly correlated. That is, an object with a high score on one observation tends to also have a high score for the other observations. Observations that assess different attributes tend to be uncorrelated. This matrix of intercorrelations may be computed directly from the objects-by-observations matrix generated by the measurement study. Pearson product-moment correlations are customarily used for this purpose.* Each correlation may be computed using the following for two attributes, denoted x and y, with measurements of both attributes performed on i objects:

$$r = \frac{\sum_i (x_i - \bar{x})(y_i - \bar{y})}{\sqrt{\sum_i (x_i - \bar{x})^2 \sum_i (y_i - \bar{y})^2}}$$

where x_i and y_i are values of the individual observations of x and y, and $\bar{x}$ and $\bar{y}$ are the mean values of x and y over all objects in the study sample. This formula looks imposing but is a built-in function in all spreadsheet and statistical programs.

Observations that are "well behaved" should be at least modestly and positively correlated with all other observations. The well-behaved observations should be retained in the measurement process, as each observation works to increase the reliability of the measurement of the attribute. (As discussed in Chapter 5, a set of observations that is well behaved as a group can be said to comprise an index, or scale.) When a measurement study reveals that a specific observation is not well behaved, and thus does not belong with the others in the group of observations, it should be revised or deleted from the measurement process. Recall that we are using the term *observations* here generically to refer, for example, to judges observing some kind of performance, or the items on a test or questionnaire.

In practice, dealing with all of the pairwise correlations among observations is cumbersome. A set of N observations has $N(N - 1)/2$ unique correlation coefficients that must be inspected, and the pattern among these correlations inferred. Analysis of 10 items, for example, involves inspection of 45 coefficients. There are, however, some shortcuts that make the process more tractable. The most basic shortcut is to compute and then inspect the

---

* When the purpose of computing the coefficients is to inspect them to determine if the observations are "well behaved," the Pearson coefficient is widely used and is the only coefficient discussed explicitly here. The Pearson coefficient assumes that the variables are both measured with interval or ratio properties and normally distributed. Even though both assumptions are frequently violated, the Pearson coefficient provides useful guidance to the investigator performing measurement studies. A helpful discussion of the various correlation coefficients and their use in measurement is found in a concise book by Isaac and Michael.[1] Note also that we are using as a criterion for "good measurement" only that independent observations be correlated: that when one observation is higher, the other is higher, and vice versa. Under this somewhat relaxed criterion, the observations do not have to agree to be well behaved, and the measurement errors of interest result from lack of correlation. This limitation is consistent with the classical measurement theory that has underpinned our discussions of measurement to this point. The more comprehensive theory of measurement, introduced later as generalizability theory, allows consideration of errors that result from lack of agreement in addition to errors that result from lack of correlation.

TABLE 6.1. "Typical measurement result" with corrected part–whole correlations.

Object	Results of five observations					Total score
	1	2	3	4	5	
A	4	5	3	5	5	22
B	3	5	5	3	4	20
C	4	4	4	4	5	21
D	3	2	3	2	3	13
Corrected part–whole correlation	0.62	0.83	0.11	0.77	0.90	

"corrected part–whole" correlation coefficients for each observation. A corrected part–whole correlation is computed for each observation, and is the correlation between that observation and the object's total score *after excluding that observation*. The process for computing this correlation is described below. Using corrected part–whole correlations, only N correlations need be inspected for N observations to determine if the observations are well behaved. Typically, an observation exhibiting a corrected part–whole correlation below 0.4 should be modified or deleted. Always keep in mind that modifying an observation or eliminating it from a set can change what the scale is assessing and can affect the validity of the measurement.

To see how this works computationally, examine Table 6.1, which portrays the "typical measurement result" previously shown in Table 5.2. Recall that the reliability coefficient for these results is 0.81.

To compute the corrected part–whole correlation for each observation, it is necessary to create ordered pairs of numbers representing the score for each observation and the total score for each object, excluding that observation. Table 6.2 illustrates computation of the corrected part–whole correlation for Observation 1 from Table 6.1. The ordered pairs used to compute the correlation consist of each object's score for Observation 1 paired with the object's total score summed across all observations but excluding observation 1. Because Object A has a total score of 22, excluding Observation 1 yields a corrected total score of 18. The correlation

TABLE 6.2. Computing the corrected part–whole correlation for observation 1.

Object	Score for Observation 1	Corrected total score, excluding Observation 1
A	4	18
B	3	17
C	4	17
D	3	10

TABLE 6.3. Correlations between observations for the
"typical measurement result".

Item	1	2	3	4	5
1	—	0.41	**−0.30**	0.89	0.91
2		—	**0.49**	0.73	0.74
3			—	**−0.13**	**0.09**
4				—	0.94

coefficient of 0.62, as shown in the bottom row of Table 6.1, is computed from these four ordered pairs.

The other corrected part–whole correlations are computed by creating analogous ordered pairs for each of the other observations: the scores on Observation 2 paired with the total scores excluding Observation 2, which yields a correlation of 0.83; the scores on Observation 3 paired with the total scores excluding Observation 3, which yields a correlation of 0.11; and so on. These calculations are relatively straightforward on a spreadsheet.

Having seen how the short-cut method of part–whole correlations works in practice, we now explore the full matrix of correlations among all pairs of observations. Table 6.3 displays these correlations for the measurement results given in Table 6.1. Overall, there are $5(5-1)/2$, or 10, correlation coefficients to inspect. The correlation between observations i and j is found at the intersection of the ith row and jth column. Because this matrix of intercorrelations is symmetrical about the diagonal, and the diagonal elements are equal to 1.0, only the values of elements above the diagonal are shown.

In this example, Observation 3 is not well behaved. This is seen several ways. From Table 6.1, it can be seen that an object with the highest total score (A) has a relatively low score on Observation 3. The object with the second lowest total score (B) has the highest score on Observation 3. We also see evidence of Observation 3's misbehavior because the corrected part–whole coefficient is less than 0.4 whereas the others are high. In Table 6.3 the correlations between Observation 3 and the other observations, seen in boldface type, show no consistent pattern: two are negative, and two are positive. Deleting Observation 3 increases the reliability of measurement (in this case, from 0.81 to 0.89), even though the number of observations in the measurement process is decreased. Observations can also fail to be well behaved if their mean values (across all objects observed) are close to either the high or low extremes, or if they display no variability across objects. Such observations add no useful information to the measurement process and should be modified or deleted.

What Corrected Part–Whole Correlations Can Reveal

In later sections of this chapter we discuss specific ways to improve measurement technique for specific situations that arise frequently in informatics studies. Here we consider general strategies that may be followed from a diagnostic process using part–whole correlations. For brevity's sake, we refer to corrected part–whole correlations simply as part–whole correlations:

1. *If all part–whole correlations are reasonably large but the reliability is too low:* Add equivalent observations to the measurement process.

2. *If many part–whole correlations are low:* Something affecting all observations is fundamentally amiss. There are likely to be only small differences in the scores among objects. Check aspects of the measurement process that relate to all observations; for example, if human judges are using a rating form, the items on the form may be phrased misleadingly.

3. *If one (or perhaps two) observations display low part–whole correlations:* First try deleting the misbehaving observation(s). The reliability may be higher and the entire measurement process more efficient if so pruned. Alternatively, try modifying or replacing the misbehaving observation(s), but always keep in mind that selectively deleting observations can affect what is being measured.

4. *If two or more observations display modest part–whole correlations while the others are high:* This situation is ambiguous and may indicate that the observations as a group are measuring two or more different attributes. In this case, each subset displays high intercorrelation of its member observations, but the observations from different subsets are not correlated with each other. This possibility cannot be fully explored using part–whole correlations and requires either careful inspection of the full intercorrelation matrix or use of more advanced statistical techniques, such as principal component or factor analysis.[2,3] If the investigator expected the observations to address a single attribute and in fact they address multiple discrete attributes, the entire measurement process is not performing as intended and should be redesigned. There is no evidence in this situation that the attribute hypothesized to be measured exists as such. (To play out an example in detail, complete Self-Test 6.2, below.)

If a specific observation is not well behaved (see Outcome 3 above), several things may be happening, and it will be necessary to pinpoint the problem in order to fix it. For example, consider items on a questionnaire as a set of observations. A misbehaving item may be so poorly phrased that it is not assessing anything at all, or perhaps the particular objects—in this case, questionnaire respondents used for the measurement study—lack some specific knowledge that enables them to respond to the item. In this case an improved part–whole correlation may be observed if the item is tested on a different sample of objects. Alternatively, the item may be well phrased but, on logical grounds, does not belong with the other items on the scale. This situation can be determined by inspecting the content of the item, or, if possible, talking to the individuals who completed it to see how it was interpreted. Because it is usually necessary to collect new measurement data after making major revisions to any set of observations, developing measurement procedures is an iterative and time-consuming process. (The illustrative examples presented here employed unrealistically few objects and observations, and as such, they may have underrepresented the work required to conduct a rigorous measurement study.) As a rule, an investigator should borrow from other investigators and other studies whenever possible, particularly if data exist to suggest that the scales have good measurement properties; that is, they have been demonstrated to be reliable and valid when used with objects (people or resources) similar to those proposed for the investigator's own study. The Web site for this volume (http://springeronline.com/0-387-25899-2) will provide links to compendia of validated measurement instruments that address attributes of interest in biomedical informatics.

In addition to computation of part–whole correlations, the data resulting from measurement studies may be analyzed using one of the many statistical techniques for grouping of observations. The most popular is exploratory factor analysis and its many close relatives.[2,3] These techniques suggest which of the observations are well behaved, in a way that can be more precise and informative than inspecting part–whole correlations or values of correlations between observations. The mechanics of these methods are beyond the scope of this discussion. The reader is advised to consult a local statistician or psychometrician, or to read one of the books, cited above, that addresses these techniques.

Self Test 6.2

1. Consider the following measurement result, with a reliability of 0.61. What is your diagnosis of this result? What would you do to improve it?

Object	Results of six observations					
	1	2	3	4	5	6
A	4	3	5	2	1	4
B	2	4	5	3	2	2
C	3	4	3	4	4	3
D	2	3	1	2	1	2
E	3	3	2	2	4	3
Part–whole correlation						
	0.49	0.37	0.32	0.37	0.32	0.49

2. Consider the following measurement result, for which the reliability is 0.72.

Object	Results of six observations					
	1	2	3	4	5	6
A	4	5	4	2	2	3
B	3	3	3	2	2	2
C	4	4	4	4	5	4
D	5	5	4	2	2	1
Part–whole correlation						
	0.21	0.13	0.71	0.76	0.68	0.51

The matrix of correlations among items for these observations is as follows.

	1	2	3	4	5	6
1	—	0.85	0.82	0	0	−0.32
2			0.87	−0.17	−0.17	−0.13
3				0.33	0.33	0.26
4					1	0.78
5						0.78

How would you interpret these results? What would you do to improve this measurement process?

3. Refer to the data in Table 5.5. Using corrected part–whole coefficients, determine who is the best judge in terms of agreement with his or her colleagues. Who is the worst? What would happen to the reliability if the worst judge's ratings were removed from the set?

New Terminology: Facets and Levels

Until now, we have considered measurement situations where only one source of error—one type of independent observation—is under explicit consideration. In the more general case of measurement, multiple sources of error may be explored simultaneously.

Consider a more complicated version of the example earlier in the chapter, where the investigator is interested not only in the effects on measurement of the number of judges employed but also in the effects of the way the patient history is abstracted for purposes of generating the ratings. The investigator divides the judges into two groups. The judges in the first group are assigned to rate all patients using a long abstract, whereas the other group of judges uses a shorter version. In this situation, the measurement study is doing double duty. Two aspects of the measurement process (judges and abstracting methods) are being investigated simultaneously. The objects-by-observations matrix takes on a third dimension, as two characteristics of the observation have been purposefully included in the measurement study. From this more complex study, the investigator can draw conclusions about not only the necessary number of judges but also the adequacy for measurement purposes of abstracts of varying lengths.

Each aspect of the measurement process that is purposefully explored in a measurement study is called a *facet*. In our example developed earlier in this chapter, "judges" is the single facet of the measurement study. In the more complex version of the example, there are two facets: "judges" and "abstract length." Each facet has a number of levels corresponding to the number of independent observations it contributes to the measurement process. In the two-facet example, with six judges used in the measurement study, the "judges" facet is said to have six levels, and with two abstract lengths, the facet "abstract length" is said to have two levels. In the previous chapter's discussion, we said that reliability is improved by increasing the number of independent observations; in this new parlance reliability is improved by increasing the number of levels of a facet. Note that the object class ("patients" in our example) is *not* considered a facet of the measurement study.

As shown in Figure 6.2, the analytical process in a measurement study determines how much of the total variability of the measurement result is statistically attributable to the objects, to the facets purposefully included in the study, and to other factors including random errors. The specific methods developed in Chapter 5 and earlier sections of this chapter allow us to analyze the results of measurement studies that have one facet, and where all observations are made on all objects. These methods also tell us how to prognosticate the effects on reliability of changing the number of levels of that facet. These techniques serve the needs of many investigators. We introduce in the next section more complex measurement situations that employ multiple facets simultaneously. Appendix A briefly introduces the methods of generalizability theory[4,5] as a way to analyze these more complex problems.

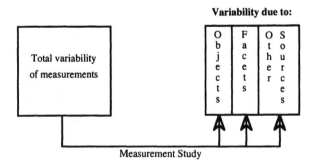

FIGURE 6.2. Analytical process of a measurement study.

Self-Test 6.3

In Chapter 4 we introduced, as an example, a study of a new admission-discharge-transfer (ADT) system for hospitals and the challenge of measuring the attribute of "time to process a new admission," with human observers completing a paper rating form as the "instruments." A measurement study may be designed with measurements taken simultaneously by five observers, at three different times of day, in each of four hospitals. The same five observers are employed for the entire measurement study. What is the object class for this measurement? What are the facets of the measurement study? How many levels does each facet have?

Key Objects and Facets of Measurement in Informatics

We turn now to the range of measurement issues encountered in the real world of informatics. We will consider four specific categories of object classes that are often of primary interest in informatics research and evaluation studies: (1) professionals who may be health care providers, researchers, or educators; (2) clients of these professionals, usually patients or students; (3) biomedical information resources themselves; and (4) work groups or organizations that conduct research or provide health care and education. Similarly, we will consider four categories of measurement facets—tasks, judges, items, and logistical factors—that arise frequently in our work. A specific measurement process can involve one and only one class of objects, but it may have multiple facets. The investigator can choose how many facets to include in a formal measurement study. In many situations a one-facet study suffices because the measurement errors attributable to that facet are often of dominant interest.

Among the classes of objects, *professionals* are important in informatics because attributes of these individuals influence whether and how information resources are used.[6,7] Attributes of professionals that are important to measure include their domain-specific biomedical knowledge; their attitudes toward information technology, the work environment, and change itself; their experience with information technology; and many others.

Clients emerge as objects of interest for many reasons. When clients are patients receiving health care, their health problems are complex and the attributes of these problems, central to the conduct of evaluation studies of information resources designed to improve their care, are difficult to assess. Important attributes of patients that often require measurement are diagnosis, prognosis, appropriateness of actual or recommended management, the typicality of their disease presentation, as well as their own beliefs and attitudes about health and disease. As patients increasingly access health information and some health services directly from the Internet, many of the attributes of professionals, as listed above, assume increased importance for patients as well. When clients are students receiving training in the health professions or biomedical research, measured attributes about them can be important determinants of what they have learned and what they are capable of learning.

Information resources have many attributes (e.g., data quality, speed of task execution, ease of use, cost, reliability, and degradation at the limits of their domain) that are of vital interest to informatics investigators.

Finally, *work groups and organizations* have many attributes (e.g., mission, age, size, budget structure, complexity, and integration) that determine how rapidly they adopt new technology and, once they do, how they use it.

The four categories of facets of frequent interest for measurement in informatics are defined as follows:

1. *Tasks:* In many studies, measurement is made by giving the members of an object class something to do or a problem to solve. Different information resources (objects) may be challenged to process sets of microarray data (tasks) to determine speed of processing or usefulness of results (measured attributes). Alternatively, health care professionals or students (objects) may be asked to review sets of clinical case summaries (tasks) to develop a diagnosis or treatment plan (measured attributes). Within these kinds of performance-based assessment, which occur often in informatics, the challenges or problems assigned to objects are generically referred to as tasks. As will be discussed later in this chapter and revisited in Chapter 7, the credibility of objectivist studies often hinges on the way the investigator manages the task facet in measurement and demonstration study design.

2. *Judges:* Many measurement processes in informatics employ judges—humans with particular expertise who provide their informed opinions, usually by completing a rating form, about behavior they observe directly or review, in retrospect, from some record of that behavior. Judges are necessary to measurement in informatics when the attribute being assessed is complex or where there is no clear standard against which performance may be measured.

3. *Items:* These are the individual elements of a form, questionnaire, or test that is used to record ratings, knowledge, attitudes, opinions, or perceptions. On a knowledge test or attitude questionnaire, for example, each individual question would be considered an item.

4. *Logistical factors:* Many measurement processes are strongly influenced by procedural, temporal, or geographic factors, such as the places where and times when observations take place.

The most general measurement process in informatics includes simultaneously all four of the key facets, as illustrated in Figure 6.3. Recalling that each facet usually has multiple levels, this general process entails multiple judges completing a rating form with multiple items to rate each object completing multiple tasks under differing logistical conditions. To assign each object a single score for the attribute of interest, we would average

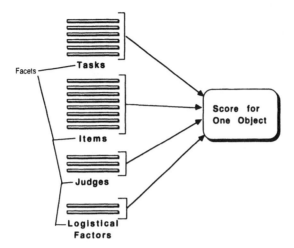

FIGURE 6.3. General (four-facet) measurement problem. A score for one object is obtained by averaging over all levels of each facet and then averaging across the facets. Note that in this example the task facet has five levels, the items facet has eight levels, the judges' facet has three levels, and the logistical factors facet has two levels.

across judges, items, tasks, and conditions (thus averaging across the levels of each facet), as shown in Figure 6.3. For a correspondingly general measurement study, we would conduct the complete measurement process with a representative set of objects and determine how much variability is statistically attributable to each of the four facets. We would also learn from such a study how many levels of each facet would be necessary to achieve an adequate level of reliability. The methods of generalizability theory (see Appendix A) are required to work analytically with a multifacet measurement problem. Generalizability theory has been applied to measurement problems in biomedical informatics.[8]

We discuss in the following section the practical aspects of the three facets that arise most frequently in measurement studies: tasks, judges, and items. Although we do not discuss logistical factors explicitly, they may be important facets of some measurement processes. As seen in the earlier example of an ADT system, the measured time to process a patient admission could depend on logistical factors, such as the general state of the clinic, which in turn could depend on the time of day, time of year, and other factors. We emphasize that the choice of specific facets to include in a measurement study rests completely with the investigator. If a facet is included, the amount of variation (error) it contributes to the measurement process can be quantified. If a facet is excluded, its contribution to measurement error is combined with all "other sources," as illustrated in Figure 6.2, and cannot be separately identified.

Self-Test 6.4

For the measurement problem and study described in Self-Test 6.3, to what category does each facet belong?

Pragmatics of Measurement Using Tasks, Judges, and Items

In this section, we decompose the multifacet general measurement problem and focus separately on each important facet of measurement in informatics. We address these pragmatics of measurement one facet at a time, for several reasons. First, each facet raises its own unique set of pragmatic issues for measurement. Second, as was noted earlier, many measurement problems in informatics are dominated by a single facet as a source of measurement error, and in these common cases, a one-facet measurement study based on the classical theory is sufficient. For each facet, we explore the following: (1) in studies, why the results for a given object vary from observation to observation and how much variation to expect; (2) in practice, how many levels of the facet are needed for reliable measurement; and (3) what can be done to improve this aspect of measurement. We discuss each facet using applicable object classes (professionals, clients, information resources) as examples. We focus first on tasks as the facet of interest, then on judges, and then on items. The three decomposed measurement problems are illustrated in Figure 6.4.

Task Facet

Many evaluation studies in informatics are performed using real-world tasks or laboratory simulations of these tasks. The relevant object classes—the entities undertaking these tasks—may be persons (professionals, students, or patients) as actual or potential users of information resources, the information resources themselves, or groups of persons. In field studies (see Chapter 3), the tasks are naturally occurring within the work environment; in laboratory studies the tasks may be invented, simulated, or abstracted for purposes of control. How these persons or resources perform these tasks depends on the goals of the study. They may be asked to diagnose, interpret, analyze, predict, retrieve pertinent literature or molecular structures, propose management, or critique the performance of others. For many reasons, selection and design of these tasks, for measurement as well as demonstration studies, is the most challenging aspect of objectivist study design.

Sources of Variation Among Tasks

The performance of persons and information resources is highly dependent on the content of the material with which they are challenged. For informa-

When Tasks are the Key Facet:

Observations: Tasks (problems, cases)

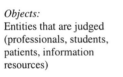
Objects:
Performers of the tasks
(professionals, students,
information resources)
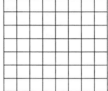

When Judges are the Key Facet:

Observations: Judges (human experts)

Objects:
Entities that are judged
(professionals, students,
patients, information
resources)

When Items are the Key Facet:

Observations: Items (elements of a form or test)

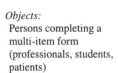
Objects:
Persons completing a
multi-item form
(professionals, students,
patients)
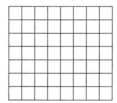

FIGURE 6.4. The general measurement problem decomposed into three one-facet problems.

tion resources, which are programmed to perform specific tasks within specific domains, this statement is hardly surprising. However, in studies involving persons as problem solvers, one might believe that intelligence could extend problem solving abilities across biomedical domains, allowing these persons to accomplish tasks for which they were not explicitly prepared. Under this assumption, a theoretical physicist could apply general physical principles to novel biological problems without knowing much about biology, or an excellent medical diagnostician specializing in gastrointestinal problems might almost equally well diagnose problems of the brain. However appealing this conception of human intelligence may be, the classic study of medical problem solving by Elstein and colleagues[9] and subsequent studies substantiating this work have documented a high level of "case dependence" of humans as problem solvers. Putting this into our measurement framework, suppose a sample of persons is given two diagnostic problems to work. If we compute the correlation between performance on the first problem with performance on the second, the magnitude of this correlation is typically small. High performance on one problem does not strongly imply a high performance on another. For this reason, "task dependence" or "case specificity" of biomedical expertise is now a central issue in research and evaluation, and the tasks or case problems used in any study are a key feature of that study's design. Typically, the results of the study apply only to that sample of tasks used in the study, or to a real or hypothetical population from which these tasks were systematically sampled.

In the context of our measurement theory, it should not be surprising that studies employing only one task are intrinsically weak. They are analogous to the archer shooting a single arrow. In such instances, the results of the study are an artifact of the features of that single task, and the effect of task specificity on the measurement process cannot be estimated. To make a statement in a demonstration study that one group of participants performs better than another group, it is necessary to challenge each member of each group with a large number of carefully selected tasks. Determining how many tasks are required for acceptable measurement is, of course, the major goal of a measurement study.

Whether the objects of measurement are persons or machines, the inter-observation correlation for tasks increases in proportion to the similarity of the tasks themselves. However, the features that contribute to making tasks similar are highly idiosyncratic to the task and objects involved in that particular study, and often are not predictable in advance. This point holds particularly with persons as objects, because humans vary enormously in their personal knowledge and how that knowledge is organized. Human ability to solve a scientific or clinical problem is best predicted by each individual's experience with problems of exactly that type and only weakly predicted by individual traits such as innate intelligence.[10] Therefore, two clinicians of equal intelligence and seniority may differ dramatically in their performance on the same case, according to their levels of problem-specific experience. The features of a problem that make it familiar, and thus easy for an individual to address, are also not readily predictable.

Similarly, when information resources are the objects of measurement, neither the performance of the resource on a specific task nor the intertask variability in performance can be predicted in advance once these systems reach a certain level of complexity. This is a restatement of the fact that system function cannot in general be predicted from its structure, as first introduced in Chapter 3. Generalizations about the performance of information resources and human problem solvers must be made with the same care. Measurement studies to determine how many tasks (cases) are required for reliable measurement are necessary whether the objects are information resources or people.

In practice, investigators can exercise control over the task facet in two ways: first, by sampling problems carefully from some real or hypothetical population; and second, by employing sufficient problems to achieve acceptable reliability when the performance is averaged across them. In accordance with our measurement theory, use of large numbers of problems is analogous to shooting a large number of arrows to ensure that the effects of idiosyncratic factors "average out."

A clear trade-off is built into measurement processes with tasks as the primary facet of interest. For a fixed number of levels (the number of tasks included in the measurement study), making the domain spanned by the included tasks larger increases the generalizability of the measurement process. However, again with the number of levels fixed, broadening the domain works to decrease the reliability of the measurement because the tasks will differ to a greater degree from one another. Making the domain smaller has the opposite effect of decreasing the generalizability while increasing the reliability. The dilemma for investigators designing evaluation studies may be rephrased as: "Do you want to know more about less, or less about more?"

Number of Tasks Needed

Much research on problem solving in clinical medicine has clarified the number of cases necessary for reliable measurement of human performance in that domain. The best research has been performed using standardized patient-actors. To reach a reliability of 0.70, six to 24 cases must be assigned to each person (object). Whether the required number of cases falls at the low or high end of this range depends on the attribute of performance under study. For diagnostic problems, 24 cases may be required.[11] This requirement creates a challenge for investigators to include relatively large numbers of time-consuming tasks in their studies, but there are some ways, addressed in the following section, to streamline the process. Although it is not always clear what makes tasks similar, the more similar the tasks that comprise a set, the higher are the performance intercorrelations between them and thus the higher the reliability of a measurement process comprising a given number of tasks. For some situations, a highly homogeneous mix, such as differing presentations of the same disease or scientific problem, might be appropriate and fewer such tasks may be required. This represents the "small domain" resolution of the trade-off described above. If we include cases of diabetes mellitus in a clinical task set, a relatively small number of cases will be needed to achieve a target level of reliability, but we would only learn from a measurement study how well the measurement process works for diabetes cases. Generalization to other disease domains would be risky and speculative. In general, the choice of the test set of tasks should follow logically from the ultimate purposes of the demonstration study anticipated by the investigator.

For studies of information resource performance (where one or more resources themselves are the objects of measurement), it is difficult to give an analogous figure for the required number of tasks, because few measurement studies have been performed. Swets,[12] for example, pointed to the need for "large and representative samples" but did not quantify "large." In domains other than medicine, for example weather forecasting, it is common to test prognostic systems with thousands of cases. Jain's[13] otherwise thorough discussion of work loads for computer system performance testing did not directly address the size of the work load necessary for reliable measurement. Lacking guidelines for the number of tasks to use for studying information resource performance in biomedical domains, the most sensible approach is to conduct measurement studies in advance, and resolve the problem empirically. If the results of an appropriately designed measurement study yield unacceptable reliability, the investigator should change the measurement process as indicated by the results of the study.

Improving Measurement with the Task Facet

When persons are the objects of measurement, it is important to challenge these persons with a set of tasks that is large enough for adequate measurement, but no larger than necessary. The longer the task set, the greater the risk of fatigue, noncompliance, or half-hearted effort; data loss through failure to complete the task set; or expense if the individuals are compensated for their work. The inherent task-to-task variability in performance cannot be circumvented, but many other steps can be taken to ensure that every task in a set is adding useful information to a study. The approaches to improve measurement in this domain are multiple: (1) careful abstracting of case data, (2) sampling a large number of tasks from a known domain, (3) attention to how performance is scored, and (4) systematic assignment of tasks to objects.

Abstracting

Much of the published research in informatics is based on case or problem abstractions of various types to provide a representation of a case that is completely consistent wherever and whenever it is employed. Typically, a subset of findings from a clinical case is extracted from the patient's chart and summarized in a concise written document, creating the ubiquitous "paper cases" that embody the tasks for a study.[14] Yet, care providers in the real world work with live patients who provide verbal and nonverbal cues about their condition. These cues are revealed over time in ways that a paper abstract cannot capture. The systematic effects of these abstractions on biomedical informatics studies represent a validity issue from a measurement perspective, and are largely unexplored.[15] However, it is clear that inconsistent abstracting diminishes the intercorrelations between cases comprising a set, and thus increases measurement error. To address this problem, the rules to select findings for inclusion in the summary should be clearly stated, even if the same person is doing all of the abstracting. Otherwise, abstracters' inconsistent judgments about what is important could substantially skew the results of a study. These rules should also be carefully reviewed to ensure that they are free of an evident bias, such as consistent omission of the information key to successful completion of the task by person or machine. Paper problems drawn from scientific domains such as biology and physics are subject to the same considerations as clinical cases. Each paper problem is an abstraction of a more comprehensive situation, and these abstractions need to be created with consistency to establish a problem set for measurement purposes.

The need for consistency goes beyond the choice of which findings to include. These findings must be represented in a consistent fashion, so they will have the same meaning within the set and across all who encounter the task. Using an example from clinical domains, an abstracter may decide to represent a laboratory test result as "normal" or "abnormal" instead of giving the quantitative value of the result. This is an effective strategy to counteract the tendency for persons who see only the quantitative value to come to different interpretations because of different standards for normalcy that exist across institutions. The abstracters must also decide how much interpretation of findings to provide and take steps to ensure that they do it consistently.

There are, of course, alternatives to the paper representations of cases, but they are time-consuming and expensive. At the extreme of high fidelity is the simulated patient, a human actor trained to sound, look, and—on physical examination—even feel like the actual patient with a particular disease.[11] A lower-fidelity compromise is representation of a case via computer simulation of a case, which could allow access to all clinical findings via a natural language interface, visual representation of the patient, and access to many clinical findings such as radiographs in uninterpreted form. Computer simulations themselves vary in ornateness,[16] and the simplest simulation that meets the needs of a study should be selected. Although possibly expensive to set up initially, the recurring cost of using a computer simulation is low. In both of these formats, the general problem of abstraction of information from the full case remains. The actor is trained to know a finite set of clinical information, and a computer simulation cannot present more than it is programmed to present.

Sampling

Task selection can be addressed by two major strategies: (1) building controlled variability into the set by purposeful sampling, and (2) including tasks that occur naturally in the study setting. To the extent that the investigator knows which case features are important for determining performance, he or she can map these features into a sampling grid and subsequently select cases to ensure balanced representation of these features. With this approach the investigator can control the amount of variability in the case set, but must do so with recognition that it invokes the trade-offs introduced earlier. Constraining the variability too much (making the cases too similar) leads to high reliability of measurement but does not allow generalization beyond that homogeneous set. On the other hand, purposeful building of a highly diverse case set inevitably requires a larger number of cases for reliable measurement.

Although building a case set from such a blueprint gives the investigator a great deal of control, it generates a sample of cases that is contrived and may be difficult to describe. With the second strategy, the investigator selects cases based on natural occurrence, for example using consecutive admissions to a hospital, or consecutive calls to the help desk, as the criterion. The resulting set of cases has a clear reference population, but the variability in the case mix is not under the investigator's control. In a study of a clinical decision support or biosurveillance system, for example, cases that invoke the capabilities of this resource may not appear with sufficient frequency in a naturally occurring sequence of cases.

Whichever strategy is followed, the key to this process is to have a defensible selection plan that follows from the purposes of the study and in turn allows the investigator to identify the population from which the cases were selected. The implications of these strategies for demonstration study design are discussed in Chapter 7.

Scoring

The execution of many tasks generates a result that can be scored by formula or algorithm, with no human judgment required to generate a score after the formula itself is established. This is often the case when the task has a generally acknowledged reference standard or the problem has an unambiguous correct answer. For example, the accuracy of a resource performing protein structure prediction can be computed as the mean displacement of the atoms' predicted location from their known actual locations as established experimentally. A task in clinical diagnosis may be scored in relation to the location of the correct diagnosis on the hypothesis list provided by the clinician, assuming that the correct diagnosis is known with a high degree of certainty. In other circumstances, where there is no reference standard or correct answer, the task does not lend itself to formulaic scoring, and in these circumstances human judges must be employed to render an opinion or a verdict that becomes the performance score. This almost always generates a two-facet measurement problem that includes both tasks and judges.

Even when tasks can be scored formulaically, the development of scoring methods may not be straightforward and merits care. For example, the apparently simple assignment of a score to a clinician's diagnostic hypothesis list, for cases where the true diagnosis is known, can be undertaken in a variety of ways, each with advantages and disadvantages. Scientists confronting technical problems may be assigned partial credit for key elements of a solution, with some omissions carrying higher penalties than others. The effects on reliability and validity of alternate scoring schemes can be built into measurement studies.[17,18]

Assignment

Many techniques can be used to assign tasks (cases) to objects in measurement studies, but whenever possible this assignment should be done by preordained design rather than chance encounter. As shown in Figure 6.5, two common assignment modes include the "fully crossed" approach, where every object is challenged by every case in the sample, and a "nested" approach, where specific subsamples of objects are assigned to specific subsamples of cases. The nested approach is especially helpful when the investigator is studying persons as objects, and wishes to include a large number of cases in the full study, but does not want to burden any single person with the entire case set. In informatics, the persons employed in studies are typically busy scientists, trainees, or care providers. Their time is scarce or expensive (or both). Using a nested approach, 15 cases can be randomly divided into three groups. If each person is assigned to work one group of cases, each works only five cases (a more manageable task than 15), and the investigator is not seriously limited in the conclusions he or she can draw from the study. Nested designs are useful in both measurement and demonstration studies. In situations where large numbers of cases are available, nested designs should be considered a way to take advantage of the ability

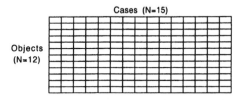

Fully Crossed Design: All Cases Assigned to All Objects

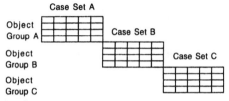

Nested Design: Sets of 5 Cases Assigned to Groups of Objects

FIGURE 6.5. Assignment of tasks (cases) to objects.

to generalize from that large number of cases without having to expose every object to every case. In measurement studies, generalizability theory (see Appendix A) provides a way to estimate sources of measurement errors for nested designs.

Judges Facet

The judges facet enters into a measurement problem whenever informed human judges assess specific aspects of the quality of an activity or a product they are observing. Judges become central to measurement in informatics for situations where there are no reference standards or correct answers for the attribute(s) under study. In these situations, the considered opinions of human experts are the best option to generate a measured score. A study might employ experts to judge the quality of the interactions between patients and clinicians, as the clinicians enter patient data into an information resource during the interaction. In another example, observers may assess key aspects of the interaction of end users with a new information resource during a beta test. As with any measurement process, the primary concern is the correlation among the independent observations—in this situation, the judges—and the resulting number of judges required to obtain a reliable measurement. A set of "well-behaved" judges, all of whom correlate with one another to an acceptable extent when rating a representative sample of objects, can be said to form a scale. A large literature on performance assessment by judges speaks in more detail to many of the issues addressed here.[18–20]

Sources of Variation Among Judges

Ideally, all judges of the same object, using the same criteria and forms to record their opinions, should render highly correlated judgments. All variation should then be among objects. Many factors that erode interjudge agreement are well known and have been well documented[21]:

1. *Interpretation or logical effects:* Judges may differ in their interpretations of the attribute(s) to be rated and the meanings of the items on the forms on which they record their judgments. They may give similar ratings to attributes that are logically related in their own minds.

2. *Judge tendency effects:* Some judges are consistently overgenerous or lenient; others are consistently hypercritical or stringent. Others do not employ the full set of response options on a form, locating all of their ratings in a narrow region, which is usually at the middle of the range. This phenomenon is known as a "central tendency" effect.

3. *Insufficient exposure:* Sometimes the logistics of a study require that judges base their judgments on less exposure to the objects than is necessary to come to an informed conclusion. This may occur, for example, if investigators schedule 10 minutes of observation of end users working with

a new information resource, but the users require 20 minutes to complete an assigned task.

4. *Inconsistent conditions:* Unless multiple judges make their observations simultaneously, the phenomena observed can vary from judge to judge. One judge may observe completion of a task in the morning, when the persons completing the task are alert and energetic, while another judge may observe in the evening when everyone is tired.

Number of Judges Needed

Although steps can be taken to reduce the effects of the factors listed above, it is not possible to completely eliminate objectivist measurement errors seen as differences among judges' ratings of the same performance. As with the other facets of measurement, multiple observations (in this case multiple judges) are necessary. The upper bound on reliability that can be expected from a one-judge study is on the order of 0.5.[22] In Chapter 5 we saw that van der Lei and colleagues obtained a reliability of 0.65 when using eight judges in the study of Hypercritic. In the self-test below, we see that three judges may be sufficient for some situations. There is, however, no precise way to determine this number in advance. A measurement study is necessary to verify that acceptable reliability is obtained for any particular situation.

Improving Measurement Using Judges

The general approach is to increase the number of judges to improve reliability or to improve the measurement process itself, affecting both reliability and validity, by training the judges or designing better instruments for them to use. Increasing the number of judges helps only if the added judges perform equivalently to, the judges already included. If they do, the Spearman-Brown prophecy formula estimates how much improvement can be obtained. What makes a human judge intrinsically "good," aside from having expert knowledge of the performance domain being assessed, is rarely clear to the investigator.

To improve the quality of a measurement process employing judges, the investigator can ensure that each judge observes a representative sample of the phenomena of interest. A nested design can be helpful when there is danger of asking each judge to do more observation than is reasonable. The phenomena to be observed can be sectioned by time, or by other naturally occurring criteria presented by the setting of the study. (For example, Judge 1 observes on Monday the first week, Tuesday the second week, etc.) Such a nested design also allows for a greater range of phenomena to form the basis of the ratings, leading to greater generalizability of the results. Laboratory studies, as opposed to field studies, give the investigator greater control of the logistics of study, making it easier to implement these approaches.

Additional benefit can derive from formal training or orientation of the judges.[22] Many strategies can be useful here. In advance of any formal observation by the judges, a meeting where the judges discuss their personal interpretations of the attributes to be rated can increase reliability. A more formal training activity where the judges watch a videotaped or live sample of the phenomena to be rated can also be helpful. Here, judges first observe the phenomenon, which might be a representative interaction of a user with an information resource, and make their ratings independently. Then the individual ratings are collected and summarized in a table, so all can see the aggregate performance of the group. This step is followed by a discussion among the judges, in which they share their reasons for rating as they did, and subsequently agree on definitions or criteria for making judgments. The lessons learned from this training activity can be folded into the actual measurement procedures employed when the study begins. (At that point, the judges must work independently.)

Some simple logistical and practical steps, often overlooked, can also improve measurement using judges. First, eliminate judges who, for a variety of reasons, are inappropriate participants in the study. An individual with a position of authority in the environment where the study is undertaken, such as the director of a lab or clinic, should not participate as a judge. Do not use unwilling conscripts, who might have been "cordially required" by their supervisors to serve as judges. Second, make the work of the judges as brief as possible, with a minimum of complications. Most judges have a fixed amount of time to devote to their task. The more time they devote to administrative aspects, such as making their own copies of forms to record their judgments, the less time they can devote to the substantive task at hand. In some studies, under appropriate conditions, the activity to be judged can be videotaped, and the judges can work asynchronously—as long as they do not informally discuss their ratings before all judgments have been rendered and as long as the videotape captures all key elements of task performance.

In informatics, judges are often used with patients as the object class of measurement, for example to obtain the closest approximation to the optimal management for each patient. This is a key measurement problem in informatics because, clinically, it is essential to assess the performance of an information resource functioning as a decision support tool in the context of the closest possible approximation to "best practice." Applying to this specific problem several of the principles introduced above, the patients should be followed for as long as is ethically and practically possible so the judges have a large amount of information on which to base their ratings. To increase the reliability and validity of measurement, several medical domain experts, preferably from different clinical centers, should be recruited. To preserve the independence of observations, judges should review case data independently.

In many instances, the attribute to be assessed by judges has interval or ratio properties, such as a rating of the quality of care provided to each of a set of patients. In these instances the best approximation to the true value of the attribute is obtained by averaging the judges' ratings. In other situations the attribute to be assessed has nominal properties: for example, the final diagnosis of a case or the correct answer to a problem. In these cases it may be necessary to first obtain a shortlist of possible diagnoses/answers from a set of judges and subsequently ask these judges or others to rate each member of the list. If the disagreement is too great among the judges, it may be that a sufficiently good approximation to the "truth" is unobtainable for this case and should be omitted from any subsequent demonstration study. In cases where judges disagree, it may be appealing to refer the case to a senior judge for a deciding vote.[23] Although this is a useful expedient, there is no guarantee that the truth resides with this individual. Also, once the final decision is vested in a single individual and not the mean of a set of independent judges, the error in the measurement process is no longer estimable using the methods introduced here.

Self-Test 6.5

The TraumAID system[24] was developed to provide minute-by-minute advice to trauma surgeons in the management of patients with penetrating wounds to the chest and abdomen. As part of a laboratory study of the accuracy of TraumAID's advice, Clarke and colleagues[24] asked a panel of three judges—all experienced surgeons from the institution where TraumAID was developed—to rate the appropriateness of management for each of a series of cases that had been abstracted to paper descriptions. Ratings were on a scale of 1 to 4, where 4 indicated essentially flawless care and 1 indicated serious deficiencies. Each case appeared twice in the set: (1) as the patient was treated, and (2) as TraumAID would have treated the patient. The abstracts were carefully written to eliminate any cues as to whether the described care was computer generated or actually administered.

Overall, 111 cases were rated by three judges, with the following results:

Condition	Corrected part–whole correlations			Reliability of ratings
	Judge A	Judge B	Judge C	
Actual care	0.57	0.52	0.55	0.72
TraumAID	0.57	0.59	0.47	0.71

Condition	Mean ± SD ratings		
	Judge A	Judge B	Judge C
Actual care	2.35 ± 1.03	2.42 ± 0.80	2.25 ± 1.01
TraumAID	3.12 ± 1.12	2.71 ± 0.83	2.67 ± 0.95

1. What are the dimensions (number of rows and number of columns) of the two objects-by-observations matrices used to compute these results?
2. Is there any evidence of rater tendency errors (leniency, stringency, or central tendency) in these data?
3. Viewing this as a measurement study, what would you be inclined to conclude about the measurement process? Consider reliability and validity issues.
4. Viewing this as a demonstration study, what would you be inclined to conclude about the accuracy of TraumAID's advice?

Items Facet

As defined earlier, items are the individual elements of an instrument used to record ratings, opinions, knowledge, or perceptions of an individual we generically call a "respondent." Items usually take the form of questions. The instruments containing the items can be self-administered, read to the respondent in a highly structured interview, or completed interactively at a computer. For the same reason that a single task cannot be the basis for reliable assessment of performance of an information resource, a single item cannot be used to measure reliably the respondent's beliefs or degree of knowledge. The measurement strategy to obtain accurate measurement is always the same: use multiple independent observations (in this case, items) and pool the results for each object (in this case, respondents) to obtain the best estimate of the value of the attribute for that object. If the items forming a set are shown to be "well behaved" in an appropriate measurement study, we can say that they comprise a scale.

When people (health care providers, researchers, students, or patients) are the object class of interest, investigators frequently use multi-item forms to assess the personal attitudes, beliefs, or knowledge of these people. This technique generates a basic one-facet measurement problem with items as the observations and persons as the objects. Items can also form a facet of a more complex measurement problem when, for example, multiple judges complete a multi-item form to render their opinions about multiple case problems. A vast array of item types and formats is in common use. In settings where items are used to elicit beliefs or attitudes, there is usually no correct answer to the items; however, in tests of knowledge, a particular response is identified by the item developer as correct. We explore a few of the more common item formats here and discuss some general principles of item design that work to reduce measurement error.

Almost all items consist of two parts, whether they are used to assess knowledge or personal beliefs, or to judge performance. The first part is a stem, which elicits a response; the second provides a structured format for the individual completing the instrument to respond to the stem. Responses can be elicited using graphical or visual analog scales, as shown in Figure 6.6. Alternatively, responses can be elicited via a discrete set of options, as shown in Table 6.4. The semantics of the response options themselves may

This patient was managed:

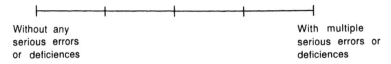

| Without any serious errors or deficiences | | | | With multiple serious errors or deficiences |

FIGURE 6.6. Rating item with a graphical response scale.

be unipolar or bipolar. Unipolar response options are anchored at the extremes by "none" and "a lot," for example, "I never do this" vs. "I always do this." Bipolar response options are anchored at the extremes by semantic opposites, for example, "good" vs. "bad," "strongly agree" to "strongly disagree." The literature does not reveal a great deal of difference among these

TABLE 6.4. An "optimism" scale for medical informatics.[25]

Effect of computers on	Highly detrimental	Detrimental on the whole	Neither detrimental nor beneficial	Beneficial on the whole	Highly beneficial
Cost of health care	1	2	3	4	5
Clinician autonomy	1	2	3	4	5
Quality of health care	1	2	3	4	5
Interactions within the health care team	1	2	3	4	5
Role of the government in health care	1	2	3	4	5
Access to health care in remote or rural areas	1	2	3	4	5
Management of medical/ ethical dilemmas	1	2	3	4	5
Enjoyment of the practice of medicine	1	2	3	4	5
Status of medicine as a profession	1	2	3	4	5
Continuing medical education	1	2	3	4	5
Self-image of clinicians	1	2	3	4	5
Humaneness of the practice of medicine	1	2	3	4	5
Rapport between clinicians and patients	1	2	3	4	5
Personal and professional privacy	1	2	3	4	5
Clinicians' access to up-to-date knowledge	1	2	3	4	5
Patients' satisfaction with the quality of care they receive	1	2	3	4	5
Generalists' ability to manage more complex problems	1	2	3	4	5

item formats in terms of the quality of the measurement information obtained.[22,26] Instrument designers choose formats largely based on the goodness of fit to the attribute being assessed, and the mechanics of the measurement process.

We now explore how multiple items can be used to form a scale. Table 6.4 contains an excerpt from a longer questionnaire that assesses the attitudes of academic physicians toward information technology.[27] Each of the items in Table 6.4 addresses the perceived effects of computers on a particular aspect of health care, but the items can be seen as having something deeper in common. Each reflects, in part, a sense of optimism about the future role of information technology in health care. The response options form a bipolar axis. We might expect an individual who responds favorably to one item to have a tendency to respond favorably to the other items in the set because of this general belief or outlook. In this sense, each item can be seen as an observation of the attribute "optimism." The assumption can be tested via an appropriate measurement study, and if the assumption holds, a person's level of optimism may be assessed using the sum (or average) of the responses to the set of items.* Across a set of items that address the same underlying attribute, it is assumed that the idiosyncratic reactions to the individual items cancel out and the average reflects the individual's true belief.

We already know how to test such an assumption using a measurement study, by examining the distributions of the responses to the individual items and the correlations among them, after administering the items to a representative sample of respondents. Perfect correlation among the different items is not expected. In this particular set of items, all but one of the items were found to be well behaved. The reliability of the scale with the poorly behaved item removed was 0.86. Of course, showing that the items form a well-behaved cluster does not demonstrate that they combine to assess optimism. Additional studies of the validity of the scale are required for that purpose.

Scales to measure attitudes and beliefs are typically developed through an iterative process where the investigators first clearly identify the attribute to be assessed and the populations of respondents who will be completing the ultimate form. They then create an initial set of items. To do this, they might conduct open-ended interviews or focus groups, or develop an initial item set from their own personal experience. The scale developers then conduct measurement studies, administering the scale to samples of persons and identifying, revising, or replacing items that are not well behaved. Over what is often a succession of measurement studies, the reliability of the scale usually improves to acceptable levels. The validity of the

---

* Summing and averaging items yield equivalent results as long as the respondent completes all the items composing the scale.

scale—content, criterion-related, construct—must also be established using methods discussed in Chapter 5.

Similar challenges are presented by other measurement situations requiring the use of multiple items to measure some shared underlying attribute. For example, a knowledge test might contain individual items that appear very different, but in fact all belong to the general knowledge domain addressed by the test. By the same token, items addressing different aspects of a laboratory procedure have in common the attribute of competence in performing that particular task.

Sources of Variation Among Items

Some variability from item to item is purposefully built into the way knowledge and beliefs are measured because the respondents are being asked multiple questions that have something fundamental in common. Careful item design can ensure that this variability is controlled (thus maximizing reliability), and that the averaged responses to this set of items capture the attribute of interest (maximizing validity). If items are ambiguously phrased, if the stems and response options are not logically matched, or if the response options do not accurately mirror the range of beliefs the respondents hold, the result will be measurement error seen as low levels of inter-item correlation. Specific ways to address these problems are described below.

The "halo effect" is a well-known problem that occurs when items are the key facet of measurement. Respondents to an instrument, in the process of completing a series of items addressing the same attribute, may quickly form an overall impression causing them to respond in an automatic way to each item in the set, rather than giving independent thought to each one. If the overall impression formed is positive, all items are completed positively regardless of the respondent's true beliefs about each item. If the overall impression is negative, the opposite occurs. Halo effects result in artificially inflated reliability, since all items are answered as if they were exactly the same, and dubious validity. Ways to reduce halo effects are also discussed below.

Number of Items Needed

This depends on the attribute being measured and the purposes of the measurement. Typically, a minimum of eight to 10 items is needed to measure a belief or an attitude. The 16-item computer optimism scale (Table 6.4) had a reliability of 0.86. The Spearman-Brown formula suggests that an eight-item version of the same scale would still have a reliability of 0.75, but removal of some of the items would raise concerns about validity by altering the meaning of the now-modified item set. In extreme cases such as high-stakes standardized tests, where very high reliability is necessary to make decisions about each individual's competence, more than 100 knowledge questions (items) are routinely used within a knowledge domain. In this situation, large numbers of items are required both to attain the high reliability necessary to generate a small standard error of measurement and to sample adequately a broad domain of knowledge. For ratings of performance by expert judges, fewer items on a form may be necessary because the attribute to be rated is often specific. For any particular measurement situation, a measurement study can determine how many items are necessary and which items should be deleted or modified to improve the performance of the item set hypothesized to comprise a scale.

Improving Measurement with Items

We offer here several practical suggestions to minimize measurement errors through attention to item design. We focus here on ratings and elicitations of attitudes and beliefs because these applications arise frequently during the evaluations that are the focus of this book.

1. *Make items specific.* Perhaps the single most important way to improve items is to make them as specific as possible. The more information the respondents get from the item itself, about what exactly is being asked for and what the response options mean, the greater is the consistency and thus the reliability of the results. Consider a basic item that may be part of a multi-item rating form (Figure 6.7A). As a first step toward specificity, the item should offer a definition of the attribute to be rated, as shown in Figure 6.7B. The next step is to change the response categories from broad qualitative judgments to behavior or events that might be observed. As shown in Figure 6.7C, we might change the logic of the responses by specifically asking for the opinion as to how frequently the explanations were clear.

2. *Match the logic of the response to that of the stem.* This step is vitally important. If the stem—the part of the item that elicits a response—requests an estimate of a quantity, the response formats must offer a range of reasonable quantities from which to choose. If the stem requests a strength of belief, the response formats must offer an appropriate way to express the strength of belief, such as the familiar "strongly agree" to "strongly disagree" format.

3. *Provide a range of semantically and logically distinct response options.* Be certain that the categories span the range of possible responses and do not overlap. When response categories are given as quantitative ranges, novice item developers often overlap the edges of the response ranges, as in the following example.

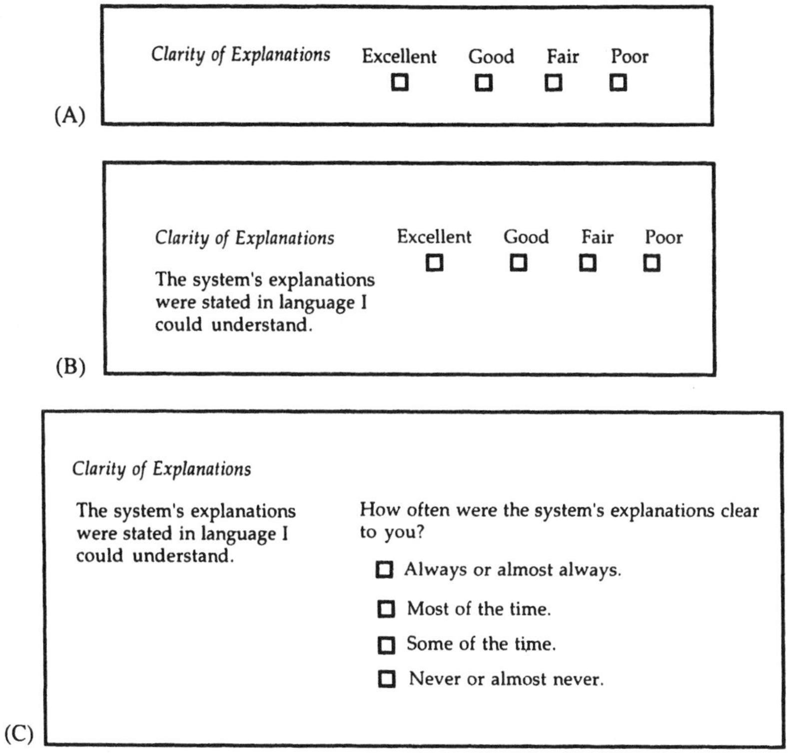

(A)

(B)

(C)

FIGURE 6.7. A: Basic rating item. B: One improvement: define the attribute. C: Second improvement: make the response categories correspond to what is directly observable.

Bad Example 1

In your opinion, with what fraction of your clinic patients this month has the resource offered useful advice?

☐ 0–25%   ☐ 25–50%   ☐ 50–75%   ☐ 75–100%

Clearly it is necessary to begin the second option with 26%, the third with 51%, and the fourth with 76%.

Similarly, when response categories are stated verbally, the terms used should be carefully chosen so the categories are as equally spaced, in a semantic sense, as possible. Consider another mistake commonly made by novice item writers:

Bad Example 2

How satisfied are you with the new resource, overall?

☐ Extremely   ☐ Very   ☐ Generally   ☐ Not at all

In this example, there is too much semantic space between "generally" and "not at all." There are three response options that reflect positive views of the resource and only one option that is negative. To rectify this problem, a response option of "slightly" or "modestly" might be added to the existing set.

4. *Include an appropriate number of response options.* Although it may seem tempting to use a large number of response options to create at least the appearance of precise measurement, the results might prove illusory. In general, the number of response options should be limited to a maximum of seven.[26]* For most purposes, four to six discrete options suffice. Using a five-option response format with a bipolar semantic axis allows a neutral response. We can offer arguments for and against neutral responses. A potential benefit is that a respondent whose true belief is neutral has a response option reflective of that belief. In the opposing view, a neutral response option plays to the central-tendency problem. It provides a way to respond that is safe and noncommittal, even though it may not be reflective of the respondent's actual belief.

5. *Invite a nonresponse.* Giving respondents permission to decline to respond to each item also contributes to successful measurement. When using rating forms, for example, respondents may offer uninformed opinions based on insufficient experience because they feel they are expected to complete every item on the form. If an "unable to respond" category is explicitly available, respondents are more likely to omit items on which they do not feel confident or competent, which of course is what they should do. If an "unable to respond" category is offered, it should be in a different typeface or otherwise visually apart from the continuum of informed responses.

6. *Request elaborations.* Asking respondents specifically for verbal elaborations or justifications of their responses can serve multiple purposes. It often forces them to be more thoughtful. Respondents may check off a specific option and then, when trying to elaborate on it, realize that their deeper beliefs differ from what a first impression suggested. Elaborations are also a source of valuable data, particularly helpful when the items are part of a rating form that is in the early stages of development, to help validate the form. Elaboration can also be informative as a source of evaluation data. If the purpose of a study is to understand "why," in addition to "how much," these verbal elaborations may even be essential. Chapters 9 and 10, where we discuss subjectivist approaches to evaluation, indicate that these verbal comments can become the data of primary interest to the investigator.

7. *Address halo effects.* There are two major ways to minimize halo effects through item design. The first is to include, within a set of items

---

* It is generally known that humans can process about seven (plus or minus two) items of disparate information at any one time.[27] The practical upper limit of seven response options may be attributable to this feature of human cognition.

composing a scale, roughly equal numbers phrased positively and negatively. For example, the set might include both of the following:

My ability to be productive in my job was enhanced by the new computer system.

☐ Strongly agree   ☐ Agree   ☐ Neither agree nor disagree
☐ Disagree   ☐ Strongly disagree

The new system slowed the rate at which I could complete routine tasks.

☐ Strongly agree   ☐ Agree   ☐ Neither agree nor disagree
☐ Disagree   ☐ Strongly Disagree

In this example, the co-presence of items that can be both endorsed and not endorsed if the respondent feels positively about the system forces the respondent to attend more closely to the content of the items themselves. This strategy increases the chance that the respondent will evaluate each item on its own terms, rather than responding to a global impression. When analyzing the responses to such item sets, the negatively phrased items should be reverse coded before each respondent's results are averaged, so that calculations to estimate reliability give correct results.

A second strategy, useful in situations where one instrument is being used to assess multiple attributes, is to intermix items that measure different attributes. This practice is common on psychological instruments to conceal the attributes measured by the instrument so respondents respond more honestly and spontaneously. It may not, however, be an advisable strategy for an instrument used by judges to rate performance. In this case the rating form should be organized to make the rating process as easy as possible, and items addressing the same attribute should be clustered together. If a form is being used to rate some behavior occurring in real time—for example, the performance by a technician of a lab procedure—it is particularly important that the form be arrayed as logically as possible so respondents do not have to search for the items they wish to complete.

The Ratings Paradox

There are profound trade-offs involved in making the items on a rating form more specific. A major part of the art of measurement using ratings is to identify the right level of specificity or granularity. The greater the specificity of the items, the less judgment the raters exercise when offering their opinions, and this will usually generate higher reliability of measurement. However, rating forms that are highly specific in the interest of generating interrater consistency can become almost mechanical. In the extreme, raters are merely observing the occurrence of atomic events ("The end user entered a search term that was spelled correctly"), and their expertise is judges are not being involved at all.

As attributes rated by individual items become less specific and more global, agreement among raters is more difficult to achieve; as they become more atomic, the process becomes mechanical and possibly trivial. This can also be viewed as a trade-off between reliability and validity. The more global the ratings, the more valid they are likely to be, in the sense that the world believes that the attributes being rated are important and indicative of what should be measured in a subsequent demonstration study. This may, however, come at a price of low (possibly unacceptably low) interrater agreement and thus low reliability.

Self-Test 6.6

Using the guidelines offered in the previous section, find and fix the problems with each of the following items.

Item 1

Accuracy of system's advice

☐ Excellent   ☐ Good   ☐ Fair   ☐ Poor

Item 2

Indicate on a 1–10 scale your satisfaction with this system.

Item 3

The new system is easier to use than the one it replaced.

☐ Strongly agree   ☐ Agree   ☐ Neither agree nor disagree
☐ Disagree   ☐ Strongly disagree

Item 4

How frequently have you used the new laboratory system?

☐ Most of the time   ☐ Some of the time   ☐ Never

Other Measurement Designs

We introduce briefly here two more complex measurement approaches that have appeared in the informatics literature. With one of these approaches, the blinded mutual audit, the perceptions by the judges remain independent so an error rate for the measurement can be computed. The other, the Delphi approach, uses consensus building, whereby the responses of judges are deliberately shared, discussed, and then revised. Although this approach is appealing because it leads to an apparently settled consensus, from a methodological viewpoint it suffers by allowing no rigorous estimate of the error inherent in the result.

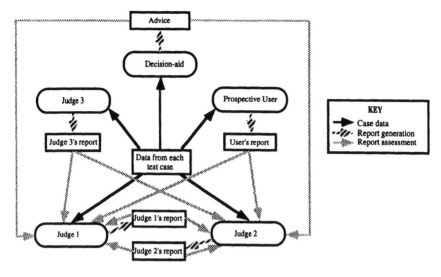

FIGURE 6.8. Possible design for blinded mutual audit.

Mutual Audit

With the blinded mutual audit design, each judge reviews data from some fraction of the objects (usually test cases), giving his or her response. Data from each object are reviewed by at least two judges. Each opinion then is graded for correctness either by the same group of judges[28] or by a second group,[29] without knowing who originally provided it. This technique allows evaluators to calculate the inter- and intrajudge agreement (and thus error) rates and to ensure efficient use of the judges' time. Although we used a simplified version of it in the exercise in Chapter 5, the study of Hypercritic employed a variant of the mutual audit technique.

The mutual audit can be used in a pure measurement study, or, as shown in Figure 6.8, it can be employed in a hybrid measurement/demonstration study where a set of test cases is reviewed by a set of expert judges, an information resource, and the persons who provided the actual care on these cases.

Delphi Technique

The Delphi technique, as it applies to developing a consensus judgment of some attribute of a clinical case, is illustrated in Figure 6.9. Each judge reviews the data from all cases independently and records his or her opinion on a report form. The forms are passed to a moderator, who extracts the consensus opinion for each case and returns them and the case data to the judges for a second opinion, usually without informing them of their

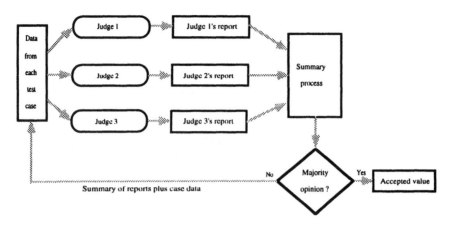

FIGURE 6.9. Delphi technique.

previous opinion. Judges continue to be asked for their opinions on each case until a convergence criterion is met. This technique is well established in a variety of fields[30] and is now being applied successfully in biomedicine.[31]

Conclusion

This completes our excursion into the world of objectivist measurement. In this chapter and its two predecessors we have demonstrated the importance of measurement to sound objectivist study. The attention in the previous chapter to measurement theory, and in this chapter to technique, was motivated by the chronic paucity of measurement instruments in biomedical informatics, resulting in the need for investigators to develop and validate their own measurement approaches. We close almost where we began, by encouraging investigators who develop measurement methods to publish their measurement studies, so other investigators may benefit from their labors. We move in the following chapters to exploration of objectivist demonstration studies. Everything that follows in Chapters 7 and 8 assumes that measurement issues have been resolved, in the sense that the reliability and validity of all measurement instruments employed in demonstration studies are known.

Answers to Self-Tests

Self-Test 6.1

1. Predicted reliability is 0.432, which is not usually acceptable.
2. The standard error of measurement is 0.34.

3. Content validity is somewhat built into the study through the choice of expert raters. It could be further ensured by asking the judges to write the rationale for their ratings for a subset of the patients and checking these rationales against published standards of care where possible. Criterion-related validity could be explored by selecting a subset of patients for whom the system's advice had been followed and comparing clinical outcomes seen in patients for whom the advice had been highly rated in comparison with those patients for whom the advice was poorly rated. Construct validity might be assessed by examining some case properties with which the system's correctness might be hypothesized to be correlated. For example, cases that are more complex, as measured by the number of clinical variables they include, might be hypothesized to be truly more difficult and thus expected to generate lower scores from the raters. Cases with diagnoses that are more prevalent might be hypothesized to be less difficult and expected to generate higher scores.

Self-Test 6.2

1. More observations are needed to increase the reliability. The observations in the set are generally well behaved.

2. It appears that two attributes are being measured. Items 1 to 3 are measuring one attribute, and items 4 to 6 are measuring the other.

3. Judge H displays the highest corrected part–whole correlation (0.55) and thus can be considered the "best" judge. Judge E is a close second with a part–whole correlation of 0.50. Judge C may be considered the worst judge, with a part–whole correlation of –0.27. Removing judge C raises the reliability from 0.29 to 0.54 in this example. Such a large change in reliability is seen in part because the number of objects in this example is small. Judges B and D can in some sense be considered the worst, as they rendered the same result for every object and their part–whole correlations cannot be calculated.

Self-Test 6.3

The object class comprises patients who are to be admitted. In this case, "observers" (five levels), "times of day" (three levels), and "hospitals" (four levels) are facets of the measurement study.

Self-Test 6.4

The "observer" facet belongs to the "judges" category. The "times of day" and "hospitals" facets belong to the "logistical factors" category.

Self-Test 6.5

1. Each (of two) objects-by-observations matrixes would have 111 rows (for cases as objects) and three columns (for judges as observations). One matrix would be generated for actual care cases and the other for TraumAID's recommendations.
2. There is no compelling evidence for rater tendency errors. The mean ratings of the judges are roughly equal and near the middle of the scale. Central tendency effects can be ruled out because the standard deviations of the ratings are substantial.
3. From a reliability standpoint, the ratings are more than adequate. However, the validity of the ratings must be questioned because the judges are from the institution where TraumAID was developed.
4. The data seem to suggest that TraumAID's advice is accurate, as the judges preferred how TraumAID would have treated the patients over how the patients were actually treated. However, the concern about validity of the ratings would cast some doubt on this conclusion.

Self-Test 6.6

Item 1: Accuracy should be defined. The response categories should be replaced by alternatives that are more behavioral or observable.

Item 2: Ten response options are too many. The respondent needs to know whether 1 or 10 corresponds to a high level of satisfaction. The numerical response options have no verbal descriptors.

Item 3: "No opinion" does not belong on the response continuum. Having no opinion is different from having an opinion that happens to be midway between "strongly agree" and "strongly disagree."

Item 4: The logic of the response options does not match the stem. There are not enough response options, and they are not well spaced semantically.

References

1. Isaac S, Michael WB. Handbook in Research and Evaluation. San Diego: EdITS, 1995.
2. Cureton EE, D'Agostino RB. Factor Analysis, an Applied Approach. Hillsdale, NJ: Lawrence Erlbaum, 1983.
3. Kim J, Mueller CW. Factor Analysis: What It Is and How to Do It. Newbury Park, CA: Sage, 1978.
4. Brennan RL, Fienberg S, Liveseley D, Rolph J. Generalizability Theory. Newbury Park, CA: Sage, 2001.
5. Shavelson RJ, Webb NM. Generalizability Theory: A Primer. Newbury Park, CA: Sage, 1991.
6. Anderson JG, Jay SJ, Schweer HM, et al. Why doctors don't use computers: some empirical findings. J R Soc Med 1986;79:142–144.

7. Brown SH, Coney RD. Changes in computer anxiety and attitudes related to clinical information system use. J Am Med Inf Assoc 1994;1:381–394.

8. Hripcsak G, Kuperman GJ, Friedman C, et al. A reliability study for evaluating information extraction from radiology reports. J Am Med Inf Assoc 1999;6: 143–150.

9. Elstein AS, Shulman LS, Sprafka SA. Medical Problem Solving. Cambridge, MA: Harvard University Press, 1978.

10. Schmidt HG, Norman GR, Boshuizen HPA. A cognitive perspective on medical expertise: theory and implications. Acad Med 1990;65:611–621.

11. Stillman P, Swanson D, Regan MB, et al. Assessment of clinical skills of residents using standardized patients. Ann Intern Med 1991;114:393–401.

12. Swets JA. Measuring the accuracy of diagnostic systems. Science 1998;240: 1285–1293.

13. Jain R. The Art of Computer Systems Performance Analysis. New York: Wiley, 1991.

14. Friedman CP, Elstein AS, Wolf FM, et al. Enhancement of clinicians' diagnostic reasoning by computer-based consultation: a multisite study of 2 systems. JAMA 1999;282:1851–1856.

15. Carey TS, Garrett J. North Carolina Back Pain Project. Patterns of ordering diagnostic tests for patients with low back pain. Ann Intern Med 1996;125: 807–814.

16. Friedman CP. Anatomy of the clinical simulation. Acad Med 1995;70: 205–208.

17. Friedman CP, Elstein AS, Wolf F, Murphy G, et al. Measuring the quality of diagnostic hypothesis sets for studies of decision support. Ninth World Congress on Medical Informatics, 1998:864–868.

18. Berk RA, ed. Performance Assessment: Methods and Applications. Baltimore: Johns Hopkins Press, 1986.

19. Murphy KR, Cleveland JN. Understanding Performance Appraisal: Social, Organizational, and Goal-Based Perspectives. Thousand Oaks, CA: Sage, 1995.

20. Hripcsak G, Wilcox A. Reference standards, judges, and comparison subjects: roles for experts in evaluating system performance. J Am Med Inf Assoc 2002;9:1–15.

21. Guilford JP: Psychometric Methods. New York: McGraw-Hill, 1954.

22. Thorndike RL, Hagen E. Measurement and Evaluation in Psychology and Education. New York: Wiley, 1977.

23. Wyatt J. A method for developing medical decision-aids applied to ACORN, a chest pain advisor. DM thesis, Oxford University, 1991.

24. Clarke JR, Webber BL, Gertner A, Rymon KJ. On-line decision support for emergency trauma management. Proc Symp Comput Applications Med Care 1994;18:1028.

25. Landy FJ, Farr JL: Performance rating. Psychol Bull 1980;87:72–107.

26. Detmer WM, Friedman CP. Academic physicians' assessment of the effects of computers on health care. Proc Symp Comput Applications Med Care 1994; 18:558–562.

27. Miller GA. The magical number seven, plus or minus two: some limits on our capacity for processing information. Psychol Rev 1956;63:46–49.

28. Quaglini S, Stefanelli M, Barosi G, Berzuini A. A performance evaluation of the expert system ANAEMIA. Comp Biomed Res 1987;21:307–323.

29. Yu VL, Fagan LM, Wraith SM, et al. Antimicrobial selection by computer: a blinded evaluation by infectious disease experts. JAMA 1979;242:1279–1282.
30. Delbecq AE. Group Techniques for Program Planning: A Guide to Nominal Group and Delphi Processes. New York: Scott, Foresman, 1975.
31. Kors JA, Sittig A, van Bemmel JH. The Delphi method used to validate diagnostic knowledge in a computerised ECG interpreter. Methods Inf Med 1990;29:44–50.

Appendix A: Generalizability Theory

Using an approach known as generalizability theory,[4,5] investigators can address multifacet measurement studies. They can analyze multiple potential sources of error and model the relations among them. This additional power is of potential importance in biomedical informatics because it can mirror the complexity of almost all measurement problems addressed in the field. Generalizability theory (G-theory) allows computation of a generalizability coefficient, which is analogous to a reliability coefficient in classical theory.

Although the specific computational aspects of G-theory are beyond the scope of this discussion, the theory has great value as a heuristic for measurement study design. If an informatics researcher can conceptualize and formulate a measurement problem in terms appropriate to study via G-theory, a psychometrician or statistician can handle the details. The basic idea is the same as in classical theory but with extension to multiple facets, whereas classical theory is limited to one facet. The basic strategy employed is portrayed in Figure 6.2. Analytical methods derived from the analysis of variance (ANOVA) are used to decompose the total variability of the measurements made on the objects included in the study. The basics of ANOVA are discussed in Chapter 8 of this volume. The total variability is decomposed into variability due to objects, variability due to the multiple facets and their statistical interactions, and variance due to other sources not explicitly modeled by the facets included by the investigator in the measurement study.

The generalizability coefficient is represented by:

$$\rho = \frac{V_{\text{objects}}}{V_{\text{total}}} = \frac{V_{\text{objects}}}{V_{\text{objects}} + V_{\text{facets}} + V_{\text{other}}}$$

Formally, the subscripted V's in the above formula are variance components, which can be computed using methods derivative from ANOVA. V_{facets} and V_{other} are taken to represent sources of measurement error. Expressions for V_{facets} explicitly involve the number of levels of each facet, which makes it possible to use G-theory to model the effects on reliability of changing the number of levels of any of the facets that are part of the measurement process. For example, for the basic one-facet models that have been developed throughout this chapter, the formula for the generalizability coefficient is:

$$\rho = \frac{V_{\text{objects}}}{V_{\text{objects}} + (V_{\text{objects} \times \text{observations}} / N_{\text{observations}})}$$

This equation is exactly equivalent to the Spearman-Brown prophecy formula.

A major value of G-theory derives from its applicability to more complex measurement problems than classical theory allows. In addition to measurement studies with multiple facets, more complex designs can be considered, including nested designs of the type portrayed in Figure 6.5. By building into V_{facets} an error component related to the absolute agreement among individual observations in addition to error related to the degree of correlation among them, errors related to disagreement can figure into the estimate of generalizability. In general, the more errors considered in a G-theory measurement model, the lower the generalizability coefficient, because these errors appear in the denominator of the calculation of this coefficient.

7
The Design of
Demonstration Studies

Demonstration studies answer questions about an information resource, exploring such issues as the resource's value to a certain professional group or its impact on the processes and outcomes of health care, research, and education.[1] Recall from Chapter 4 that measurement studies are required to test, refine, and validate measurement processes before they can be used to answer questions about a resource or its impact. Chapters 5 and 6 explained these ideas and how to conduct measurement studies in more detail. In this chapter we assume that measurement methods are available and have been verified as reliable and valid (in the measurement sense) by appropriate measurement studies.* To answer questions via a demonstration study, appropriate evaluation strategies and study designs must be formulated, the sample of participants and tasks defined, any threats to validity (in the demonstration sense) identified and either eliminated or controlled for, and the results analyzed.[2,3] These issues are discussed in this chapter.

In Chapter 3, we discussed the attributes of information resources and their users that can be important to study. We also introduced nine kinds of studies that can be used to verify the need for the resource; validate its design and structure, test its function in laboratory and field settings, study its effects on users' behavior, and examine its impact on the original problem through relevant outcomes in field settings. These various studies may invoke different generic approaches to evaluation, as described in Chapter 2, and may entail different formal demonstration study designs, as described in Chapter 4. For example, validation of resource design and structure requires inspection of design documentation and the resource components by a panel of judges. It invokes a subjectivist "professional review" approach to evaluation and has no formal objectivist demonstration study design. By contrast, studying the impact of the resource on care providers or patient care invokes a comparison-based approach using

---

* As we will see later in this chapter, "validity" takes on very different meanings when discussed in the contexts of measurement and demonstration. All we can do is apologize for this confusion. We did not invent this terminology.

controlled, "experimental" demonstration studies. This chapter primarily addresses the more complex, controlled studies concerned with resource function and impact.

We discussed in Chapter 2 how different stakeholders in the evaluation process often have different questions they wish to answer and in Chapter 3 how the questions of interest tend to hinge on the resource's current stage in the developmental life cycle. In Chapter 4 we saw that demonstration study questions may be classed broadly as pragmatic (What is the impact of the information resource on working practices?) or explanatory (Why does the information resource change working practices?).[4] Studies of an information resource at any early stage of development are usually designed to answer pragmatic questions. The needs of a pragmatic question may be well served by a relatively simple study design. To answer an explanatory question about why a mature information resource changes working practices—with possible impact on health care, research, and education—usually requires study designs that are more ornate.

Study Designs

In the following sections we start with a method for classifying demonstration study designs and describing their components before illustrating the kinds of studies that are possible. We use the running example of a clinical antibiotic reminder system, of the kind commonly integrated into computer-based prescribing or order communication systems. A brief paragraph at the end of each study design section illustrates how the particular design can be described using the language developed in this first section. Expressing a study design using appropriate language can be useful when communicating with statisticians and other experimental scientists or methodologists; it also helps the investigator to step back from the details of the study to see what is being planned.

Descriptive, Correlational, and Comparative Studies Revisited

Recall from Chapter 4 that objectivist demonstration studies can be divided into three kinds: descriptive, correlational, and comparative.

A *descriptive* design seeks only to estimate the value of a variable or set of variables in a selected sample of participants. For example, to ascertain the ease of use of a nursing information resource, a group of nurses could be given a rating form previously validated through a measurement study. The mean value of the "ease of use" variable would be the main result of this demonstration study. Descriptive studies can be tied to the objectives-based approach to evaluation described in Chapter 2. When an investigator seeks to determine if a resource has met a predetermined set of performance objectives, the logic and design of the resulting study are often descriptive.

Correlational studies explore the relationships or association between a set of variables the investigator measures but does not manipulate in any way. Correlational studies can be seen as primarily linked to the decision facilitation approach to evaluation discussed in Chapter 2, as they are linked to pragmatic questions and cannot typically settle issues of cause and effect. For example, a correlational study may reveal a statistical relationship between users' clinical performance at some task and the extent they use an information resource to accomplish those tasks, but it cannot tell us which is the direction of causation, or whether the association is due to a third, unidentified and thus unmeasured, factor.*

In a *comparative* study, the investigator typically creates or exploits a pre-existing contrasting set of conditions to compare the effects of one with another. Usually the motive is to correctly attribute cause and effect or to further explore questions raised by earlier studies. Extending the example from the previous paragraph, a comparative study can address whether use of the information resource *causes* improved performance. After identifying a sample of participants for the study, the investigator assigns each participant, often randomly, to one or more sets of conditions. Here, the conditions would perhaps be "no use of information resource" and "use of information resource." Some variable of interest is then measured for each participant. The aggregated values of this variable are then compared across the conditions. Comparative studies are aligned with the comparison-based approach to evaluation introduced in Chapter 2.

Terminology for Demonstration Studies

In this section we develop a terminology and several ideas necessary to design studies of information resources. At this point, the reader may wish to refer to Chapter 4, where terminology for measurement and demonstration studies was first introduced. For the purposes of the immediate discussion, the terms of most importance are as follows:

Participants: Participants in a study are the entities about whom data are collected. A specific study employs one sample of participants, although this sample might be subdivided if, for example, participants are assigned to conditions in a comparative design. It is key to emphasize that although participants are often people—care providers or care recipients—they also may be information resources, groups of people, or even organizations. Confusingly, participants in a demonstration study are sometimes called subjects, and can be the equivalent of objects in a measurement study!

---

* "Data mining" of previously collected data are also a form of correlational study.

Variables: Variables are specific characteristics of participants that are purposefully measured by the investigator, or are self-evident properties of the participants that do not require measurement. Each variable in a study is associated with a level of measurement, as described in Chapter 4. In the simplest descriptive study, there may be only one variable. In comparative and correlational studies, there must be at least two variables, and there may be many more.

Levels of variables: A categorical (nominal or ordinal) variable can be said to have a discrete set of levels corresponding to each of the measured values the variable can have. For example, in a hospital setting, physician-members of a ward team can be classified as residents, fellows, or attending physicians. In this case, the variable "physician's level of qualification" is said to have three levels.

Dependent variables: The dependent variables are a subset of the variables in the study that capture the outcomes of interest to the investigator. For this reason, dependent variables are also called "outcome variables" or just "outcomes." A study may have one or more dependent variables. Studies with one dependent variable are referred to as univariate, and studies with multiple dependent variables are referred to as multivariate. In an informatics study, the measured value of the dependent variable is often computed for each participant as an average over a number of tasks.

By definition, the participants in a study are the entities on which the dependent variables are measured. This point is important in informatics because almost all professional practice—including health care, research, and education—is conducted in hierarchical settings with naturally occurring groups (a doctor's patients, care providers in a ward team, students in a class). This raises challenging questions about the level of aggregation at which to measure the dependent variables for a demonstration study.

Independent variables: The independent variables are those included in a study to explain the measured values of the dependent variables. Note that a descriptive study has no independent variables, whereas comparative and correlational studies can have one or many independent variables.

Measurement challenges of the types discussed in Chapters 5 and 6 almost always arise during assessment of the outcome or dependent variable for a study. Often, for example, the dependent variable is some type of performance measure such as "the quality of a medication plan" or the "precision of information retrieval" that invokes all of the concerns about reliability and validity of measurement. Depending on the study, the independent variables may also raise measurement challenges. When the independent variable is gender, for example, the measurement process is relatively straightforward. However, if the independent variable is an attitude, level of experience, or extent of resource use, significant measurement challenges can arise.

Study Types Further Distinguished

Using our terminology, we can now sharpen the differences among descriptive, correlational, and comparative studies. Studies of all three types are, in a profound sense, designed by the investigator. In all three, the investigator chooses the participants, the variables, the measurement methods and the logistics used to assign a value of each variable to each participant. In a descriptive study, however, there are no further decisions to be made. The defining characteristic of a descriptive study is the absence of independent variables. The state of a set of participants is described by measuring one or more dependent variables. Although a descriptive study may report the relations among the dependent variables, there is no attempt to attribute variation in these variables to some cause.

In correlational studies, the investigator hypothesizes a set of relations among variables that are measured for a group of participants in the study but are not manipulated. The variability in these measures is that which occurs naturally in the sample of participants included in the study. Correlational studies can be retrospective, involving analyses of archival data, or prospective, involving data collected according to a plan generated in advance of the study. Some investigators believe that assertions of cause and effect can occasionally be derived from the pattern of statistical relations observed in correlational studies, although this topic remains controversial.[5,6] Note that measurement studies that explore the construct validity of a new measure, as discussed in Chapter 5, also employ the logic of correlational studies.

The defining characteristic of a comparative study is the purposeful manipulation of independent variables to enable sound inference of cause and effect from the data collected. To this end, the investigator creates at least one new independent variable that defines the study groups. The value of this variable, for each participant, describes that participant's group membership, with values such as "intervention," "control," or "placebo." The investigator usually assigns participants randomly to different levels of this independent variable. If all sources of variation in the dependent variables are controlled, either by random allocation or specific assignment to groups, cause-and-effect relations among the independent and dependent variables can be rigorously attributed. When the dependent variable is continuous (with interval or ratio properties), this can be achieved by employing methods such as analysis of variance (ANOVA) to demonstrate differences among the levels of the independent variables that are explicitly part of the design. When the dependent variable is discrete (binary or categorical), contingency table analysis and receiver operating characteristics (ROC) curves are customarily used. There is an extensive literature on the design of comparative studies,[7–9] and this chapter contains an exploration of some of the most important study designs. Note that random allocation of participants to different levels of the independent variable is

TABLE 7.1. Summary of descriptive, correlational, and comparative studies.

Parameter	Descriptive study	Correlational study	Comparative study
Goal of study	To describe a resource in terms of variables	To explore the relations between variables	To assign causality to the relation between variables
Independent variables	None	One or more as selected by investigator	One or more, with at least one created by the investigator
Dependent variables	One or more	One or more as selected by the investigator	One or more as selected by the investigator
Logic of data analysis	Descriptive statistics about dependent variables	Analysis of patterns of relationships among variables	Continuous variables: ANOVA Discrete variables: contingency table, ROC analyses

ANOVA, analysis of variance; ROC, receiver operating characteristics.

completely different from selecting a random sample of participants for a survey, for example. These concepts are often confused.

The contrasts between descriptive, correlational, and comparative studies are summarized in Table 7.1. Readers are also referred to Figure 4.3 in Chapter 4.

Generic Issues in Demonstration Study Design

As we move into a more technical discussion of study design, we introduce three key issues that always arise: defining the intervention, choosing the participants, and selecting the tasks for the participants to undertake. When evaluating therapeutic technologies such as drugs, the participants are usually patients. For evaluating interventions such as health education, practice guidelines, or information resources, the participants can be care providers, departments, or even hospitals.[10,11] In studies where the care providers are participants, we usually consider the patients these care providers treat to be tasks and average the performance of each care provider over a set of tasks.

When studying an information resource, evaluators should be aware that its performance or impact may vary greatly among participants (e.g., clinicians may vary greatly in the information they obtain from the clinical laboratory system, perhaps because of differing prior experience) or between different kinds of tasks (e.g., the resource may only improve the management of certain groups of patients, such as those in intensive care, irrespective of which clinician is looking after them). This means that evaluators should be aware of both the range of participants and the range of tasks to be included in their study. In laboratory studies the investigator often can directly control both the participants included in the study and the tasks with which they are challenged. In field studies, this level of control may not be possible or desirable, as the identity of care providers who work in clinical units and the patients who receive care in these units cannot often be manipulated. Even when the participants and tasks are out of the investigator's direct control, she should carefully document the samples that were involved in the study, so others know how far the results can be generalized.

Defining the Intervention

Recall that an explanatory question is one that seeks to understand why, rather than simply ask if something happens or not. One way to answer an explanatory question is to split the information resource up into its components and evaluate them separately. When we use the phrase *information resource*, we have deliberately not defined precisely what the resource or system includes. However, particularly when trying to answer questions such as "How much difference is the resource likely to make in a new setting?" it is important to isolate the effects due to the information resource itself from effects due to other activities surrounding its development and implementation. For example, if a department were to implement a set of computer-based practice guidelines, a considerable amount of time might be spent on developing the guidelines before any implementation took place. Changes in clinical practice following the implementation of the information resource might be largely due to this guideline development process, not to the computer technology itself.[12] Transplanting the computer-based guidelines to a new hospital without repeating the guideline development process at the new site might yield inferior results to those seen at the development site. When implementing new information resources it is usually necessary to offer training, feedback, and other support to resource users; these could also be considered part of the intervention.

An example from the literature is the Leeds Abdominal Pain Decision Support System. Various components of this resource were tested for their effects on the diagnostic accuracy of 126 junior doctors in a multicenter trial in 12 hospitals.[13] Table 7.2 shows the average percentage improvement due to each component of the system. The data are extracted from a 2-year

TABLE 7.2. Effects due to components of an information resource.

Intervention	Change in diagnostic accuracy from baseline (%)	
	End of month 1	End of month 6
None	0	+1
Data collection forms	+11	+14
Monthly feedback and data collection forms	+13	+27
Computer advice, feedback, and forms	+20	+28

Source: Data calculated from Adams et al.[13]

study of four groups of junior doctors working for 6 months in 12 emergency rooms, each group being exposed to a different level of implementation of decision support. The investigators measured diagnostic accuracy after the doctors had been in place for 1 and 6 months. The first row shows that there was minimal improvement over the 6-month period when no information resource was in place. The second row shows the sustained improvement in diagnoses due to what may be called a checklist effect, described in more detail later in the chapter. Decision making improved when structured forms were used to assist clinical data collection. In the third group the doctors were given monthly feedback about their diagnostic performance as well as using the forms, and marked learning is seen. The fourth group received diagnostic probabilities calculated by a computer-based advisory system at the time of decision making as well as monthly feedback and using data collection forms.

The advice apparently aided diagnoses during the early months only, because in later months diagnostic accuracy in the third and fourth groups was similar. Also, the computer advice is contributing less to improving diagnostic accuracy than either the data collection forms or the individual feedback. If the information resource is defined as the computer advice alone, it is contributing only one third of the 20% improvement in diagnostic accuracy seen at month 1, and 1/30th of the 28% improvement at month 6. (Of the 20% improvement seen at month 1, only the difference between row 3 and row 4, which is 7%, is attributable to the computer advice. Of the 28% improvement seen at month 6, only 1% appears due to the computer advice.)

Thus, careful definition of the information resource and its components is necessary in demonstration studies to allow the evaluator to answer the explanatory question: "Which component of the information resource is responsible for the observed effects?" It is critical that the investigator define the resource before the study begins and use that definition consistently through the entire effort.

Selection of Participants

The participants or resource users selected for demonstration studies must resemble those to whom the evaluator and others responsible for the study wish to apply the results. For example, when attempting to quantify the likely impact of an information resource on clinicians at large, there is no point in studying its effects on the clinicians who helped develop it, or even built it, as they are likely to be technology enthusiasts and more familiar with the resource than average practitioners. Characteristics of participants that typically need to be taken into account include age, experience, clinical role, attitude toward computerized information resources, and extent of their involvement in the development of the resource. These factors can be formalized as a set of selection criteria that include only a certain class of participants in the study, or they can be made into explicit independent study variables if their effects are to be explored.

Volunteer Effect

A common bias in the selection of participants is the use of volunteers. It has been established in many areas that people who volunteer as participants, whether to complete questionnaires,[14] participate in psychology experiments, or test-drive new cars or other technologies, are atypical of the population at large, being more intelligent, open to innovation, and extroverted. Although volunteers make willing participants for measurement studies or pilot demonstration studies, they should be avoided in definitive demonstration studies, as they considerably reduce the generality of findings. One strategy is to include all participants meeting the selection criteria in the study. However, if this would result in too many participants, rather than asking for volunteers, it is better to randomly select a sample of all eligible clinicians, following up invitation letters with telephone calls to achieve as near 100% recruitment of the selected sample as possible. Note again that this random selection is not the same as random allocation of participants to groups, as discussed later in this chapter.

Number of Participants Needed

The financial resources required for an evaluation study depend critically on the number of participants needed. The required number in turn depends on the precision of the answer required from the study and the risk investigators are willing to take of failing to detect a significant effect (discussed later). Statisticians can advise on this point and carry out sample size calculations to estimate the number of participants required. Sometimes, in order to recruit the required number of participants, some volunteer effect must be tolerated; often there is a trade-off between obtaining a sufficiently large sample and ensuring that the sample is representative.

Selection of Tasks

In the same way that participants must be carefully selected to resemble the people likely to use the information resource, any tasks or test cases the participants complete must also resemble those that will generally be encountered. Thus when evaluating a clinical order entry system intended for general use, it would be unwise to use only complex patient cases from, for example, a pediatric endocrinology practice. Although the order entry system might well be of considerable benefit in endocrine cases, it is inappropriate to generalize results from such a limited sample to the full range of cases seen in ambulatory care. An instructive example is provided by the study of Van Way et al.,[15] who developed a scoring system for diagnosing appendicitis and studied the resource's accuracy using, exclusively, patients who had undergone surgery for suspected appendicitis. Studying this group

TABLE 7.3. Guidelines for selection of tasks or test cases.

- Cases should be representative of those in which the information resource will be used; consecutive cases or a random sample are superior to volunteers or a hand-picked subset
- There should be a sufficient number and variety of cases to test most functions and pathways in the resource
- Case data should be recent and preferably from more than one, geographically distinct site
- Include cases abstracted by a variety of potential resource users
- Include a percentage of cases with incomplete, contradictory, or erroneous data
- Include a percentage of normal cases
- Include a percentage of difficult cases and some that are clearly outside the scope of the information resource
- Include some cases with minimal data and some with comprehensive data

of patients had the benefit of allowing the true cause of the abdominal pain to be obtained with near certainty as a by-product of the surgery itself. However, in these patients who had all undergone surgery for suspected appendicitis the symptoms were more severe and the incidence of appendicitis was five to 10 times higher than for the typical patient for whom such a scoring system would be used. Thus the accuracy obtained with postsurgical patients would be a poor estimate of the system's accuracy in routine clinical use.

If the performance of an information resource is measured on a small number of hand-picked cases, the functions may appear spuriously complete. This is especially likely if these cases are similar to, or even identical with, the training set of cases used to develop or tune the information resource before the evaluation is carried out. When a statistical model that powers an information resource is carefully adjusted to achieve maximal performance on training data, this adjustment may worsen its accuracy on a fresh set of data due to a phenomenon called overfitting.[16] Thus it is important to obtain a new set of cases and evaluate performance on this test set.

Sometimes developers omit cases from a sample if they do not fall within the scope of the information resource, for example, if the final diagnosis for a case is not represented in a diagnostic system's knowledge base. This practice violates the principle that a test set should be representative of all cases in which the information resource will be used, and will overestimate its effectiveness with unseen data. Some guidelines for the selection of test cases are given in Table 7.3.

Control Strategies for Comparative Studies

One of the most challenging aspects of comparative study design is how to monitor all the other changes taking place that are not attributable to the information resource, or, in technical language, to obtain control. In clinical medicine it is sometimes possible to predict patient outcome with good accuracy from a handful of initial clinical findings, for example the survival of patients in intensive care.[17] In these unusual circumstances where we have a close approximation to an "evaluation machine" (see Chapter 2) that can tell us what would have happened to patients if we had not intervened, we can compare what actually happens with what was predicted to draw tentative conclusions about the impact of the information resource. Such accurate predictive models, however, are unusual across all of biomedicine,[16] so it is generally impossible to determine what students, health workers or investigators would have done, or what the outcome of their work would have been, had no information resource been available. Instead, we must use various types of controls. A control, most generally, is a group of observations (such as a distinct group of participants, tasks or measures on those tasks) that are unlikely to be influenced by the intervention of interest or that are influenced by a different intervention.

In the following sections we review a series of specific control strategies, using as an anchor point the least controlled approach, a purely descriptive study, and moving to increasingly more sophisticated approaches. We employ, as a running example, an information resource that prompts doctors to order prophylactic antibiotics for orthopedic patients to prevent postoperative infections. In this example, the intervention is the installation and commissioning of the reminder system, the participants are the physicians, and the tasks are the patients cared for by the physicians. The dependent variables include physicians' rate of ordering antibiotics (an effect measure, in the parlance of Chapter 3) and the rate of postoperative infection averaged across the patients cared for by each physician (an outcome measure). The independent variables in each example below are an inherent feature of the study design and derive from the specific control strategies employed. Although they are not explicitly discussed in what follows to keep the presentation as focused as possible, measurement issues of the types addressed in Chapters 5 and 6 (e.g., determining whether each patient's infection can be accurately judged a postoperative infection) abound in this situation.

Descriptive (Uncontrolled) Studies

In the simplest possible design, a descriptive or uncontrolled study, we install the reminder system, allow a suitable period for training, then make our measurements. There is no independent variable. Suppose we discover that the overall postoperative infection rate is 5% and that physicians order prophylactic antibiotics in 60% of orthopedic cases. Although we have two measured dependent variables, it is difficult to interpret these figures without any comparison; it is possible that there has been no change attributable to the resource. This point is of course the weakness of the descriptive study.

One way to understand the significance of these figures is to compare them with the same measurements made using the same methods in a comparison group, which transforms the study from a descriptive to a comparative one. Two types of comparison groups are possible: (1) historical controls, comprising the same patient care environment (doctors and their patients) before the system was installed; or (2) simultaneous controls, comprising a similar patient care environment not provided with the reminder system.

Historically Controlled Studies

As a first improvement to the uncontrolled or descriptive study, let us consider a historically controlled experiment, sometimes called a before–after study. The investigator makes baseline measurements of antibiotic ordering and postoperative infection rates before the information resource is installed and then makes the same measurements some time after the information resource is in routine use. The independent variable is "time" and has two levels: before and after resource installation. Let us say that at baseline the postoperative infection rate was 10% and doctors ordered prophylactic antibiotics in only 40% of cases; the postintervention figures are the same as before (Table 7.4).

After reviewing these data, the evaluators may claim that the information resource is responsible for halving the infection rate, especially because this was accompanied by a 20% increase in doctors' prophylactic antibiotic prescribing. However, many other factors might have changed in the interim to cause these results, especially if there was a long interval between the baseline and postintervention measurements. New staff could have taken over the care of the patients, the case mix of patients on the ward could have altered, new prophylactic antibiotics might have been introduced, or clinical audit meetings might have highlighted the infection problem causing greater medical awareness of it. Simply assuming that the reminder system alone caused the reduction in infection rates is naive. Other factors, known or unknown, could have changed meanwhile, making untenable the assumption that the intervention is responsible for all of the observed effects.

The weakness of crediting all benefit to the information resource in a historically controlled study is highlighted by considering the likely response of the resource developers to a situation where performance of clinicians *worsens* after installing the information resource. Most developers, partic-

TABLE 7.4. Hypothetical results of a historically controlled study of an antibiotic reminder system.

Time	Antibiotic prescribing rate (%)	Postoperative infection rate
Baseline (before installation)	40	10
After installation	60	5

ularly those directly involved in the creation of the resource, would search long and hard for other factors to explain the deterioration. However, there would be no such search if performance improved, even though the study design has the same faults.

Evidence for the bias associated with before–after studies comes from a paper that compared the results of many historically controlled studies of antihypertensive drugs with the results of simultaneous randomized controlled trials carried out on the same drugs.[18] About 80% of the historically controlled studies suggested that the new drugs evaluated were more effective, but this figure was confirmed in only 20% of the randomized studies that evaluated the same drugs.

No assignment or manipulation of the participants or their environment is involved with before-and-after studies, other than introduction of the information resource itself. For this reason, some methodologists label these studies correlational, not comparative. Equally, we usually reserve the word *experiment* for studies in which intentional manipulation is done rather than making baseline and follow-up measurements.

Simultaneous Nonrandomized Controls

To address some of the problems with historical controls we might instead use simultaneous controls, making additional outcome measurements in doctors and patients not influenced by the prophylactic antibiotic reminder system but who are still subject to the other changes taking place in the environment. If these measurements are made both before and after intervention, it strengthens the design by providing an estimate of the changes due to the nonspecific factors taking place during the study period.

This study design is a parallel group comparative study with simultaneous external controls. Table 7.5 gives some hypothetical results of such a study, focusing on postoperative infection rate as a single outcome measure or dependent variable. The independent variables are "time," as in the above example, and "group," which has the two levels of intervention and control. There is the same improvement in the group where reminders were available, but no improvement (indeed slight deterioration) where no reminders were available. This design provides suggestive evidence of an improvement that is most likely to be due to the reminder system. This

TABLE 7.5. Hypothetical results of a simultaneous nonrandomized controlled study of an antibiotic reminder systems.

Time	Postoperative infection rate (%)	
	Reminder group	Control group
Baseline	10	10
After intervention	5	11

inference is stronger if the control doctors worked in the same wards during the period the resource was introduced, and if similar kinds of patients, subject to the same nonspecific influences, were being operated on during the whole time period.

Even though the controls in this example are now simultaneous, skeptics may still refute our argument by claiming that there is some systematic unknown difference between the clinicians or patients in the reminder and control groups. For example, if the two groups comprised the patients and clinicians in two adjacent wards, the difference in the infection rates could be attributable to systematic or chance differences between the wards. Perhaps hospital staffing levels improved in some wards but not others, or there was cross-infection by a multiply resistant organism but only among patients in the control ward. To overcome such criticisms, we could expand the study to include all wards in the hospital—or even other hospitals—but this requires many more measurements, which would clearly take considerable resources. Such externally and internally controlled before–after studies are described later. We could try to measure everything that happens to every patient in both wards and build complete psychological profiles of all staff to rule out systematic differences, but we are still vulnerable to the accusation that something we did not measure—did not even know about—explains the difference between the two wards. A better strategy is to ensure that the controls are truly comparable by randomizing them.

Simultaneous Randomized Controls

The crucial problem in the previous example is that, although the controls were simultaneous, there may have been systematic, unmeasured differences between the participants in the control group and the participants receiving the intervention. A simple, effective way to remove systematic differences, whether due to known or unknown factors, is to randomize the assignment of participants to control or intervention groups. Thus we could randomly allocate half of the doctors on both wards to receive the antibiotic reminders, and the remaining doctors could work normally. We would then measure and compare postoperative infection rate in patients managed by doctors in the reminder and control groups. Providing that the doctors never look after one another's patients, any difference that is statistically significant can reliably be attributed to the reminders, as the only way other differences could have emerged is by chance. We discuss the concept of statistical significance in the following chapter.

Table 7.6 shows the hypothesized results of such a study. The baseline infection rates in the patients managed by the two groups of doctors are similar, as would be expected because they were allocated to the groups by chance. There is a greater reduction in infection rate in patients of reminder physicians than those treated by the control physicians. The only systematic

TABLE 7.6. Results of a simultaneous randomized controlled study of an antibiotic reminder system.

Time	Postoperative infection rate (%)	
	Reminder physicians	Control physicians
Baseline	11	10
After intervention	6	8

difference between the two groups of patients is receipt of reminders by their doctors. Provided that the sample size is large enough for these results to be statistically significant, we can conclude with some confidence that giving doctors reminders *caused* the reduction in infection rates. One lingering question is why there was also a small reduction, from baseline to postinstallation, in infection rates in control cases. Four explanations are possible: chance, the checklist effect, the Hawthorne effect, and contamination. These possibilities are discussed in detail in later sections.

When analyzing studies in which doctors or teams are randomized but the measurements are made at the level of patients (randomization by group), data analysis methods must be adjusted accordingly. In general, when randomizing doctors or hospitals, it is a mistake to analyze the results as if patients had been randomized—known as the "unit of analysis error."[11,19] This problem and potential methods for addressing it are discussed in the section on hierarchical or nested designs (later in this chapter).

Externally and Internally Controlled Before–After Studies

An alternative approach to randomized simultaneous controls is to add internal controls to an externally controlled before–after study. Using internal controls, we add to the study some new observations or dependent variables that would not be expected to be affected by the intervention. We already discussed the benefits of external controls—comparing the rates of infection and antibiotic prescribing with those in another ward where the resource has not been implemented. However, the situation is strengthened further by measuring one or more appropriate variables in the same ward to check that nothing else in the clinical environment is changing during the period of a before–after study. As long as this works out, and there are no unexpected changes in the external site, one really can then begin to argue that any change in the measurement of interest must be due to the information resource.[20] However, the risk one takes in this kind of study design is that the results often turn out to be hard or impossible to interpret because of unforeseen changes in the dependent variable in the external or internal controls.

TABLE 7.7. Hypothetical results of an internally controlled before–after study of an antibiotic reminder system.

Time	Antibiotic prescribed (%)		Postoperative infections	Postoperative DVT
	Prophylactic	Chest infections		
Baseline	40	40	10	5
After intervention	60	45	5	6

DVT, deep venous thrombosis.

Pursuing our antibiotic reminder system example, for our internal controls we need to identify actions by the same doctors and outcomes in the same patients that are not affected by the reminders but would be affected by any of the confounding, nonspecific changes that might have occurred in the study ward. An internal clinical action that would reflect general changes in prescribing is the prescribing rate of antibiotics for chest infections, whereas an internal patient outcome that would reflect general postoperative care is the rate of postoperative deep venous thromboses (DVTs).* This is because DVTs in pre- and postoperative patients can usually be prevented by appropriate heparin therapy and other measures. Any general improvements in clinical practice in the study ward should be revealed by changes in these measures. However, providing reminders to doctors about prescribing prophylactic antibiotics to orthopedic patients should not affect either of these new measures, at least not directly. Table 7.7 shows the hypothetical results from such an internally controlled before–after study.

The increase in prescribing for chest infections (5%) is much smaller than the increase for prophylaxis of wound infections (20%), and the postoperative DVT rate increased, if anything. The evidence suggests that antibiotic prescribing in general has not changed much (using prescribing for chest infections as the internal control), and that postoperative care in general (using DVT rate as the internal control) is unchanged. Although less convincing than randomized simultaneous controls, the results rule out major confounding changes in prescribing or postoperative care during the study period, so the observed improvement in the target measure, postoperative infections, can be cautiously attributed to introduction of the reminder system. This argument is strengthened by the 20% increase in prophylactic antibiotic prescribing observed. Unfortunately, interpretation of the results of internally controlled before–after studies that are performed in the real world is often more difficult than in this hypothetical example; adding in an external control as well may help.[20]

---

* DVTs are blood clots in the leg or pelvic veins that cause serious lung problems or even sudden death if they become detached.

TABLE 7.8. Hypothetical results of a randomized crossover study of an antibiotic reminder system.

Period	Postoperative infection rate (%)	
	Group A	Group B
First	5 (reminders)	10 (control)
Second	7 (control)	5 (reminders)

Randomized Crossover Studies

In crossover studies, measurements are made on the same participants with and without access to the information resource. In our example, this would mean dividing up the study period into two equal halves—perhaps each 2 months long. Half of the doctors working on both wards (group A) would then be randomized to use the reminders for the first 2 months only, followed by 2 months without the reminders. The doctors who had no access to the reminders during the first 2-month period (group B) would then get access during the second period (Table 7.8). However, for this crossover design to be valid, evaluators must assume that the participant has not changed except for gaining (or losing) access to the information resource— that there is no carryover. Thus in a crossover study of our antibiotic reminder system, evaluators must assume that the user's performance is not subject to learning, an assumption that usually needs to be tested. In this example, learning from the decision support system is suggested by the lower postoperative infection rates in group A during their control period (which followed use of the reminder system) compared to group B during their control period, which came before their exposure to any reminders.

So long as there is no carryover, the crossover design overcomes the imperfections of historically controlled studies by arranging that there are simultaneous randomized controls during all phases of the experiment. Making each participant act alternately as intervention and control also gives greater statistical power than a simple parallel group study, and avoids the difficulty of matching control and information resource participants or institutions. However, the crossover study can be used only with interventions that achieve a temporary improvement in the attribute being measured, so this approach cannot be employed to evaluate information resources that have significant carryover or educational effects. Proving that the intervention causes no carryover can actually require more participants and tasks than conducting a more convincing randomized parallel group study. Because withdrawing the information resource from participants who have previously had free access to it may antagonize them if they believe it is beneficial, the crossover may have to be synchronized with staff changeover. To be valid, it requires the assumption that the next group of staff closely resembles the previous group. On the other hand, for studies where it may be unacceptable for participants to be denied access to the information resource altogether—as often happens in educational set-tings—the crossover may be the only feasible randomized design, and may overcome refusal to participate because it allows all participants access, albeit for only half of the study period. Note that the statistical analysis needs to take account of the crossover design by using paired tests.

Matched Controls as an Alternative to Randomization, and the Fallacy of Case-Control Studies

The principle of controls is that they should sensitively reflect all the non-specific influences and biases present in the study population, while being isolated in some way from the effects of the information resource. As argued earlier, it is only by random assignment that equivalence of the groups can be achieved. Allocation of participants to control and intervention groups may be done by other methods, such as matching, when randomization is not feasible. When this is done, participants and tasks in the control and intervention groups should be matched on all the features likely to be relevant to the dependent variable. Usually, a pilot correlational study is needed to identify which participant factors are most important. Let us assume that participant age and prior use of information resources turn out to be important predictors of participant use of an information resource. In that case, the participants for a study could be divided up into two groups, taking care that each older person with or without experience in the group who are to be given access to the resource is matched by a similar person in the control group.

However, matching controls prior to allocation in the way just described is definitely not the same as carrying out a case-control study. In a case-control study, investigators try to infer whether a dependent variable is associated with one or more independent variables by analyzing a set of data that has already been collected, so it is a retrospective study design. For example, investigators could measure attitudes to computers in partic-ipants who happened in the past to use the information resource ("cases") and compare them to attitudes of participants who, in the past, did not ("controls"). This is an invalid comparison, as the fact that certain partici-pants chose to use the resource is a clear marker of different levels of skill, attitude, experience, uncertainty, etc., compared to those who ignored it. Thus, any differences in outcome between participants in the two groups are much more likely to follow from fundamental differences between the participants involved than from use of the information resource. As a result, case-control studies suffer from the most serious kinds of confounding and bias, as discussed later in more detail.

One published example is a study that tried to attribute reduced length of stay in hospital inpatients to use by their physician of the medical library.[21] In the study, patient lengths of stay were compared in two groups of patients: those for whose physicians a literature search had been conducted, and a control group consisting of patients with the same disease and severity of illness. The length of stay was lower in those patients for whom an early literature search had been conducted, suggesting that this caused a lower length of stay. However, an alternative explanation is that those doctors who request literature searches may also be more efficient in their use of hospital resources, and so discharge their patients earlier. This would imply that the literature search was a *marker* that the patient was being managed by a good doctor, rather than a *cause* of the patient spending less time in hospital. A cynic might even argue that the study shows that doctors who order literature searches want to spend more time in the library and less time with their patients, and thus tend to discharge the patients earlier! All these explanations are consistent with the data, showing the dangers of such a case-control study.

Summary

To summarize this section on controls and study designs, although investigators may be tempted to use either no controls or historical controls in demonstration studies, we have illustrated, using a running example, why such studies are seldom convincing.[22] If the goal of a demonstration study is to show cause and effect, simultaneous (preferably randomized) controls are required.[20] Using both internal and external controls within a before–after study design may be an alternative, but exposes the evaluators to the risk that their results will be impossible to interpret. The risk of other designs—most clearly the case control design—is that there is no way of quieting those who inevitably, and appropriately, point out that confounding factors, known or unknown, could account for all of the improvements the investigator might wish to attribute to the information resource.

Self-Test 7.1

For each of the scenarios given below, (a) name the independent variables and the number of levels of each, (b) identify the dependent variables and the measurement strategy used to assess them, (c) identify the participants, and (d) indicate the control strategy employed by the study designers.

1. A new admission/discharge/transfer resource is purchased by a major medical center. Evaluators administer a 30-item general attitude survey about information technology to staff members in selected departments 6 months before the resource is installed, 1 week before the resource is installed, and 1 and 6 months after it is installed.

2. A diagnostic decision support system in an early stage of development is employed to offer advice on a set of test cases. A definitive diagnosis for each test case had previously been established. The investigators measure the accuracy of the resource as the proportion of time the computer-generated diagnoses agree with the previously established diagnosis.

3. At each of two metropolitan hospitals, 18 physicians are randomized to receive computer-generated advice on drug therapy. At each hospital, the first group receives advice automatically for all clinic patients, the second receives this advice only when the physicians request it, and the third receives no advice at all. Total charges related to drug therapy are measured by averaging across all relevant patients for each physician during the study period, where relevance is defined as patients whose conditions pertained to the domains covered by the resource's knowledge base.

4. A new reminder system is installed in a hospital that has 12 internal medicine services. During a 1-month period, care providers on six of the services, selected randomly, receive reminders from the system. On the other six services the reminders are generated by the system but not issued to the care providers. An audit of clinical care on all services is conducted to determine the extent to which the actions recommended by the reminders were in fact taken.

5. A new computer-based educational tool is introduced in a medical school course. The tool covers pathophysiology of the cardiovascular (CV) and gastrointestinal (GI) systems. The class is divided randomly into two groups. The first group learns CV pathophysiology using the computer and GI pathophysiology by the usual lecture approach. The second group learns GI pathophysiology by the computer and CV pathophysiology by the lecture approach. Both groups are given a validated knowledge test, covering both body systems, after the course. (Example drawn from Lyon et al.[23])

Validity and Inference

Internal vs. External Validity

We all want our demonstration studies to be valid and therefore credible.* There are two aspects to study validity: internal and external. If a study is internally valid, we can be confident in the conclusions drawn from the specific circumstances of the study: the population of participants actually studied, the measurements made, and the interventions provided. We are justified in concluding that the differences observed are due to the attributed causes. However, there are many potential threats to internal validity, such as confounders, misclassification bias, and selection bias, which we discuss later. Even if all these threats to internal validity are overcome to our satisfaction, we also want our study to have external validity. This means that the conclusions can be generalized from the specific setting,

---

* Note again the difference in the terminology of measurement and demonstration studies. Validity of a demonstration study design, discussed here, is different from validity of a measurement method, discussed in Chapter 5.

participants, and intervention studied to the broader range of settings others encounter. Thus, even if we demonstrate convincingly that our antibiotic reminder system reduces postoperative infection rates in our own hospital, it is of little interest to others unless we can show them that the results can safely be generalized to other reminder systems in other hospitals. Some threats to what we are now calling external validity have already been mentioned under the topics of selecting participants and measures and deciding on the nature of the intervention. (For example, testing a predictive model on the same cases on which it was trained, as opposed to a new test set.). The remaining aspects are discussed on p. 215.

Inference and Error

When we conduct a demonstration study, there are four possible outcomes. We illustrate these outcomes in the context of a demonstration study exploring the effectiveness of an information resource using an appropriate comparative design. The four possible outcomes are:

1. The information resource was effective, and our study shows this.
2. The information resource was ineffective, and our study shows this.
3. The information resource was effective, but for some reason our study mistakenly failed to show this—a type II error.
4. The information resource was ineffective, but for some reason our study mistakenly suggested it was effective—a type I error.

Outcomes 1 and 2 are gratifying from a methodological viewpoint; the results of our study mirror reality. Outcome 3 is a false-negative result, or type II error. In the language of inferential statistics, we mistakenly accept the null hypothesis. Type II errors can arise when the size of the sample of participants included in the study is small relative to the size of the information resource's effect on the measure of interest.[24] Risks of type II errors relate to the concept of study power discussed in the following section. In outcome 4 we have concluded that the resource is valuable when in reality it is not: a false-positive result, or type I error. We have mistakenly rejected the null hypothesis. When we accept, for example, the value of $p < .05$ as a criterion for statistical significance, we are consciously accepting a 5% risk of making a type I error as a consequence of using randomization as a mechanism of experimental control.

Study Power

Every demonstration study has a probability of detecting a difference of particular size between the groups. This probability is known as the statistical power of the design. All other things remaining equal, a larger number of participants is required in a demonstration study to detect a smaller effect. So by increasing the number of participants, the power can be increased, though the relationship is nonlinear—four times as many participants are typically needed to double the study power. One challenge when designing studies is to decide how much of a difference to look for. Ideally, the study should be powered to look for a difference that would be just enough to lead to a change in practice—the "minimum worthwhile difference." For example, although looking for a 30% improvement in student knowledge scores after using a new resource would take very few students to demonstrate, the minimum worthwhile difference that might cause a university to adopt the resource could be 15%. This means planning a larger study to detect this smaller but still useful effect.

Power is an important consideration in study design as it is closely linked to the number of participants needed. A study with insufficient participants is unlikely to detect the minimum worthwhile difference between the groups, and will make poor use of the participant time and the investigators' resources.[24] While a detailed discussion of statistical power and sample size is beyond the scope of this volume, a clear and comprehensive discussion is found in the text by Cohen.[25] In general, the formulas used to compute sample size take account of the degree of difference between the groups the study is designed to detect and some measure of the dispersion of the results per task, typically the standard deviation. If the calculation reveals that more participants are required than are likely to be available to the investigator, a number of strategies are possible:

- Study each case for longer, to allow the outcome more time to develop.
- Use a more sensitive measure of the outcome, such as a laboratory test rather than a patient outcome. However, such surrogate outcomes may be criticized for their poor external validity.
- Use a more powerful study design (e.g., a crossover study, assuming that there is no carryover effect).
- Contact potential collaborators and set up a multicenter study.

For simple two-group studies with equal numbers of participants allocated to each group, nomograms give a convenient indication of the required sample size (e.g., p. 456 in Altman[7]). When more certainty is needed, when the study is designed to demonstrate equivalence (as opposed to differences), when the intent is to measure the time until an event occurs, or when there are more than two groups or one outcome variable, investigators are advised to consult a statistician for advice. In Chapter 12, where we discuss the writing of evaluation proposals, we will stress again the importance of exploring statistical power.

Threats to Internal Validity: Biases and How to Avoid Them

The motive for conducting demonstration studies is to provide reliable conclusions that are of interest to those making decisions. Our primary interest is to inform decisions about the particular information resource in the context in which it was studied. To this end, we want our results to be free from threats to internal validity. In the sections that follow, we examine many of the potential sources of bias that work to jeopardize internal validity.

Assessment Bias

It is important to ensure that no one involved in a demonstration study can allow his or her own feelings and beliefs about an information resource, whether positive or negative, to affect the results. Simply asking study participants to ignore their feelings so as to avoid biasing the study is unrealistic; we must ensure that they cannot affect the results, consciously or unconsciously. The people who could bias a study include those designing it, those recruiting participants, those using the information resource, those collecting follow-up data, and those who participate as judges in making measurements of dependent or independent variables.

Consider a study in which the users of an antibiotic reminder system also collect data needed for determining whether the advice generated by the system was correct. If they were skeptics about the value of the resource, they might subconsciously collect additional data to prove themselves right and the reminder system wrong. Thus, despite believing themselves to be unbiased, they might become more likely to record that a patient was suffering from chest symptoms to justify an antibiotic prescription that the reminder system had not advised, or to collect bacteriological specimens from a wound infection in such a way that the laboratory was unable to culture any pathogens in a patient in whom the system reminded them to prescribe an antibiotic but they had ignored its advice.

In many studies, judges are employed to ascertain the quality of a process or outcome for cases or problems in which the information resource was and was not used. A concern is that the judges might be prejudiced, particularly if they participated in the development of the information resource, or if the criteria used for judging the correctness of decisions or outcome are poorly formulated.

To eliminate these potential biases, everyone involved in such judgments should be blinded to whether the information resource was used in each case. If follow-up data about a case are necessary to render a judgment, these data should ideally be obtained after an independent person removes any evidence of information resource use that may exist.[26,27]

Allocation and Recruitment Bias

Studies of information resources conducted early in the life cycle often take place in the environment in which the resource was developed and frequently arouse strong positive (or negative) feelings among study participants. In a study where patients are randomized and the clinicians have strong beliefs about the information resource, two biases may arise. In clinical studies, investigators may, subconsciously perhaps, but still systematically allocate easier (or more difficult) cases to the information resource group (allocation bias), or they may avoid recruiting easy (or difficult) cases to the study if they know in advance that the next patient will be allocated to the control group (recruitment bias).[28] These biases can either over- or underestimate the information resource's value. In a study in which care providers or departments are randomized, bias can arise if the care providers' enthusiasm for the information resource is inversely correlated with their level of experience or competence. Thus inexperienced care providers might drop out of a study less often if they are in the information resource group, confounding the benefit of the information resource with the care providers' inexperience and reducing the information resource's apparent benefit. To address these potential biases, it is helpful to define carefully the population of participants eligible for the study, screen them strictly for eligibility, randomize them as late as possible before the information resource is used, and conceal the allocation of participants to intervention or control groups until they have firmly committed to participate in the study.[28]

The Hawthorne Effect

The Hawthorne effect—the tendency for humans to improve their performance if they know it is being studied—was discovered by psychologists measuring the effect of ambient lighting on workers' productivity at the Hawthorne factory in Chicago.[29] Productivity increased as the room illumination level was raised, but when the illumination level was accidentally reduced, productivity increased again, suggesting that it was the study itself, rather than changes in illumination, that caused the increase. During a study of a biomedical information resource, the Hawthorne effect can lead to an improvement in the performance of all participants in all study groups, in reaction to their knowing they are being studied. This "global" Hawthorne effect is particularly likely to occur when performance can be increased relatively easily, for example by acquiring a small amount of knowledge or a simple insight.[26] The net result is to increase performance in both control and information resource groups, potentially causing the benefit from the information resource to be underestimated. To quantify a global Hawthorne effect requires a preliminary low-profile study of the performance of participants before any large-scale study. Disguising the true intention of this baseline study may take some ingenuity, but is a necessary evil if the Hawthorne effect is not to bias this study too. Life is much easier if the baseline performance of decision makers can be measured from data that are routinely collected, which is increasingly the case in the clinical world. Thus, for example, analysis of prescribing data over a 6-month period before the start of a trial can be used to determine the baseline rate of prescribing errors, free of the Hawthorne effect.

TABLE 7.9. Hypothetical results of a balanced incomplete block design of two antibiotic reminder systems.

	Postoperative infection rate (%)	
Patients	Orthopedic reminders	Cardiac reminders
Orthopedic	5	10
Cardiac	18	11

In rare cases where the Hawthorne effect is known to be a major threat to a successful study, one approach is to ensure that it acts on all participants' activities by using an alternative study design. Investigators introduce two similar interventions and allocate each participant randomly to one of them. The investigators make two sets of measurements: One set measures the effects of the first intervention on the first group of participants and uses the second group as control; the other measurements assess the effects of the second intervention on the second group, using the first group as the controls. Participants are randomized to the two groups, so there is no systematic difference between groups. Because both groups of participants experience what appears to be an important experimental intervention, the Hawthorne effect is equal, and each group can safely act as a control for the other. The two interventions is this "balanced incomplete block design" should be made similar, for example providing anesthetists with reminders about prophylactic antibiotics for preoperative orthopedic patients or for preoperative cardiac patients (Table 7.9). The postoperative infection rates in orthopedic patients whose doctors received orthopedic reminders was half that of patients whose doctors received reminders about cardiac patients. Both groups of doctors were receiving reminders about some of their patients, so the Hawthorne effect is not responsible. Equally, the postoperative infection rates in cardiac patients whose doctors received cardiac reminders were nearly half that of patients whose doctors received reminders about orthopedic patients, suggesting that the cardiac reminders were also effective.

Data Collection Biases

While the potential biases discussed above relate primarily to the design of a demonstration study, the following biases relate to the process of data collection itself.

Checklist Effect

The checklist effect is the improvement observed in performance due to more complete and better-structured data collection about a case or problem when paper- or computer-based forms are used. Most information resources require that data be well structured and consistently represented. Perhaps it is the structuring of the data, rather than any computations that are performed, that generates performance improvement. As shown earlier (Table 7.1), the impact of forms on decision making can equal that of computer-generated advice,[13] so it must either be controlled for, quantified, or ignored as described below. To control for the checklist effect, the same data can be collected in the same way in control and information resource conditions, even though the information resource's output is only available for the latter group.[26] To quantify the magnitude of this effect, a randomly selected "data collection only" group of patients can be recruited.[13] Sometimes the checklist effect is ignored by defining the intervention to include both the revised data collection methods and the computation performed on the data after it is collected. While this approach may be scientifically unsatisfying, for purposes of evaluation it may be entirely satisfactory if the stakeholders have no interest in separating the issues.

Data Completeness Effect

In some studies, the information resource itself may collect the data used to assess a dependent variable. Thus more data are available in intervention cases than in controls. The data completeness effect may cut both ways in influencing study results. For example, consider a field study of an intensive care unit (ICU) information resource where the aim is to compare recovery rates from adverse events, such as transient hypotension between patients monitored by the information resource with those allocated to traditional methods. Because the information resource logs adverse episodes that may not be recorded by the manual system, the recovery rate may apparently *fall* in this group of cases, because more adverse events are being detected. To detect this bias, the completeness and accuracy of data collected in the control and information resource groups can be compared against some third method of data collection, perhaps in a short pilot study. Alternatively, clinical events for patients in both groups should be logged by computer even though the information resource's output is available only for care of patients in the invention group. Subsequently, all data from control patients would be reviewed for evidence of hypotensive episodes.

Feedback Effect

As mentioned in the earlier discussion, one interesting result of the classic 1986 study of the Leeds Abdominal Pain System[13] was that the diagnostic accuracy of the control house officers spending 6 months in a training level failed to improve over the period, whereas the performance of the doctors given both data collection forms and monthly feedback did improve, starting at 13% above control levels at month 1 and rising to 27% above control levels at month 6 (Table 7.1). Providing these doctors with the opportunity to capture their diagnoses on a form and encouraging them to audit their performance monthly improved their performance, even though they did not receive any decision support per se. Many information resources provide a similar opportunity for easy audit and feedback of personal performance. If investigators want to distinguish the effects of any decision support or advice from the effects of audit or feedback, control participants can be provided with the same audit and feedback as those in the intervention group. Alternatively, the study could include a third "audit and feedback only" group to quantify the size of the improvement caused by these factors alone, as was done in the Leeds study.[13] As was the case with the checklist effect, investigators also have the option of ignoring it by considering audit and feedback to be components bundled in the overall intervention. If this is consistent with what stakeholders want to know, and the investigators are aware they are ignoring this effect, ignoring it can be a defensible strategy.

Carryover Effect

The carryover effect is a contamination of the management of the control condition by care providers who also have, or who have previously had, access to the information resource. It is most likely to occur with information resources that have an intentional or unintentional educational effect, as would be the case for decision support systems. A carryover effect reduces the measured difference in performance between information resource and control conditions. To eliminate the carryover effect, it is probably best to randomize at the level of the care provider instead of the patient[22] or department instead of care provider.[13] This creates what is called a hierarchical or nested study design. To quantify the carryover effect, investigators can conduct a crossover study with alternating information resource and control periods.[30] Such a design allows carryover after the information resource is withdrawn to be quantified.

Placebo Effect

In some drug trials, simply giving patients an inactive tablet, or placebo, causes them to recover. This placebo effect may be more powerful than the drug effect itself and may even obscure a complete absence of therapeutic benefit. Placebo effects can occur in biomedical informatics studies. For example, in a clinical information resource study, patients who watch their doctors use impressive technology may believe they are receiving better or additional care. This can potentially overestimate the value of the information resource. (But this can also go the other way: some patients may believe that a care provider who needs a workstation is less competent.) The problem is most likely to arise when the attributes being measured are attitudes or beliefs (e.g., the patients' satisfaction with therapy) or when the technology is used in front of the patient. Possible remedies are for all care providers to leave the patient for the same brief period (when some would use the information resource) or for all care providers to use computers but the resource output would be available only to intervention care providers.

Measuring features of the patients' condition that are less dependent on the patients' perceptions makes the study more immune to the placebo effect.

The Hawthorne effect and the placebo effect can be difficult to distinguish. The Hawthorne effect is more likely to be in play when the study participants, those on whom measurements are made, are professionals who are reacting to the perception of being studied. Placebo effects are more likely to be in play when the participants are clients, care recipients, or students, who believe that they may be receiving exceptional or special treatment.

"Second-Look" Bias

When conducting a laboratory study of the effects of an information resource on clinical decision making using written case scenarios, a common procedure is to ask clinicians to read a problem or case scenario and state their initial decision. They are then allowed to use the information resource (e.g., a decision support system) and are asked again for their decision.[31,32] Any improvements in decision making might then be credited to the decision support system. However, there is a potential bias here. The participants are being given a second opportunity to review the same case scenario, which allows them more time and further opportunities for reflection, which can itself improve decision making. This second-look bias can be reduced or eliminated by increasing the interval between the two exposures to the stimulus material to some weeks or months[33] or by providing a different set of case data, matched for difficulty with the first, for the second task.[34] Alternatively, the size of the effect can be quantified by testing participants on a subset of the test data a second time without providing them access to the information resource. Another approach is to examine whether the information resource provided participants with any information of potential value, and determine if the increase in performance was correlated with the utility of the information resource's advice.

External Validity Revisited

Even if we believe that the study findings are internally consistent and the conclusions are correct, evaluators and recipients of evaluation reports (see Chapter 2) are often interested in generalizing from the specific details of the study to a range of other, similar settings. This requires the study to demonstrate external validity. Possible threats to external validity are discussed below.

Generalizing from the Sample

We have already mentioned the risks of using homogeneous sets of selected tasks (cases or problems) and participants when conducting demonstration studies. Unless the evaluators have sampled cases and participants to reflect the variability to be expected everywhere,[35] the results of the study will apply to narrow circumstances only and fail attempts at replication.[16] A classic example is a prognostic model to predict relapse from asthma that performed very well in the physical location where it was developed but had near-zero discriminatory power in a second, similar location.[36]

When the Resource Developers also Evaluate the Resource

If the developers of an information resource also attempt to evaluate it, and human judgment is required to decide whether the resource is correct, they may be influenced in subtle ways by their understandable, preexisting belief in the value of the resource to give it the benefit of the doubt. This event is a special problem during early-stage laboratory studies of resource function (see Chapter 3) when test cases (or problems) are input, and the information resource's output may be recorded by a member of the development team. If data items for a test case are missing or ambiguous, the developer may know how to persuade the information resource to produce the "right" output. In sum, the developers and their associated professionals know how to use the information resource to best effect; others outside the center of development do not, so study results that paint the resource in a very positive light may not apply elsewhere.

Also, biomedical information resources seldom encompass every aspect of the domain in which they operate, even in a subarea, so it is common for a given information resource to be confronted with novel combinations of data when tested on a new set of cases or problems. If these novel challenges appear to require modifications in the software, developers sometimes suspend a study while the information resource is modified and then quote its accuracy on the whole series, neglecting that the modifications may now cause the information resource to fail on some of the previous cases. An impartial evaluation would report the performance of one version of the resource over the whole case series, without modification.

Of course, there is an opposite side to this argument. Developers of the resource know it better than anyone else, and perhaps understand better than anyone else its shortcomings and weaknesses. If so inclined, they can use this knowledge to identify what would be the most stringent test of the resource. So depending on the inclination of the persons involved, the developer who is also the evaluator could bias the studies in either direction.

The Evaluation Paradox

In a demonstration study conducted in the context of real professional work, users are understandably reluctant to employ and act on the output of an information resource until its value has been established. However, to establish the information resource's value, its output must be acted on. This evaluation paradox applies especially to so-called black box information resources, which provide little if any insight into the reasons for their output,[37] for example an expert system that could not "explain" its reasoning or a sequencing program that could not reveal the underlying algorithm. This could cause professionals to ignore the information resource's output and lead to its benefits being underestimated. Although one strategy to promote use might be to deliberately exaggerate the benefits of using the resource, it is preferable to give professionals an honest account of the resource's scope and performance in laboratory tests; the differences between its computational method and that of other resources, or how the same tasks would be performed "by hand", and specific examples of cases where the resource was helpful and where it was not. This approach encourages professionals to treat the information resource as an aid, not as a black-box dictator. There is little reason to require them to always follow the information resource's output during a demonstration study, as this will certainly not be the case when the resource is available more widely.

Analysis by "Intention to Provide Information"

In a demonstration study, there are many instances when the information resource is not used as intended[26,38] or when its output is ignored. When analyzing the results of the study, it may be tempting to exclude such cases, thereby increasing the difference between control and information resource groups. There is a close analogy when analyzing the results of drug trials: To which group should one assign participants who were randomized to a drug but failed to take it, or who took it but were found not to absorb it? If one excludes from analysis all patients who did not take the drug, the *average* benefit of giving the drug to patients described by the study entry criteria is overestimated, as we know that in real life a certain percentage of patients are noncompliant. Thus when analyzing drug trials, participants are included in the group to which they were originally randomized. This method is called analysis by the principle of *intention to treat*.

The same argument should apply to studies of biomedical information resources: The aim of demonstration studies is usually to measure the *average* impact of the information resource on professionals and their clients to whom it is made available, not its *maximum* potential for benefit after excluding nonusers. Indeed, this is the motivation for conducting demonstration studies. Thus we must analyze the study according to the principle of *intention to provide information*. Employing this principle helps the investigator make decisions about which participants to include in or exclude from a study. Three illustrative scenarios that might arise in studies of clinical information resources follow. In each scenario, it is appropriate to retain the case in the study despite what might appear to be a justification to delete it.

Scenario 1: A care provider uses the information resource for a case that was in the control group (i.e., for whom the resource was not supposed to be used).

If the care provider had been sufficiently uncertain about the patient's care to consult the information resource, he or she might have sought information from elsewhere had the information resource not been available. (The analogy here is to self-medication by patients in a drug trial). Verdict: *retain the case in the control group.*

Scenario 2: For a patient assigned to the control group, a care provider consulted someone else to obtain the same information that could have been obtained from the information resource.

If the care provider had been sufficiently uncertain to consult someone else, this would probably have happened regardless of whether there was a study in progress. Again, the analogy is self-medication. Verdict: *retain the case in the control group.*

Scenario 3: A case in which the care provider was supposed to use the information resource but failed to use it, used it incorrectly, or ignored its output or advice.

If the care provider was unwilling to use the information resource, failed to use it correctly, or ignored its output under the conditions of a trial when their performance was under scrutiny, he or she would probably not have used it in a real setting. The analogy is patient noncompliance or failure to absorb the drug. Verdict: *retain the case in the information resource group.*

Conclusion

We have explored in this chapter the three major kinds of demonstration studies: descriptive, correlational and comparative. We have also defined the kinds of variables that are encountered in demonstration studies: dependent and independent variables. This has allowed us to describe the anatomy of demonstration studies and to identify the key areas on which we need to focus to ensure that the study results are useful to us, and preferably to others.

The problem of validity has been explored with respect to external validity or generalizability, and internal validity or truthfulness of the results. There are many threats to internal validity and the various ways in which these can be overcome using a variety of study designs have been described.

This chapter should equip you with the necessary knowledge and understanding to design a rigorous, useful demonstration study. The aim of the next chapter is to explore issues arising during the analysis of data from such studies.

Self-Test 7.2

For each of the following short study scenarios, try to identify any of the potential biases or threats to validity discussed in this chapter. Each scenario may contain more than one bias or threat to validity. Then consider how you might alter the resource implementation or evaluation plans to reduce or quantify the problem.

1. As part of its initiative to improve patient flow and teamwork, a family practice intends to install an electronic patient scheduling resource when it moves to new premises in 3 months' time. Evaluators propose a 1-month baseline study of patient waiting times and phone calls between clinicians, starting at 2 months and conducted prior to the move, to be repeated immediately after starting to use the new resource in 3 months.

2. A bacteriology laboratory is being overwhelmed with requests for obscure tests with few relevant clinical data on the paper request forms. It asks the hospital information system director to arrange for electronic requesting and drafts a comprehensive three-screen list of questions clinicians must answer before submitting the request. The plan is to evaluate the effects of electronic test ordering on appropriateness of requests by randomizing patients to paper request forms or electronic requests for the next year. The staff members intend to present their work at a bacteriology conference.

3. A renowned chief cardiologist in a tertiary referral center on the West coast is concerned about the investigation of some types of congenital heart disease in patients in her unit. A medical informatics expert suggests that her expertise could be represented as reminders about test ordering for the junior staff looking after these patients. She agrees, announces her plans at the next departmental meeting, and arranges system implementation and training. Each patient is managed by only one junior staff member; there are enough staff members to allow them to be randomized. After the trial, the appropriateness of test ordering for each patient is judged by the chief cardiologist from the entire medical record. It is markedly improved in patients managed by the doctors who received reminders. Based on these results, the hospital chief executive agrees to fund a start-up company to disseminate the reminder system to all U.S. cardiology units.

Answers to Self-Tests

Self-Test 7.1

1. (a) Independent variables: time period before and after resource installation (four levels).
   (b) Dependent variables and measurement strategy: attitude to information technology—30-item survey.

    (c) Participants: hospital staff members.

    (d) Control strategy employed: before–after.

2. (a) Independent variables: none; this study is descriptive.

    (b) Dependent variables and measurement strategy: accuracy of the resource—the proportion of time the computer-generated diagnoses agree with the previously established diagnosis, measured perhaps by an expert panel.

    (c) Participants: none.

    (d) Control strategy employed: none.

3. (a) Independent variables: hospital (two levels), advice mode (three levels).

    (b) Dependent variables and measurement strategy: total drug charges, averaged across all relevant patients for each physician during the study period.

    (c) Participants: physicians.

    (d) Control strategy employed: simultaneous randomized study.

4. (a) Independent variables: receipt of advice (two levels).

    (b) Dependent variables and measurement strategy: extent to which the actions recommended by the reminders were in fact taken, measured by a case notes audit.

    (c) Participants: the 12 internal medicine services and the staff employed in them.

    (d) Control strategy employed: simultaneous randomized trial.

5. (a) Independent variables: body system (cardiovascular or gastrointestinal) and version of the resource accessed (two levels).

    (b) Dependent variables and measurement strategy: knowledge scores for both disease areas, measured by a validated written test.

    (c) Participants: students.

    (d) Control strategy employed: randomized crossover design.

Self-Test 7.2

1. Potential biases or threats to validity: Proposed study confounds impact of new premises on patient flow and teamwork with impact of new patient scheduling resource; fails to allow time for staff to train on new resource before making measures. Baseline measurement period ends on the day that move takes place, so last week or so may be disrupted by preparations for the move.

Improvements to implementation/plan: Start 4-week baseline data collection at least 6 weeks before move. Postpone later data collection periods until at least 4 weeks after move. Ideally, carry out a second data collection period before new resource implemented, to measure impact of new premises on patient flows and communication, followed by a third data collection period once staff are familiar with new resource to quantify additional benefit of the resource on top of the move. Take care not to credit any improvements with the resource itself—other unknown changes may also have been associated with the move.

2. Potential biases or threats to validity: The trial may fail because the clinicians may refuse to fill out the three screens of data to request a test. It will be hard to compare the appropriateness of paper-based and detailed electronic requests relying on the supplied data alone, as there will be much more data once the electronic requesting resource is in place. There may be a carryover effect if patients are randomized—it would be better to randomize doctors. The study results may be specific to the tests, electronic requesting resource, and clinicians studied, so the generalizability of the study results to others attending the bacteriology conference may be limited.

Improvements to implementation/plan: Carry out a pilot study to ensure that the new electronic test request resource is usable and is likely to be used before the trial. Determine whether a request was appropriate or not by reference to case notes, not the data supplied. Randomize doctors, not patients, to eliminate the carryover effect; analyze at the level of doctors. Generalize from the study results to other settings with caution. Ideally, recruit other labs and conduct a multicenter study.

3. Potential biases or threats to validity: The generalizability of the findings from the study seem low, as this is a tertiary referral center handling particularly challenging cases, and attracting high-flying staff. The benefits therefore may not be replicated when the resource is rolled out to settings where most patients have simpler problems and the staff are less able to respond to the requests and interpret the resulting tests. The attention drawn to the study by an announcement at a departmental meeting could lead to a marked Hawthorne effect, thus reducing the apparent benefit from the reminders. The judgment of appropriate test ordering is carried out by a single cardiologist, whose views may not be shared by the community. The judge of appropriate ordering is the same person as the source of the rules, so the evaluation is circular: the testing is judged appropriate if it was done as she said it should be done.

Improvements to implementation/plan: Recruit a variety of hospitals to the study with a more typical case mix and staffing to enhance generalizability. Ignore the first 2 to 3 weeks of data during the trial to reduce the impact of Hawthorne effects. Carry out some kind of consensus process to develop broadly acceptable criteria of appropriate test ordering in cases such as these. Rather than the circular process above, measure a patient outcome, to see if more appropriate ordering actually helps the patients.

References

1. Donabedian A. Evaluating the quality of medical care. Millbank Mem Q 1966;44:166–206.
2. Wasson JH, Sox HC, Neff RK, Goldman L. Clinical prediction rules: applications and methodological standards. N Engl J Med 1985;313:793–799.

3. Wyatt J, Spiegelhalter D. Evaluating medical expert systems: what to test and how? Med Inf (Lond) 1990;15:205–217.
4. Schwartz D, Lellouch J. Explanatory and pragmatic attitudes in therapeutic trials. J Chronic Dis 1967;20:637–648.
5. Anderson C. Measuring what works in health care. Science 1994;263:1080–1081.
6. Byar DP. Why data bases should not replace randomized controlled clinical trials. Biometrics 1980;36:337–342.
7. Altman D. Practical Statistics for Medical Research. London: Chapman & Hall, 1991.
8. Cochran WG, Cox GM. Experimental Designs. New York: Wiley, 1957.
9. Winer BJ. Statistical Principles in Experimental Design. New York: McGraw-Hill, 1991.
10. Buck C, Donner A. The design of controlled experiments in the evaluation of non-therapeutic interventions. J Chronic Dis 1982;35:531–538.
11. Diwan VK, Eriksson B, Sterky G, Tomson G. Randomization by groups in studying the effect of drug information in primary care. Int J Epidemiol 1992;21:124–130.
12. Grimshaw JM, Russell IT. Effect of clinical guidelines on medical practice: a systematic review of rigorous evaluations. Lancet 1993;342:1317–1322.
13. Adams ID, Chan M, Clifford PC, et al. Computer aided diagnosis of acute abdominal pain: a multicentre study. BMJ 1986;293:800–804.
14. Myers DH, Leahy A, Shoeb H, Ryder J. The patient's view of life in a psychiatric hospital: a questionnaire study and associated methodological considerations. Br J Psychiatry 1990;156:853–860.
15. Van Way CW, Murphy JR, Dunn EL, Elerding SC. A feasibility study of computer-aided diagnosis in appendicitis. Surg Gynecol Obstet 1982;155:685–688.
16. Wyatt JC, Altman DG. Prognostic models: clinically useful, or quickly forgotten? BMJ 1995;311:1539–1541.
17. Knaus W, Wagner D, Lynn J. Short term mortality predictions for critically ill hospitalized patients: science and ethics. Science 1991;254:389–394.
18. Sacks H, Chalmers TC, Smith H. Randomized vs. historical controls for clinical trials. Am J Med 1982;72:233–240.
19. A: Cornfield J. Randomization by group: a formal analysis. Am J Epidemiol 1978;108:100–102.
20. Wyatt J, Wyatt S. When and how to evaluate health information systems? Int J Med Inf 2003;69:251–259.
21. Klein MS, Ross FV, Adams DL, Gilbert CM. Effect of online literature searching on length of stay and patient care costs. Acad Med 1994;69(6):489–495.
22. Tierney WM, Overhage JM, McDonald CJ. A plea for controlled trials in medical informatics. J Am Med Inf Assoc 1994;1:353–355.
23. Lyon HC Jr, Healy JC, Bell JR, et al. PlanAlyzer, an interactive computer-assisted program to teach clinical problem solving in diagnosing anemia and coronary artery disease. Acad Med 1992;67:821–828.
24. Freiman JA, Chalmers TC, Smith H, Kuebler RR. The importance of beta, the type II error and sample size in the design and interpretation of the randomised controlled trial. N Engl J Med 1978;299:690–694.
25. Cohen J. Statistical Power Analysis for the Behavioral Sciences. Hillsdale, NJ: Lawrence Erlbaum, 1988.

26. Wyatt J. Lessons learned from the field trial of ACORN, an expert system to advise on chest pain. In: Barber B, Cao D, Qin D, eds. Proceedings of the Sixth World Conference on Medical Informatics, Singapore. Amsterdam: North Holland 1989:111–115.

27. Yu VL, Fagan LM, Wraith SM, et al. Antimicrobial selection by computer: a blinded evaluation by infectious disease experts. JAMA 1979;242:1279–1282.

28. Schultz KF, Chalmers I, Hayes RJ, Altman DG. Dimensions of methodological quality associated with estimates of treatment effects in controlled trials. JAMA 1995; 273:408–412.

29. Roethligsburger FJ, Dickson WJ. Management and the Worker. Cambridge, MA: Harvard University Press, 1939.

30. Pozen MW, d'Agostino RB, Selker HP Sytkowski PA, Hood WB. A predictive instrument to improve coronary care unit admission in acute ischaemic heart disease. N Engl J Med 1984;310:1273–1278.

31. Murray GD, Murray LS, Barlow P, et al. Assessing the performance and clinical impact of a computerized prognostic system in severe head injury. Stat Med 1986;5:403–410.

32. deBliek R, Friedman CP, Wildemuth BM, Martz JM, Twarog RG, File D. Information retrieval from a database and the augmentation of personal knowledge. J Am Med Inf Assoc 1994;1:328–338.

33. Cartmill RSV, Thornton JG. Effect of presentation of partogram information on obstetric decision-making. Lancet 1992;339:1520–1522.

34. Suermondt HJ, Cooper GF. An evaluation of explanations of probabilistic inference. Comput Biomed Res 1993;26:242–254.

35. Horrocks JC, Lambert DE, McAdam WAF, et al. Transfer of computer-aided diagnosis of dyspepsia from one geographical area to another. Gut 1976; 17:640–644.

36. Centor RM, Yarbrough B, Wood JP. Inability to predict relapse in acute asthma. N Engl J Med 1984;310:577–580.

37. Hart A, Wyatt J. Evaluating black boxes as medical decision-aids: issues arising from a study of neural networks. Med Inf (Lond) 1990;15:229–236.

38. Wellwood J, Spiegelhalter DJ, Johannessen S. How does computer-aided diagnosis improve the management of acute abdominal pain? Ann R Coll Surg Engl 1992;74:140–146.

8
Analyzing the Results of Demonstration Studies

The previous chapter described in some detail the different kinds of objectivist demonstration studies, the anatomy of a demonstration study, options in study design, and some of the many kinds of bias that may affect the validity of study results. This chapter continues the discussion of demonstration studies, focusing on how to represent and analyze the results of these studies. We begin with a general framework for approaching all such analyses, and then discuss in some depth the more specific circumstances that arise most frequently in biomedical informatics studies. The goal here is not to qualify the reader as a statistician, but rather to develop an intuitive appreciation of a number of relevant concepts as well as to provide what may approach a "cookbook" for a few common examples. We limit our discussion to univariate demonstration studies that have one dependent variable.

The available methods to analyze demonstration studies are continuously improving. Investigators who wish to do state-of-the-art analyses should consult a practicing statistician for assistance in employing methods that are perhaps better than the very conventional and basic approaches presented here—and certainly when addressing study designs not explicitly addressed here. The limitations of the methods presented in this chapter are emphasized at many points. One goal of this chapter is to facilitate communication between investigators who are primarily trained in biomedical informatics and their statistician colleagues.

Grand Strategy for Analysis of Demonstration Study Results

When the time comes to analyze the data collected during a demonstration study, the levels of measurement of the dependent and independent variables is the most important factor determining the approach taken. Even though there are four possible levels of measurement for any given variable, as introduced in Chapter 4, the discussion here requires us only to

TABLE 8.1. Indices of effect size and statistical inference tests in relation to levels of measurement of dependent and independent variables for demonstration studies.

Dependent variable level of measurement	Independent variable(s) level of measurement	
	Discrete	Continuous
Discrete	*Index of Effect Size* Sensitivity, kappa, other indices *Statistical Inference Test:* Chi-square	*Index of Effect Size* Magnitude of Regression Coefficients *Statistical Inference Test:* Tests of Significance of Coefficients
Continuous	*Index of Effect Size* Differences between group means *Statistical Inference Test:* Analysis of variance (*t*-test) *t*-test of group means	*Index of Effect Size* Magnitude of Correlation Regression Coefficients, R squared *Statistical Inference Test:* Tests of Significance of Coefficients

Note: Shaded cells of table are examples discussed in the text.

dichotomize levels of measurement as either discrete (nominal/ordinal) or continuous (interval/ratio). Turning our attention for the moment just to the structure of Table 8.1, we can envision four types of analytic situations, depending on whether the dependent and independent variables are continuous or discrete. So the first step in study analysis is to understand into which cell of Table 8.1 the demonstration study falls. In the material that follows in this chapter, we will explore in some detail analytic strategies for three of the four cells of Table 8.1.*

Having determined the cell of Table 8.1 that is relevant, the next step is to determine the appropriate index of the effect size for the demonstration study. The effect size is a measure of the degree of association between the dependent variable and each of the independent variables. For example, consider a simple two-group demonstration study with a continuous dependent variable. This study fits in the bottom left cell of the table, as it has a discrete independent variable ("group membership") with two levels. So the index of effect size is the difference between the mean values of the dependent variable for each group. At one extreme, if the means are the same in both groups, the effect size is zero. We will discuss specific indices of effect size in more detail as we introduce specific examples later in this chapter.

The next step in the grand strategy is to determine an appropriate test of statistical inference. Recall from the previous chapter that tests of statistical

---

* An additional situation, not explicitly represented in Table 8.1, obtains if some of the independent variables in the study are discrete and others are continuous. We do not discuss this situation explicitly here, but it can be addressed with so-called logistic regression methods that are briefly considered later in this chapter.

inference allow estimation of the probability of making a type I error, concluding that the dependent variable is related to the independent variable(s) when in truth it is not. When this probability is below a chosen threshold value (usually 0.05), we say that the results of the demonstration study are "statistically significant." All other things remaining equal, the larger the effect size in a given study, the lower the probability of making a type I error. However, the probability of making a type I error is also related to the sample size (number of participants in the study) and other factors. It is vital to maintain the distinction, both conceptually and when analyzing study results, between effect sizes and results of statistical significance testing. The two concepts are often confused, especially because many analytical techniques simultaneously generate estimates of effect sizes and statistical significance. Nonetheless, there are many reasons to keep these concepts distinct. Among them is the fact that statistically significant results, particularly for studies with large numbers of participants, may have effect sizes so small that they have no clinical or practical significance.

The choice of methods to test statistical significance is primarily guided by the levels of measurement of the dependent and independent variables. Table 8.1 suggests some of the possible methods of testing statistical significance for these combinations. For example, analysis of variance (ANOVA) or t-tests of the sample means can be used when the independent variables of a study are discrete and the outcome variable is continuous.

When following this grand strategy, it is important to ensure that a study is placed into the cell of Table 8.1 where it naturally belongs, and not forced into a cell that admits analytical procedures with which the investigator is perhaps more familiar. For example, if the dependent variable (outcome measure) lends itself naturally to measurement at the interval or ratio level, there is usually no need to categorize it (or "discretize" it) artificially. Consider a study in which mean blood pressure, a continuous variable, is the outcome measure. The directly measured value can and should be used for purposes of statistical analysis. Categorizing measured blood pressure values as low, normal, and high neglects potentially useful differences between observations that otherwise would fall into the same category, and may make the results dependent on what might be arbitrary decisions regarding the choice of thresholds for these categories.

Analyzing Studies with Discrete Independent and Dependent Variables

Contingency Tables

In biomedical informatics, many demonstration studies employ discrete dependent (outcome) variables and independent variables that are also discrete. The most common example from clinical domains compares the output of an information resource—for example, whether a patient has a given disease or not—with some type of accepted gold standard indicating whether the patient really has the disease or not. In other cases, investigators conducting demonstration studies sometimes cleave the values of what are really continuous variables into two or more discrete buckets, thus making them discrete.

The results of studies with both independent and dependent variables that are discrete (interval or ordinal) are best represented in terms of contingency tables. Contingency tables are matrices that create all combinations of the levels of the independent and dependent variables. The dimensionality of the contingency table is equal to the total number of variables in the study design. For example, a study with two independent variables and one dependent variable could be represented as a three-dimensional contingency table. If the first independent variable had two levels, the second independent variable three levels, and the dependent variable had two levels as well, the complete contingency table representing the results would have $2 \times 3 \times 2$ or 12 cells. The results of the demonstration study, for each participant, would fall uniquely into one of these 12 combinations, and the results of the study as a whole could be fully expressed as the total number of observations classified into each cell of the table.

While it is clear that the general case of this kind of study includes contingency tables with an arbitrary number of dimensions, and an arbitrary number of levels of each dimension, a very common situation in informatics is the demonstration study that has two discrete variables, each with two levels, generating a 2×2 contingency table to portray and analyze the study results. We discuss this important special case below.

Using Contingency (2 × 2) Tables: Indices of Effect Size

With contingency tables, many indices of effect size, each with its own strengths and weaknesses, can be reported. Consider a study where the output of an information resource is dichotomized as the presence or absence of some disease or other entity of interest, and this output is being compared with some kind of gold standard proxy for the truth. The results of such a study can be described in a 2×2 contingency table. One index of effect size that can be reported is the percentage of agreements between the information resource and a gold standard for a set of test cases. Citing this crude accuracy alone can cause a number of problems. First, it gives the reader no idea of what accuracy could have been obtained by chance. For example, consider a diagnostic aid designed to detect a disease D, where the prevalence (prior probability) of disease D in the test cases is 80%. If a decision support system always suggests disease D no matter which case data are input, the measured accuracy over a large number of cases is 80%. If the resource was slightly more subtle, still ignoring all input data but advising diagnoses solely according to their prevalence, it would still achieve an accuracy of around 64% by chance because it would diagnose disease D on 80% of occasions, and on 80% of occasions disease D would be present.

Citing accuracy alone also ignores differences between types of errors. If a decision support system erroneously diagnoses disease D in a healthy patient, this false-positive error may be less serious than if it pronounces that the patient is suffering from disease E, or that a patient suffering from disease D is healthy, a false-negative error. More complex errors can occur if more than one disease is present, or if the decision support system issues its output as a list of diagnoses ranked by probability. In this case, including the correct diagnosis toward the end of the list is less serious than omitting it altogether, but is considerably less useful than if the correct diagnosis is ranked among the top three.[1]

The disadvantages of citing accuracy rates alone can be largely overcome by using a contingency table to compare the output given by the information resource against the gold standard, which (as discussed in Chapter 4) is the accepted value of the truth. This method allows the difference between false-positive and false-negative errors to be made explicit.

As shown in Table 8.2,[2] errors can be classified as false positive (FP) or false negative (FN). Table 8.2 illustrates different indices based on the rates of occurrence of these errors. Sensitivity and specificity, related to the false negative and false positive rates respectively, are most commonly used. In a field study where an information resource is being used, care providers typically know the output and want to know how often it is correct, or they suspect a disease and want to know how often the information resource correctly detects it. In this situation, some care providers find the predictive value positive and the sensitivity, also known as the detection rate,[3] intuitively more useful than the false-positive and false-negative rates. The positive predictive value has the disadvantage that it is highly dependent on disease prevalence, which may differ significantly between the test cases used in a study and the clinical environment in which an information resource is deployed.

Sensitivity and positive predictive value are particularly useful, however, with information resources that issue alarms, as the accuracy, specificity, and

TABLE 8.2. Example of a contingency table.

Decision-aid's advice	Gold standard		Totals
	Attribute present	Attribute absent	
Attribute present	TP	FP	TP + FP
Attribute absent	FN	TN	FN + TN
Total	TP + FN	FP + TN	N

TP, true positive; FP, false positive; FN, false negative; TN, true negative.
Accuracy: (TP + TN)/N; false-negative rate: FN/(TP + FN); false-positive rate: FP/(FP + TN); positive predictive value: TP/(TP + FP); negative predictive value: TN/(FN + TN); detection rate (sensitivity): TP/(TP + FN); specificity: TN/(FP + TN).

TABLE 8.3. Hypothetical study results as a contingency table.

| | Panel verdict, observed results (no.) | | |
System's prediction	Disease	No disease	Total
Disease	**27** (19.6)	**14** (21.4)	41
No disease	**16** (23.4)	**33** (25.6)	49
Total	43	47	90

Numbers in parentheses are the expected results. Observed results are in boldface.

false-positive rates may not be obtainable. This is because, in an alarm system that continually monitors the value of one or more physiological parameters, there is no way to count discrete true negative events.

Chi-Square Test for Statistical Significance

The basic test of statistical significance for 2×2 tables is performed by computing the chi-square statistic. Chi-square can tell us the probability of committing type I errors (i.e., incorrectly inferring a difference when there is none). Chi-square can be computed from the following formula:

$$\chi^2 = \frac{\sum_i (O_i - E_i)^2}{E_i}$$

where the summation is performed over all i cells of the table, O_i is the observed value of cell i and E_i is the value of cell i expected by chance alone. The expected values are computed by multiplying the relevant row and column totals for each cell and dividing this number by the total number of observations in the table. For example, Table 8.3 gives the results of a hypothetical laboratory study of an information resource based on 90 test cases. The columns give the gold standard verdict of a panel as to whether each patient had the disease of interest, and the rows indicate whether the patient was predicted by the system to have the disease of interest. Observed results are in boldface type; expected frequencies for each cell, given these observed results, are in parentheses.*

The value of chi-square for Table 8.3 is 9.8. A 2×2 contingency table is associated with one so-called statistical degree of freedom. Intuitively, this can be appreciated from the fact that, once the row and column totals for

---

* The reader should confirm the calculations of expected values. For example, the expected value for the disease–disease cell is obtained by multiplying the relevant row total (41) by the relevant column total (43) and dividing the product by the total number of participants (90).

the table are fixed, changing the value of one cell of the table determines the values of all the other cells. With reference, then, to a standard statistical table, we note that the effect seen in the table is significant at about the .001 level, which means that we accept a 1 in 1000 chance of making a type I error if we conclude that there is a relation between the system's predictions and the verdict of the panel. This of course is below the standard threshold of $p < 0.05$ for statistical significance, so most investigators would report this result as statistically significant. As with any statistical test, there are cautions and limitations applying to its use. Chi-square should not be used (or should be corrected for continuity) if the expected value for any of the table's cells is less than five.

Cohen's Kappa: A Useful Effect Size Index

A very useful index of effect size is given by Cohen's kappa (κ), which compares the agreement between the variables against that which might be expected by chance.[4] The formula for calculating κ is

$$\kappa = \frac{O_{Ag} - E_{Ag}}{1 - E_{Ag}}$$

where O_{Ag} is the observed fraction of agreements (the sum of the diagonal cells divided by the total number of observations) and E_{Ag} is the expected fraction of agreements (the sum of the expected values of the diagonal cells, divided by the total number of observations). In our example above, $O_{Ag} = 0.67$ [(27 + 33)/90] and $E_{Ag} = 0.50$ [(19.6 + 25.6)/90], which makes the value of $\kappa = 0.33$. Note that even though the value of κ is corrected for chance, this index still conveys size of effect and does not directly convey the result of a formal test of statistical inference.

Kappa can be thought of as the *chance-corrected proportional agreement*,[5] and possible values range from +1 (perfect agreement) via 0 (no agreement above that expected by chance) to –1 (complete disagreement). Some authorities consider a κ above 0.4 as evidence of useful agreement, but this threshold obviously depends on the particular circumstances of the study.[5]

The weighted κ is a similar statistic to Cohen's κ (discussed above) but incorporates different weights for each kind of disagreement. Further discussion of the use of κ may be found in Altman[6] and Hilden and Habbema.[7]

Receiver Operating Characteristic Analysis

Receiver operating characteristic (ROC) analysis is a technique commonly used in biomedical informatics. From the viewpoint of the framework presented in Table 8.1, it is something of a hybrid. Consider a demonstration study with two variables: a dependent or outcome variable that is discrete and an independent or predictor variable that is continuous. In some circumstances, the purposes of the study are well served by treating the continuous variable as if it were a two-level discrete variable, allowing the results to be displayed in contingency table format. To make the continuous variable discrete, a threshold or cut-point must be selected. Since this choice is completely arbitrary, ROC analysis allows the investigator to explore the relationship between the two variables in the study across a range of choices of threshold.

For example, consider an antibiotic reminder system that predicts the probability of postoperative infection for a surgical patient and then sends an "alert" (or not) to clinicians that the patient is in danger of infection. The probability computed by the resource is a continuous variable. In a demonstration study, the investigator may want to relate the predictions of this computational resource to the "truth": whether patients develop an infection or not. The study could be done by treating the variables exactly as measured, with the patients' actual experience as a discrete outcome and the probability generated by the system as a continuous predictor. However, the reminder system, when deployed in the real world, will be programmed to either send an alert or not, so it may be more useful to see how this resource behaves over a range of choices of threshold probabilities for triggering an alert. (Should a computed probability of .5 trigger an alert, or should the threshold be higher?) If a suboptimal threshold is chosen, the information resource's accuracy may appear lower than can actually be attained and, in practice, the resource will be less useful than it can be.

In these cases, the ROC curve becomes a useful tool to assess variation in the usefulness of the resource's advice as an internal threshold is adjusted.[8] The ROC curve is a plot of the true-positive rate against the false-positive rate for varying threshold levels (Figure 8.1). Each different choice of threshold level creates a unique 2×2 contingency table from which the true-positive and false-positive rates can be computed and subsequently plotted. The ROC curve is generated when these plotted points are connected. If an information resource provides random advice, its ROC curve lies on the diagonal, whereas an ideally performing information resource would have a "knee" close to the upper left hand corner. The area under the ROC curve provides an overall measure of the predictive or discriminatory power of the information resource.[9]

The example described above represents the most basic, and common, use of ROC curves in informatics. Other uses are possible. For example, ROC curves can be plotted from results obtained as the number of input data items to an information resource is varied or the number of facts in a decision support system's knowledge base is changed.[10]

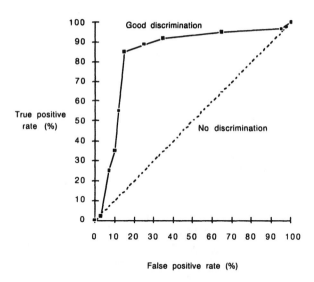

FIGURE 8.1. Sample receiver operating characteristic (ROC) curve.

Analyzing Studies with Continuous Dependent Variables and Independent Variables That Are Discrete

A Representational Scheme

Many important demonstration studies in biomedical informatics are comparative in nature. They employ a dependent (outcome) variable that is continuous in conjunction with independent variables that are discrete. Field experiments to assess resource effect and problem impact often take this form. To set the stage for a discussion of analysis of the data collected in these studies, we introduce a formal representation for comparative study designs. These representational tools help investigators describe their designs to others and enable them to step back from the study details to adapt the design to meet specific needs or features of the environment in which they are conducted.

Complete Factorial Designs

A complete factorial study is one of the designs that can be used to explore the effects of one or more independent variables on the dependent variable. "Factorial" means that each group of participants is exposed to a unique set of conditions where each condition is a specified combination of the levels of each independent variable. "Complete" means that all possible conditions (combinations of each level of each independent variable) are included in the design. Consider our example of a randomized controlled trial of the effects of an antibiotic reminder system (Chapter 7, Table

TABLE 8.4. Notation of a complete factorial design.

Physician experience level	Intervention in four subject groups (G1–G4)	
	Reminders	Control
Junior	G1	G2
Senior	G3	G4

7.6) with doctors as the participants. Let us assume that there are junior and senior doctors on the wards, and we wish to study (1) if reminders work at all and (2) the effects of seniority on the response to reminders. The dependent variable is postoperative infection rate, and the independent variables are exposure to antibiotic reminders (two levels: yes or no) and the experience of the doctors (two levels: junior or senior). No doctor is studied both with and without reminders. To run the complete factorial design, physicians at both levels of experience must be randomized to a "reminders" group or a "no reminders" group, so a unique group of physicians is exposed to each condition. This design can be represented as in Table 8.4. Note that the table expresses the plan for the study, not the results. The four unique groups of participants are denoted G1 through G4.

When data are collected for factorial designs, the logic of the analysis is to compare the means of the groups, or cells, of the study. In the example in Table 8.4, the mean and standard deviation of infection rates for each of the four groups would be computed. Using the ANOVA technique, discussed later in the chapter, it is possible to test statistically for two so-called main effects: (1) if there is a difference in infection rate attributable to the reminders, and (2) if there is difference in infection rates attributable to the grade of doctor. It is also possible to test for an interaction between the grade of doctor and availability of decision support, which tests whether the magnitude of the effect of decision support on infection rates depends on the seniority of the doctor.

Thus a complete factorial design may be thought of as a matrix with each cell occupied by a unique group of participants. Each dimension of the matrix corresponds to one independent variable. If there are N independent variables, the matrix is N-dimensional.

Nested (Hierarchical or Multilevel) Designs

Factorial designs tend to work well in laboratory settings, but investigators conducting field studies may find factorial designs unsuited to their needs because the real world presents situations where the independent variables are hierarchically related. This situation typically occurs when participants in a study are part of groups inherent to the setting in which the study is conducted and thus cannot be disaggregated. Recall that, in the earlier discussion of the antibiotic reminder system, we assumed that physicians do not look after one another's patients. More typically, clinicians are part of ward teams that work closely together in patient care. If we wanted to retain clinicians as the participants in a study conducted in this setting, a factorial design would not be acceptable, as individual clinicians within a team could not be randomly assigned to receive reminders because they work so tightly in groups. If we did randomize some team members to receive reminders and others to the control group, the differential effects attributable to the reminder system would be diluted through interactions among team members. In this setting, randomization must occur at the level of the ward team even though the dependent variable is measured for individual clinicians.

This situation calls for a nested (hierarchical or multilevel) design, as shown in Table 8.5. There are two independent variables: ward team (with six levels) and intervention (with two levels). Each participant belongs to one of six ward teams, and all participants in each team are exposed to only one level of the independent variable by random allocation of the teams. The experimental groups (G1 through G6) are not created by the experimenter. They exist as part of the natural environment of the study. G1 is ward team A. The well-known study of reminder systems by McDonald et al.[11] used a nested design similar to this example. In general, nested designs can be used when naturally occurring *groups* of participants (those on whom the dependent variables is measured) are the units of randomization.

In such a nested design, it is possible to test for a main effect for each independent variable. In the example in Table 8.5, it would be possible to determine if there is a difference attributable to the availability of reminders and if there is a difference attributable to membership of each ward team. It is not possible, however, to explore a possible statistical interaction between reminders and ward team, which could potentially tell us if some ward teams benefited more from the intervention than others. In general, factorial designs are preferable to nested designs,[12] but investigators in informatics often are presented with situations where the nested design is the only option that is both practical and rigorous.

TABLE 8.5. A nested or hierarchical design to study the effects of reminders.

Ward team	Intervention	
	Reminders	Control
A	G1	
B	G2	
C	G3	
D		G4
E		G5
F		G6

TABLE 8.6. Repeated measures design.

	Intervention	
Time	Reminders	Control
Baseline	G1	G2
After installation	G1	G2

Repeated Measures Designs

In the complete factorial design and the nested design, each participant is exposed to only one combination of the independent variables and thus appears only once in a table representing the design. By contrast, in repeated measures designs, each participant appears in two or more cells in the table and is, in effect, reused during the study. Thus in a repeated measures design, participants are said to be employed as their own controls. The hypothetical study discussed in Chapter 7 (see Simultaneous Randomized Controls), provides a perfect example of a repeated measures design. Each participant, a physician, is randomly assigned to one of two groups (G1 or G2), and all the postoperative infection rates of their patients are measured before and after any antibiotic reminders are issued. Using our design notation, this study is illustrated in Table 8.6.

Note that each group, and thus each participant in each group, appears twice in this design. In the terminology of experimental design, time is a "within subject" variable because the same participants appear at multiple levels of that variable: before and after installation. Reminder delivery method is a "between subject" variable because each participant appears in only one level of that variable: reminder or control.

Self-Test 8.1

Using the notation developed in the previous section, diagram the studies described in scenarios 1, 3, 4, and 5 of Self-Test 7.1. Scenario 4, as worded, can be interpreted two ways. For purposes of this exercise, treat it as a nested design with care providers as the participants and clinical services as the unit of randomization.

Logic of Analysis of Variance (ANOVA)

Statistical methods using analysis of variance (ANOVA), discussed briefly here, exist specifically to analyze results of studies with continuous dependent and discrete independent variables, including all the variants on the designs discussed in the previous section.

Recognizing that study design and ANOVA are the topics of entire textbooks,[12] we seek here to establish the basic principles using the results of an actual study as an example. Our example is based on preliminary and somewhat simplified results of a biomedical information retrieval study conducted at the University of North Carolina.[13] The study explores whether a Boolean search tool or Hypertext access to a text database results in more effective retrieval of information to solve biomedical problems. The biomedical information available to participants was a "fact and text" database of bacteriology information and was identical across the two access modes. With the Boolean search tool, participants framed their queries as combinations of key words joined by logical *and* or *or* statements. With the Hypertext mode, participants could branch from one element of information to another via a large number of preconstructed links.

The results to be discussed here are based on data collected from a study in which medical students were randomized to the Boolean or Hypertext access mode. Participants were also randomized to one of two sets of clinical case problems, each set comprising eight clinical infectious disease scenarios. Students were given two passes through their eight assigned problems. On the first pass they were asked to generate diagnostic hypotheses using only their personal knowledge. Immediately thereafter, on the second pass, they were asked to generate another set of diagnostic hypotheses for the same set of problems but this time with aid from the text database.

First we examine the basic structure of this study and note that it has two independent variables, each measured at the nominal level:

- The first independent variable is access mode: Boolean or Hypertext.
- The second independent variable is the particular set of eight case problems to which students were assigned, arbitrarily labeled set A and set B.

Because each of the two independent variables has two levels and is fully randomized, the study design is that of a complete factorial experiment (as discussed earlier in the chapter) with four groups as shown in Table 8.7. The table also shows the number of participants in each group. The dependent variable is the improvement in the diagnostic hypotheses from the first pass to the second—the differences between the aided and unaided scores— averaged over the eight assigned cases. This variable was chosen because it

TABLE 8.7. Structure of the example information retrieval study.

Access mode	Structure, by assigned problem set	
	A	B
Boolean	G1	G2
	($n = 11$)	($n = 11$)
Hypertext	G3	G4
	($n = 10$)	($n = 10$)

TABLE 8.8. Results of the example information retrieval study.

Access mode	Results, by assigned problem set (mean ± SD)	
	A	B
Boolean	11.2 ± 5.7	17.5 ± 7.3
	($n = 11$)	($n = 11$)
Hypertext	15.7 ± 7.2	21.8 ± 5.2
	($n = 10$)	($n = 10$)

estimates the effect attributable to the information retrieved from the text database, controlling for each participant's prior knowledge of bacteriology and infectious disease.

The logic of analyzing data from such an experiment is to compare the mean values of the dependent variable across each of the groups. Table 8.8 displays the mean and standard deviations of the improvement scores for each of the groups. For all participants, the mean improvement score is 16.4 with a standard deviation of 7.3.

Take a minute to examine Table 8.8. It should be fairly clear that there are differences of potential interest between the groups. Across problem sets, the improvement scores are higher for the Hypertext access mode than the Boolean mode. Across access modes, the improvement scores are greater for problem set B than for problem set A. The effect sizes for this study are directly related to the differences between the means in each of the cells of Table 8.8.*

Using ANOVA to Test Statistical Significance

The methods of ANOVA allow us to determine the probability that the effect sizes reflected in differences between group means, whatever the magnitude of these differences, arose due to chance alone. Group differences attributable to each of the independent variables are called *main effects*; differences attributable to the independent variables acting in combination are called *interactions*. The number of possible main effects is equal to the number of independent variables; the number of possible interactions increases geometrically with the number of independent variables. With two independent variables there is one interaction; with three

---

* A useful way of expressing effect sizes for this kind of study is Cohen's d, which, for any pair of cells of the design, is the difference between the mean values divided by the standard deviation of the observations. Use of Cohen's d allows standardized expression of effect sizes in "standard deviation units," which are comparable across studies. Traditionally, effect sizes of .8 standard deviations (or larger) are interpreted as "large" effects, .5 standard deviations as "medium" effects, and .2 standard deviations (or smaller) as "small" effects.[14]

TABLE 8.9. Analysis of variance results for the information retrieval example.

Source	Sum of squares	df	Mean square	F ratio	p
Main effects					
Problem set	400.935	1	400.935	9.716	.003
Access mode	210.005	1	210.005	5.089	.030
Interaction					
Problem set by access mode	0.078	1	0.078	0.002	.966
Error	1568.155	38	41.267		

independent variables there are four; with four independent variables there are 11.*

In our example with two independent variables, we need to test for two main effects and one interaction. Table 8.9 shows the results of ANOVA for these data. Again, a full understanding of this table requires reference to a basic statistical text. For purposes of this discussion, note the following:

1. The *sum-of-squares* is an estimate of the amount of variability in the dependent variable attributable to each main effect or interaction. All other things being equal, the greater the sum-of-squares, the more likely is the effect to be statistically significant.

2. A number of statistical *degrees of freedom* (df) is associated with each source of statistical variance. For each main effect, df is one less than the number of levels of the relevant independent variable. Because each independent variable in our example has two levels, df = 1 for both. For each interaction, the df is the product of the dfs for the interacting variables. In this example, df for the interaction is 1, as each interacting variable has a df of 1. Total df in a study is one less than the total number of participants.

3. The *mean square* is the sum of squares divided by the df.

4. The inferential statistic of interest is the F ratio, which is the ratio of the mean square of each main effect or interaction to the mean square for error. The mean square for error is the amount of variability that is unaccounted for statistically by the independent variables and the interactions among them. The df for error is the total df minus the df for all main effects and interactions.

5. Finally, with reference to standard statistical tables, a p value may be associated with each value of the F ratio and the values of df in the ANOVA table. A p value of less than .05 is typically used as a criterion for statistical significance. In Table 8.9, the p value of the effect for problem set depends

---

* With three independent variables (A, B, C), there are three two-way interactions (AB, AC, BC) and one three-way interaction (ABC). With four independent variables (A, B, C, D), there are six two-way interactions (AB, AC, AD, BC, BD, CD), four three-way interactions (ABC, ABD, ACD, BCD), and one four-way interaction (ABCD).

of the value of the F ratio ($F = 9.716$), the df for problem set ($df = 1$), and the df for error ($df = 38$).

In our example, we see that both main effects (mode of access and problem set) meet the conventional criterion for statistically significance, but the interaction between the dependent variables does not. Note that the ANOVA summary (Table 8.9) does not tell us anything about the directionality or substantive implications of these differences across the groups. Only by inspecting the mean values for the groups, as shown in Table 8.8, can we conclude that the Hypertext access mode is associated with higher improvement scores and that the case problems in set B are more amenable to solution with aid from the database than the problems in set A. Because there is no statistical interaction, this superiority of Hypertext access is consistent across problem sets.

A statistical interaction would be in evidence if, for example, the Hypertext group outperformed the Boolean group on set A, but the Boolean group outperformed the Hypertext group on set B. To see what a statistical interaction means, it is frequently useful to make a plot of the group means, as shown in Figure 8.2, which depicts the study results represented in Table 8.8. Departure from parallelism of the lines connecting the plotted points is the indicator of a statistical interaction. In this case, the lines are nearly parallel.

Special Issues

In this section it was possible only to scratch the surface of analysis of study results using ANOVA methods. To close this section of the chapter, we mention three special issues:

1. In the special case where a study has one independent variable with two levels, we have the familiar two group study where the t-test applies. Applying ANOVA to this case yields the same results as the t-test, with $F = t^2$.

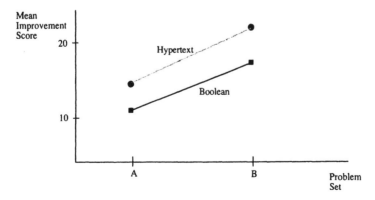

FIGURE 8.2. Graphing results as a way to visualize statistical interactions.

2. The analysis example discussed above pertains only to a completely randomized factorial design. The ANOVA methods employed for other designs, including nested and repeated measures designs, require special variants on this example.

3. Appropriate use of ANOVA requires that the measured values of the dependent variables are distributed roughly according to a "normal" distribution, and also meet other statistical requirements. If the dependent variables as measured fail to meet the assumptions, corrective actions such as transformations of the data may be required, or ANOVA methods may not be applicable.

Self-Test 8.2

1. Given below are the data from the Hypercritic study discussed in Chapter 5. For these data, compute (a) Hypercritic's accuracy, sensitivity, and specificity; (b) the value of chi-square; and (c) the value of Cohen's κ.

| Hypercritic | Pooled rating by judges | | Total |
	Comment valid (≥5 judges)	Comment not valid (<5 judges)	
Comment generated	145	24	169
Comment not generated	55	74	129
Total	200	98	298

2. Review scenario 3 in Self-Test 7.1. Hypothetical results of that study are summarized in the two tables below. The first table gives means and standard deviations of the outcome measure, charges per patient, for each cell of the experiment. Note that $n = 6$ for each cell. Interpret these results.

| Hospital | Advice mode | | |
	Advice always provided	Advice when requested	No advice
A	58.8 ± 7.9	54.8 ± 5.8	67.3 ± 5.6
B	55.2 ± 7.4	56.0 ± 4.7	66.0 ± 7.5

The second table gives the ANOVA results.

Source	Sum-of-squares	df	Mean square	F ratio	p value
Main effects					
Hospital	12.250	1	12.250	0.279	.601
Advice mode	901.056	2	450.528	10.266	<.001
Interaction					
Hospital by group	30.500	2	15.250	0.348	.709
Error	1316.500				

3. Consider an alternative, hypothetical outcome of the information retrieval study as shown below. Make a plot of these results analogous to that in Figure 8.2. What would you conclude with regard to a possible statistical interaction?

Access mode	Mean ± SD, by assigned problem set	
	A	B
Boolean	19.3 ± 5.0	12.4 ± 4.9
	(n = 11)	(n = 11)
Hypertext	15.7 ± 5.7	21.8 ± 5.1
	(n = 10)	(n = 10)

Analyzing Studies with Independent and Dependent Variables that are Continuous

Studies with One Independent Variable

Recall from Chapter 7 that in simple correlational studies, the investigator makes at least two measurements, the dependent or outcome measure and at least one independent variable. Often both of these variables are continuous in nature, such as age and usage rate for an information resource. Many readers will be familiar with the use of simple regression analysis to analyze such data. Here, the continuous dependent variable is plotted against a single continuous independent variable on an x-y graph and a regression line is fitted to the data points, typically using a least squares algorithm—see Figure 8.3 for an example. Here, the number of times each of a set of 11 users logged on to an information resource per week is plotted against the age of that user. A regression line, or line of best fit, has been added by the spreadsheet package. In addition, the package has calculated the equation of the line, showing that the predicted usage rate per week (y) is approximately $35 - 0.4$ times the user age (x). However, it is clear from the graph that there is a lot of scatter in the data, so that although the general trend is for lower log-on rates with older users, some older users (e.g., one of 47 years) actually show higher usage rates than some younger users (e.g., one of 23 years).

In this two-variable example, the slope of the regression line is proportional to the statistical correlation coefficient (r) between the two variables. The square of this correlation, seen as R^2 in Figure 8.3, is the proportion of the variation in the dependent variable (here, log-on rate) that is explained by the independent variable (here, age). In this example, the R^2 is 0.31, meaning that 31% of the variance in usage rate is accounted for by the age of the user, and the other 69% is not accounted for.

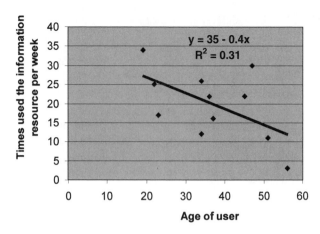

FIGURE 8.3. Simple regression analysis of user age versus the number of times each user logged on to information resource per week.

Studies with Multiple Independent Variables

If we had access to additional data about these users, such as their number of years of computer experience or their scores on a computer attitude survey, we could try to more closely predict or explain their information resource usage rate by using multiple regression analysis. This is an extension of the simple regression approach in which changes in a single continuous dependent variable are compared simultaneously with two or more continuous independent variables to identify the unique contributions of each of these variables to these changes. Such an approach allows us to generate a predictive equation of the form:

$$y = ax_1 + bx_2 + cx_3 + \text{constant}$$

where each x denotes a different independent variable and a, b, and c are coefficients that can be computed from the study data.

In our example above, we might find that 55% of the variation in usage rate can now be explained by the following equation:

Usage rate $= 45 - (0.4 \times \text{age}) + (0.2 \times \text{years of computer experience})$
$+ (0.1 \times \text{computer attitude score})$

This equation shows that user age remains a key factor (with older people generally using the resource less frequently), but that their number of years of computer experience is also an important independent factor, acting in the opposite direction. Users with more experience tend to use the resource more frequently. The user's score on a computer attitude scale is a third independent predictor. Users with a higher attitude score also tend to use the information resource more frequently.

The coefficients in these regression equations may be seen as indices of effect size. Investigators wishing to know whether the coefficients are statistically significant must undertake additional analyses.

Relationships to Other Methods

We can see from the above example that multiple regression methods can be very useful for analyzing correlational studies with continuous variables as it helps to identify which independent variables matter, and in which direction. However, the standard methods for multiple regression analysis often cannot be used when the independent variables include a mix of discrete and continuous variable types. This more general situation requires an expanded method called logistic regression that is beyond the scope of this volume and discussed in a range of texts.[15]

It is also the case that ANOVA and the regression methods discussed in this chapter belong to a general class of analytic methods known as general linear models. With appropriate transformations and mathematical representations of the independent variables, an ANOVA performed on demonstration study data can also be performed using multiple regression methods—with identical results. We introduced ANOVA and regression separately for different cells of Table 8.1 because ANOVA is better matched to the logic of experimental, comparative studies where the independent variables are discrete. Regression analysis is better matched to the logic of correlational studies where all variables tend to be continuous.

Choice of Effect Size Metrics: Absolute Change, Relative Change, Number Needed to Treat

We conclude this chapter with a discussion of alternative ways of portraying effect sizes in demonstration studies. When we conduct demonstration studies, the goal is to inform and enhance decisions about information resources. We should not try to exaggerate the effects we have observed any more than we would deliberately ignore known biases or threats to generality. Thus it is important to describe the results of the study, particularly the effect sizes, in terms that effectively and accurately convey their meaning. Consider the study results in Table 8.10, showing the rates of postoperative infection in patients managed by physicians before and after the introduction of antibiotic reminders.

We can summarize these results in three main ways:

1. *By citing the absolute difference (after intervention versus baseline) in the percentage infection rates due to the reminders (row 3 of Table 8.10).* It may appear to be 5%, but a more conservative estimate is 3%. The 5%

TABLE 8.10. Hypothetical results of a simultaneous randomized controlled study of an antibiotic reminder system.

	Postoperative Infection rate (%)	
Time	Reminder cases	Control cases
Baseline	11	10
After intervention	6	8
Absolute difference	5	2
Relative difference	−46	−20

change in the reminder group should be corrected by the 2% change due to nonspecific factors in the control cases.

2. *By citing the relative difference in the percentage infection rates due to the reminders.* It is a 46% fall, though again the more conservative estimate would be 26%: the 46% fall in the reminder group minus the 20% fall due to nonspecific factors in the control cases.

3. *By citing the "number needed to treat" (NNT).* This figure gives us an idea about how many patients would need to be treated by the intervention to produce the result of interest in one patient, in this case the prevention of an infection. The NNT is the reciprocal of the absolute difference in rates (3%, or 0.03) and is 33 for these results. To put it another way, reminders would need to be issued for an average of 33 patients before one postoperative infection would be prevented.

$$NNT = \frac{1}{rate_1 - rate_2}$$

where $rate_1$ = absolute rate of the event in group 1
$rate_2$ = absolute event rate in group 2.

Several studies have shown that clinicians make much more sensible decisions about prescribing when the results of drug trials are cited as NNT rather than absolute or relative percentage differences.[16] For studies in biomedical informatics, the NNT is often the most helpful way to visualize the effects of implementing an information resource and should be reported whenever possible.

Answers to Self-Tests

Self-Test 8.1

Scenario 1: G1 (group 1): 6 months before, 1 week before, 1 month after, 6 months after.

Scenario 3:

Hospital	Mode of receiving advice		None
	All patients	By request	
A	G1	G2	G3
B	G4	G5	G6

Scenario 4:

Services	Intervention	Control
	Reminders	
A	**G1**	
B	G2	
C	G3	
D	G4	
E	**G5**	
F	G6	
G		**G7**
H		G8
I		G9
J		G10
K		G11
L		G12

Scenario 5:

Body system	Studied by	Lecture
	Computer	
CV	G1	G2
GI	G2	G1

Self-Test 8.2

1. Accuracy = $(145 + 74)/298 = 0.73$; sensitivity = $145/200 = 0.72$; specificity = $74/98 = 0.75$. (b) chi-square = 61.8 (highly significant with $df = 1$). (c) $\kappa = 0.44$.

2. By inspection of the ANOVA table, the only significant effect is the main effect for the advice mode. There is no interaction between hospital and group, and there is no difference, across groups in mean charges for the two hospitals. Examining the table of means and standard deviations, we see how the means are consistent across the two hospitals. The mean for all

participants in hospital A is 60.3 and the mean for all participants in hospital B is 59.1. This small difference is indicative of the lack of a main effect for hospitals. Also note that, even though the means for groups vary, the pattern of this variation is the same across the two hospitals. The main effect for the groups is seen in the differences in the means for each group. It appears that the difference occurs between the "no advice" group and the other two groups. Although the F test used in ANOVA can tell us only if a global difference exists across the three groups, methods exist to test differences between levels of the dependent variables.

3. Nonparallelism of lines is clearly suggestive of an interaction. A test using ANOVA is required to confirm that the interaction is statistically significant.

References

1. Indurkhya N, Weiss SM. Models for measuring performance of medical expert systems. AI Med 1989;1:61–70.
2. Titterington DM, Murray GD, Murray LS, et al. Comparison of discriminant techniques applied to a complex data set of head injured patients (with discussion). J R Stat Soc A 1981;144:145–175.
3. Wald N. Rational use of investigations in clinical practice. In: Hopkins A, ed. Appropriate Investigation and Treatment in Medical Practice. London: Royal College of Physicians, 1990:7–20.
4. Cohen J. Weighted kappa: nominal scale agreement with provision for scaled disagreement or partial credit. Psychol Bull 1968;70:213–220.
5. Fleiss JL. Measuring agreement between two judges on the presence or absence of a trait. Biometrics 1975;31:357–370.
6. Altman D. Practical Statistics for Medical Research. London: Chapman & Hall, 1991.
7. Hilden J, Habbema DF. Evaluation of clinical decision-aids: more to think about. Med Inf (Lond) 1990;15:275–284.
8. Hanley JA, McNeil BJ. The meaning and use of the area under a receiver operating characteristic (ROC) curve. Radiology 1982;143:29–36.
9. Swets JA. Measuring the accuracy of diagnostic systems. Science 1988;240:1285–1293.
10. O'Neil M, Glowinski A. Evaluating and validating very large knowledge-based systems. Med Inf 1990;15:237–252.
11. McDonald CJ, Hui SL, Smith DM, et al. Reminders to physicians from an introspective computer medical record. A two-year randomized trial. Ann Intern Med 1984;100:130–138.
12. Winer BJ. Statistical Principles in Experimental Design. New York: McGraw-Hill, 1991.
13. Wildemuth BM, Friedman CP, Downs SM. Hypertext vs. Boolean access to biomedical information: a comparison of effectiveness, efficiency, and user preferences. ACM Trans Computer-Human Interaction 1998;5:156–183.

14. Cohen J. Statistical Power Analysis for the Behavioral Sciences. Hillsdale, NJ: Lawrence Erlbaum, 1988.
15. Kleinbaum DG. Logistic regression. New York: Springer, 1992.
16. Bobbio M, Demichelis B, Ginstetto G. Completeness of reporting trial results: effect on physicians' willingness to prescribe. Lancet 1994;343:1209–1211.

9
Subjectivist Approaches to Evaluation

As usual, the most significant results of the project are not measurable with a t-test. (M. Musen, summarizing his experience with a 5-year project, personal communication, 1996)

With this chapter we turn a corner. The previous five chapters have dealt almost exclusively with objectivist approaches to evaluation. These approaches are useful for answering some, but by no means all, of the interesting and important questions that challenge investigators in biomedical informatics. The subjectivist approaches, introduced here and in Chapter 10, address the problem of evaluation from a different set of premises, as initially discussed in Chapter 2. These premises derive from philosophical views that may be unfamiliar and perhaps even discomforting to some readers. They challenge some fundamental beliefs about scientific method and the validity of our understanding of the world that develops from objectivist investigation. They argue that, particularly within the realm of evaluation of information resources, the kind of "knowing" that develops from subjectivist studies may be as useful as that which derives from objectivist studies. While reading what follows in this chapter, it may be tempting to dismiss subjectivist methods as informal, imprecise, or "subjective." When carried out well, however, these studies are none of the above. They are equally objective, but in a different way. Professionals in informatics, even those who choose not to conduct subjectivist studies, can come to appreciate the rigor, validity, and value of this work.

Chapter 2 introduced four subjectivist approaches to evaluation: connoisseurship, quasi-legal, professional review, and illuminative/responsive. Chapters 9 and 10 focus on what we have called the illuminative/responsive approach to evaluation.* This approach is rooted in the investigative traditions of ethnography and social anthropology, traditions that emphasize observation of naturally occurring behavior in defined cultural

---

* Many proponents of these methods refer to them generically as "qualitative" methods.

settings. These investigative methods have been extensively applied to the general problem of evaluating social programs, educational programs, and information technology. Our emphasis on this approach derives from the applicability it has found in evaluation and from the extensive methodological literature that has developed for it over the past three decades.

The major goals of this chapter are to establish the scientific legitimacy of subjectivist methods and to offer a general framework for understanding how studies using these methods are conducted. Chapter 10 provides a much more detailed tour through the methods of illuminative/responsive evaluation, and seeks to provide insight into how the thought processes of those who conduct these studies must differ from that of those who do objectivist work.

Motivation for Subjectivist Studies: What People Really Want to Know

In Chapter 2 we presented some prototypical evaluation questions:

- Is the information resource working as intended?
- How can it be improved?
- Does it make any difference?
- Are the differences it makes beneficial?
- Are the observed effects those envisioned by the developers or are they different?

We also noted that we could append "Why or why not?" to each of the questions listed above. The reader should take a moment to examine these questions carefully and begin to think about how we might go about answering them. When subjected to such deeper scrutiny, the questions quickly become more ornate and intricate:

- Is the resource working as intended?
  As who intended? Were the intentions set realistically? Did these intentions shift over time? What is it really like to use this resource as part of everyday professional activity?
- How can it be improved?
  How does one distinguish important from idiosyncratic suggestions for improvement? Which suggestions should be addressed?
- Does it make any difference?
  Was it needed in the first place? What features are making the difference?
- Are the differences it makes beneficial?
  To whom? From whose point of view? Are all the pertinent views represented?
- Are the observed effects those envisioned by the developers or are they different?
  How do you detect what you do not anticipate?

These more specific, more explanatory, and more probing questions, shown in italics, are often what those who commission evaluation studies—and others with interest in an information resource—want to know. Some of these deeper questions are difficult to answer using objectivist approaches to evaluation. It may be that these questions are never discussed, or are deferred as interesting but "subjective" issues during discussions of what should be the foci of an evaluation study. These questions may never be asked in a formal or official sense because of a perception that the methods do not exist to answer them in a credible way. This chapter and Chapter 10 beg readers to suspend their own tendencies to this belief.

Many of these deeper questions derive their importance from life in a pluralistic world. As discussed in Chapters 1 and 2, information resources are typically introduced into complex organizations where there exist competing value systems: different beliefs about what is "good" and what is "right," which translate into different beliefs about whether specific changes induced by information resources are beneficial or detrimental. These beliefs are real to the people who hold them and difficult to change. Indeed, there are many actors playing many roles in any real-world setting where an information resource is introduced. Each actor, as an individual and a member of multiple groups, brings a unique viewpoint to questions about inextricably fuzzy constructs such as need, quality, and benefit. If these constructs are explored in an evaluation study, perhaps the actors should not be expected to agree about what these constructs mean and how to measure them. Perhaps need, quality, and benefit do not inhere in an information resource. Perhaps they are dependent on the observer as well as the observed. Perhaps evaluation studies should be conducted in ways that document how these various individuals and groups "see" the resource, and not in ways that assume there is a consensus when there is no reason to believe one exists. Perhaps there are many "truths" about an information resource, not just one.

Definition of the Responsive/Illuminative Approach

The responsive/illuminative approach to evaluation is designed to address the deeper questions: the detailed "whys" and "according to whoms" in addition to the aggregate "whethers" and "whats." As defined in Chapter 2, the responsive/illuminative approach seeks to represent the viewpoints of those who are users of the resource or otherwise significant participants in the environment where the resource operates. The goal is "illumination" rather than judgment. The investigators seek to build an argument that promotes deeper understanding of the information resource or environment of which it is a part. The methods used derive largely from ethnography. As such, the investigators immerse themselves physically in the environment where the information resource is or will be operational and collect data primarily through observations, interviews, and reviews of documents. The designs—the data collection plans—of these studies are not rigidly prede- termined and do not unfold in a fixed sequence. They develop dynamically and nonlinearly as the investigators' experience accumulates. The study team begins with a minimal set of orienting questions; the deeper questions that receive more thorough study evolve from initial investigation. Investi- gators keep records of all data collected and the methods used to collect and analyze them. Reports of responsive/illuminative studies tend to be written narratives. Such studies can be conducted before, during, or after the introduction of an information resource.

Support for Subjectivist Approaches

It is not surprising that endorsements for subjectivist approaches come from those who routinely undertake such studies. A more compelling endorse- ment may come from designers of information resources themselves who believe that subjectivist methods can provide a deeper understanding of their own work and thus more useful information to guide their future efforts. As suggested by the quotation that began this chapter, the results of a study, when reduced to tables and tests of statistical significance, may no longer capture what the developers see as most important. When a study is "for" the developers, this can be a serious shortcoming.

Although subjectivist approaches may run counter to many readers' notions of how one conducts empirical investigations, these methods and their conceptual underpinnings are not at all foreign to the worlds of information and computer science. The pluralistic, nonlinear thinking that underlies subjectivist investigation shares many features with modern con- ceptualizations of the information resource design process. Consider the following statements from two highly regarded works addressing issues central to resource design. Winograd and Flores[1] argued as follows:

In designing computer-based devices, we are not in the position of creating a formal "system" that covers the functioning of the organization and the people within it. When this is attempted, the resulting system (and the space of potential action for people within it) is inflexible and unable to cope with new breakdowns or poten- tials. Instead we design additions and changes to the network of equipment (some of it computer based) within which people work. The computer is like a tool, in that it is brought up for use by people engaged in some domain of action. The use of the tool shapes the potential for what those actions are and how they are conducted. . . . Its power does not lie in having a single purpose . . . but in its connection to the larger network of communication (electronic, telephone, paper-based) in which organizations operate [p. 170].

Norman[2] added:

Tools affect more than the ease with which we do things; they can dramatically affect our view of ourselves, society, and the world [p. 209].

These thoughts from the work of system designers alert us to the multiple forces that shape the "effects" of introducing an information resource, the unpredictable character of these forces, and the many viewpoints on these effects that exist. These sentiments are highly consonant with the premises underlying the subjectivist evaluation approaches.

Another connection is to the methodology of formal systems analysis, generally accepted as an essential component of information resource development. Systems analysis uses many methods that resemble closely the subjectivist methods for evaluation that we introduce here. It is recognized that systems analysis requires a process of information gathering about the present system before a design for an improved future system can be inferred. Systems analysis requires a process of information gathering, heavily reliant on interviews with those who use the existing system in various ways. Information gathering for systems analysis is typically portrayed as a cyclical, iterative process rather than a linear process.[3] In the literature of systems analysis we find admonitions, analogous to those made by proponents of subjectivist evaluation, about an approach that is too highly structured. An overly structured approach can misportray the capabilities of workers in the system's environment, misportray the role of informal communication in the work accomplished, underestimate the prevalence of exceptions, and fail to account for political forces within every organization that shape much of what happens.[4] Within the field of systems analysis, then, there has developed an appreciation of some of the shortcomings of objectivist methods and the potential value of subjectivist methods drawn from ethnography that we discuss here.[5]

Also worthy of note is the high regard in which studies using subjectivist methods are held when these studies are well conducted. In biomedicine, one prominent example is Becker's[6] classic *Boys in White*. Another is Bosk's[7] superb work, *Forgive and Remember: Managing Medical Failure*. Several valuable studies in biomedical informatics are referenced in the following section.

Are Subjectivist Studies Useful in Informatics?

It is possible to argue that subjectivist approaches are applicable at all stages of development of an information resource, but they are most clearly applicable at two points in this continuum. First, as part of the design process, a subjectivist study can document the need for the resource and clarify its potential niche within a given work environment.[8,9] Indeed, it is possible for system developers to misread or misinterpret the needs and beliefs of potential users of an information resource[10,11] in ways that could lead to failure of an entire project. Formal subjectivist methods, if applied appropriately, can clarify these issues and direct resource development toward a more valid understanding of user needs. There is already a substantial literature and sense of general support for use of subjectivist methods at the design stage of a resource.[8–12] At this point, the relation between subjectivist evaluation and the methods of formal systems analysis is most evident.

Second, after an information resource is mature and has been tested in laboratory studies, further study using subjectivist approaches can describe the impact of the resource on the work environments in which it is installed.[13–17] At this developmental stage, the insights that can derive from objectivist and subjectivist studies are different and potentially complementary.[18,19] Objectivist methods, and specifically the comparison-based approach, have dominated the literature on the impact of information resources. The randomized clinical trial has been put forward as the standard against which such studies should be measured.[20] Although the randomized trial can estimate the magnitude of an effect of interest for an information resource, this method cannot elucidate the meaning of this effect for users of the resource and other interested parties, and typically sheds little light on whether the effect of interest to the evaluation as conducted was the effect of most importance. Whether the impact of a resource is better established by objectivist methods derived from the clinical trials tradition, or by subjectivist methods derived from the ethnographic tradition, is and should be a matter of ongoing discussion with those who are commissioning the study. Overall, subjectivist study of deployed information resources remains a relatively unexploited opportunity in biomedical informatics.

Rigorous, But Different, Methodology

The subjectivist approaches to evaluation, like their objectivist counterparts, are empirical methods. Although it is easy to focus only on their differences, objectivist and subjectivist approaches to evaluation share many general features. In all empirical studies, for example, evidence is collected with great care; the investigator is always aware of what he or she is doing and why. The evidence is then compiled, interpreted, and ultimately reported. Investigators keep records of their procedures, and these records are open to subsequent audit by the investigators themselves or by individuals outside the study team. The principal investigator or evaluation team leader is under an almost sacred scientific obligation to report his/her methods in detail, ideally in enough detail to enable another investigator to replicate the study. Failure to be able to do so invalidates any study.

The two approaches also share a dependence on theories that guide investigators toward explanations of the phenomena they observe, and share a dependence on the pertinent empirical literature: published studies that address similar phenomena or similar settings. Within objectivist and subjectivist approaches, there are rules of good practice that are generally accepted. It is therefore possible to distinguish a good study from a bad one. Finally, a neophyte can learn either or both types of approaches, initially by reading textbooks and other methodological literature and ultimately by conducting studies under the guidance of experienced mentors.

There are, at the same time, many fundamental differences between objectivist and subjectivist approaches. First and foremost, subjectivist studies are "emergent" in design. Objectivist studies typically begin with a set of hypotheses or specific questions and a plan for addressing each member of this set. There is also an assumption by the investigator that, barring major unforeseen developments, the plan will be followed exactly. (When objectivist investigators deviate from their plan, they do so apologetically and view their having done it as a limitation of their study.) Not following the plan is seen as a source of bias, because the investigator who sees negative results emerging from the exploration of a particular question or use of a particular measurement instrument might change strategies in the hope of obtaining more positive findings. By contrast, subjectivist studies typically begin with some general orienting issues that stimulate the early stages of investigation. Through these initial investigations, the important questions for further study begin to emerge. The subjectivist investigator is willing, at virtually any point, to adjust future aspects of the study in light of the most recent information obtained. Subjectivist investigators are incrementalists; they live from day to day and have a high tolerance for ambiguity and uncertainty. (In this respect, they are again much like good software developers.) Also like software developers, skilled subjectivist investigators must develop the ability to recognize when a project is finished—when further benefit can be obtained only at great cost in time and effort.

A second feature of subjectivist studies is a "naturalistic" orientation—a reluctance to manipulate the setting of the study, which in most cases is the work environment into which the information resource is introduced. Because subjectivist studies avoid altering the environment in order to study it, these studies have an appealing "ecological validity." There is no question that the results apply to the exact setting, work process, and culture within which the information resource under study is deployed. The extent to which the results can be safely generalized from that specific setting to other similar settings depends very much on local circumstances. In subjectivist investigation, however, the aim is rarely to generalize to other settings, and more usually to gain better insight and understanding into the specific setting under scrutiny. Control groups, placebos, purposefully altering information resources to create contrasting interventions, and other techniques central to the construction of objectivist studies are typically not used in subjectivist work. Subjectivist studies do employ quantitative data for descriptive purposes and may additionally offer quantitative comparisons when the study setting offers up a natural experiment where such comparisons can be made without altering how work is organized or performed in that environment. Subjectivist investigators are opportunists where pertinent information is concerned; they use what they see as the best information available to illuminate a question under investigation.

A third important distinguishing feature of subjectivist studies is seen in their product or "deliverable"; they result in reports written in narrative prose. Although these reports can be lengthy and may require a more significant time investment on the part of the reader, no technical understanding of quantitative methods or statistics is required to comprehend them fully. Results of subjectivist studies are therefore accessible to a broad community—and even entertaining—in a way that results of objectivist studies are not. Reports of subjectivist studies seek to engage their audience.

Subjectivist Arguments and Their Philosophical Premises

Subjectivist studies do not seek to prove or demonstrate. They strive for insightful description—what has been called "thick description"[21]—leading to deeper understanding of the phenomenon under study. They offer an argument; they seek to persuade rather than demonstrate.[22]*

It has been emphasized that the purpose of evaluation is to be useful to various "stakeholders": those with a need to know. These needs vary from study to study, and within a given study the needs vary across the different stakeholder groups over time. A major feature of subjectivist approaches is their responsiveness to these needs.[23] The foci of a study are formulated though a process of negotiation, to ensure their relevance from the outset. These foci can be changed in light of accumulating evidence to guarantee their continuing relevance. As with objectivist methods, subjectivist methods are therefore concordant with the basic tenets of evaluation as a process that, in order to be successful, must be useful in addition to truthful.

As our discussion of subjectivist methods unfolds, it becomes clear that there are numerous features working to ensure that well-executed studies meet the dual criteria of utility and veracity. At this point, we might ask whether a method that is so open-ended and responsive can also generate confidence in the veracity of the findings. In so doing, we come immediately to the general issue of what makes evidence credible. Objectivist studies rely on methods of quantitative measurement, discussed in great detail earlier in this book, which in turn are based on the principle of intersubjectivity, what might also be called *quantitative objectivity*.[24] Simply stated,

---

* At this point, the reader is encouraged to refer to the "Evaluation Mindset" section of Chapter 2 to see the concordance between subjectivist methods and the broad purposes of evaluation as described earlier.

this principle holds that the more independent observers who agree with an observation, the more likely it is to be correct. (Recall that in Chapter 5 we developed a specific method for implementing this principle.) Indeed, within the objectivist mindset, unless we can show that several observers agree to an acceptable extent, their observations are *prima facie* not credible. One observer is not to be trusted. By contrast, the principle of *qualitative objectivity* is central to subjectivist work. It holds that an experienced, unbiased observer is capable of making fundamentally truthful observations that may, in fact, be superior to those of a panel of observers who agree but are all wrong because of some bias they share. In this light, subjectivist approaches can be seen to be as objective (i.e., truthful) as objectivist studies. They rely, however, on a different definition of objectivity.

We can also contrast objectivist and subjectivist approaches on the ways they address issues of cause and effect. How can cause-and-effect relationships be established without the experimental control customary to randomized trials? In subjectivist investigation, a case for cause and effect can be made in much the same way that a detective determines the perpetrator of a crime or a forensic pathologist infers cause of death.[25] Through detailed examination of evidence, the investigator recreates the pertinent story, often depicting in great detail a number of critical events or incidents. Via this portrayal, the investigator crafts a logical, compelling case for cause and effect. In the end, such a portrayal can be as compelling as the result of a controlled experiment that is subject to the manifold biases described in Chapter 7.

Natural History of a Subjectivist Study

As a first step in describing the method of subjectivist evaluation, Figure 9.1 illustrates the stages or natural history of a study. These stages comprise a general sequence, but, as mentioned earlier, the subjectivist investigator must always be prepared to revise his or her thinking and possibly return to earlier stages in light of new evidence. Backtracking is a legitimate aspect of this model.

1. *Negotiation of the "ground rules" of the study:* During any empirical research, and particularly for evaluation studies, it is important to negotiate an understanding between the study team and those commissioning the study. This understanding should embrace the general aims of the study; the kinds of methods to be used; access to various sources of information including health care providers, patients, and documents; and the format for interim and final reports. The aims of the study might be formulated in a set of initial "orienting questions." Ideally, this understanding is expressed in a memorandum of understanding, analogous to a contract, signed by all

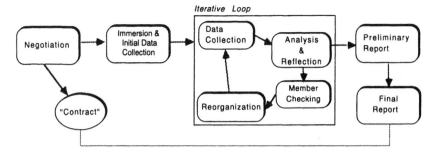

FIGURE 9.1. Natural history of a subjectivist study.

interested parties. By analogy to a contract, these ground rules can be changed during a study with the consent of all parties. (Although essential to a subjectivist study, a memo of understanding or evaluation contract is recommended for all studies, irrespective of methods employed.)

2a. *Immersion into the environment:* At this stage the investigators begin spending time in the work environment. The activities range from formal introductions to informal conversations and the silent presence of the investigators at meetings and other events. Investigators use the generic term *field* to refer to the setting, which may be multiple physical locations, where the work under study is carried out. Trust and openness between the investigators and those in the field are essential elements of subjectivist studies. If a subjectivist study is in fact to generate insights with minimal alteration of the environment under study, those who live and work in the field (clinicians, patients, researchers, students, and others) must feel sufficiently comfortable with the presence of the investigators to go about their work in the customary way. Time invested by the investigators in building such relationships pays compound interest in the future.

2b. *Initial data collection to focus the questions:* Even as immersion is taking place, the investigator is already collecting data to sharpen the initial questions or issues guiding the study. The early discussions with those in the field and other activities primarily targeted toward immersion inevitably begin to shape the investigators' views. Immersion and initial data collection are labeled "2a" and "2b" to convey their close interaction. Almost from the outset, the investigator is typically addressing several aspects of the study simultaneously.

3. *Iterative loop:* At this point, the procedural structure of the study becomes akin to an iterative loop as the investigator engages in cycles of data collection, analysis and reflection, and reorganization. Data collection involves interview, observation, document analysis, and other methods. Data are collected on planned occasions as well as serendipitously or spontaneously. The data are carefully recorded and interpreted in the context of what is already known. Reflection entails the contemplation of the new find-

ings during each cycle of the loop. Reorganization results in a revised agenda for data collection in the next cycle of the loop.

Although each cycle within the iterative loop is depicted as linear or unidirectional, even this portrayal is somewhat misleading. The net progress through the loop is clockwise, as shown in Figure 9.1, but backward steps within each cycle are both natural and inevitable. They are not reflective of mistakes or errors. An investigator may, after conducting a series of interviews and studying what participants have said, decide to speak again with one or two participants to clarify their positions on a particular issue.

An important element of the iterative loop, which can be considered part of the reflection process, is sharing of the investigator's own thoughts and beliefs with the participants themselves. (This step is called "member checking" and is discussed in more detail in Chapter 10.) Within the objectivist tradition, member checking might "unblind" the study and introduce bias. In the subjectivist tradition, the views of informed participants on the investigators' evolving conclusions are considered a key resource.

4. *Preliminary report:* The first draft of the final report should itself be viewed as a form of investigative instrument. By sharing this draft report with a variety of individuals, a major check on the validity of the findings can be obtained. Typically, reactions to the preliminary report generate useful clarification and a general sharpening of the study findings. Sometimes (but rarely if previous stages of the study have been carried out with care), reactions to the preliminary report generate needs for further data to be collected. Because the subjectivist study report is usually a narrative, it is vitally important that it be relatively concise and well written, in language understood by all intended audiences. Circulation of the report in draft can ensure that the final document communicates as intended. Liberal use of anonymous quotations from interviews and documents, distinguished typographically from the main text, makes a report highly vivid and meaningful to readers.

5. *Final report:* The final report, once completed, should be distributed as negotiated in the original memorandum of understanding. In subjectivist evaluation studies, distribution of the report is often accompanied by "meet the investigator" sessions that allow interested persons to explore the study findings interactively and in greater depth.

As shown in Figure 9.2, the natural history of a subjectivist study results in the progressive focusing of issues. Parlett and Hamilton[26] describe a transition from stage to stage, as the investigation unfolds, with problem areas becoming progressively clarified and redefined. The course of the study cannot be charted precisely in advance. Beginning with an extensive database, the investigators systematically reduce the breadth of their inquiry to give more concentrated attention to the emerging issues. This "progressive focusing" permits unique and unpredicted phenomena to be given due

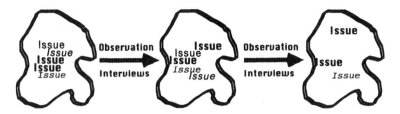

FIGURE 9.2. Process of progressive focusing.

weight. It reduces the problem of data overload and prevents the accumulation of a mass of unanalyzed material.

Data Collection Methods

What data collection strategies are in the subjectivist investigator's black bag? There are several methods, and they are typically used in combination. We discuss each one, assuming a typical setting for a subjectivist study in biomedical informatics: the introduction of an information resource into patient care activities in a hospital ward. These methods are discussed in greater detail in Chapter 10.

1. *Observation:* Investigators typically immerse themselves in the setting under study. This is done in two ways. The investigator may act purely as a detached observer, becoming a trusted, unobtrusive feature of the environment but not a participant in the day-to-day work and thus reliant on multiple "informants" as sources of information. True to the naturalistic feature of this kind of study, great care is taken during the investigator's immersion into the environment. This should diminish the possibility that the presence of the observer will skew the work activities that occur, or that the observer will be rejected outright by the ward team. An alternative approach is participant-observation, in which the investigator becomes to some degree a member of the work team. Participant-observation is more difficult to engineer, as it will require the investigator to have training in some aspect of health care. It is also much more time-consuming but can give the investigator a more vivid impression of life in the work environment. During both kinds of observation, data accrue continuously. These data are qualitative and may be of several varieties: statements by health care providers and patients, gestures and other nonverbal expressions of these same individuals, and characteristics of the physical setting that seem to affect the delivery of health care.

2. *Interviews:* Subjectivist studies rely heavily on interviews. Formal interviews are occasions where both the investigator and interviewee are aware that the answers to questions are being recorded (on paper or tape)

for direct contribution to the evaluation study. Formal interviews vary in their degree of structure. At one extreme is the unstructured interview where there are no predetermined questions. Between the extremes is the semi-structured interview where the investigator specifies in advance a set of topics he or she would like to address but is flexible as to the order in which these topics are addressed and open to discussion of topics not on the prespecified list. At the other extreme is the structured interview with a schedule of questions that are always presented in the same words and in the same order. In general, the unstructured and semi-structured interviews are preferred for subjectivist studies. Informal interviews, spontaneous discussions between the investigators and members of a ward team that occur during routine observation, are also part of the data collection process and are considered a source of important data.

3. *Document/artifact analysis:* Organized human activity produces a trail of paper and other artifacts. In biomedical informatics, these include patient charts, the original researchers' notes, various versions of computer programs and their documentation, memos prepared by the project team, and others. Unlike the day-to-day events of patient care, these artifacts do not change once created or introduced. They can be examined retrospectively and referred to repeatedly as necessary over the course of a study. Records accrued as part of the routine use of an information resource, such as automatically generated user log files, are key artifacts of biomedical informatics projects. Data from these records are often quantifiable, and are frequently analyzed quantitatively even within the framework of a subjectivist study.

4. *Anything else that seems useful:* Subjectivist investigators are supreme opportunists. As questions of importance to a study emerge, they collect the best information perceived to bear on these questions. In this way, subjectivist studies can include clinical chart analysis, questionnaires, tests, simulated patients, and other methods more commonly associated with the objectivist approaches. Rarely, however, does a subjectivist study deliberately manipulate the work setting, as is common in objectivist studies, for the purpose of collecting data and seeking to demonstrate cause and effect.

Qualitative Data Recording and Analysis

As mentioned earlier, subjectivist investigators keep careful records of their procedures and are extremely diligent in their handling of qualitative data. Data gathered from observations, interviews, and document analysis are recorded and usually reviewed within 24 hours of initial recording. In the case of interviews and other discussions with participants in the work setting, this review is particularly important if there is no permanent record of the discussion on tape and the only documentation that exists is the investigator's own notes rapidly jotted during the conversation. Even when the interview has been tape recorded, listening to the tape soon after the interview was conducted can stimulate thoughts that might not occur to the investigator later. During this review the investigator should annotate the notes, being careful to maintain the distinction between what was recorded during the interview itself and what is subsequent annotation or interpretation. Some investigators do this by writing their annotations in a different color than the original notes; others use a two-column format where original notes appear on the left, annotations on the right. A careful investigator must also distinguish between verbatim quotations and paraphrasing of what an interviewee said.

There are many systematic procedures for analyzing qualitative data. In general terms, the investigator looks for themes or insights emerging from several sources. Thus it is important to be able to collate individual statements and observations by theme as well as by source. Traditionally, investigators would transfer these observations to file cards so they could be sorted and resorted in a variety of ways, and this method is still sometimes used. However, contemporary investigators typically use software—either a standard spreadsheet or word processor, or a purpose-written application—to facilitate analysis of qualitative data.[27] Highly portable hand-held computing devices will increasingly benefit subjectivist investigators by enabling them to record in the field notes that can load directly into analytic software, avoiding the need for transcription as a separate expensive and time-consuming step.

The analysis process is fluid, with analytical goals shifting as the study becomes more mature. At an early stage the goal is primarily to identify and then focus the questions that are to be the targets of further data elicitation. At the later stages of study, the primary goal is to collate data that address these questions. The investigator must recognize that the data often raise new questions in addition to answering preexisting ones. Sometimes new data do not alter the basic conclusions of a study but reveal to the investigator how a significant reorganization of the results will lend greater clarity to their exposition. (This situation is analogous to a linear transformation in mathematics; the same information is contained in the data set but is expressed relative to a different and more revealing set of axes.)

Subjectivist study requires a frame of mind on the part of the investigator different from that in objectivist study. The agenda is never closed. The investigator must always be alert to new information that may require a systemic reorganization of everything he or she has done so far. For these reasons, many heuristic strategies and safeguards are built into the process. Just as there are well-documented procedures for collecting data while conducting subjectivist studies, there is also a set of strategies used by investigators to validate results and insights. A few are noted here and are discussed in more detail in Chapter 10.

Triangulation is a strong check on the veracity of study findings. The subjectivist investigator looks across different types of information (observation of work events, interviews of individuals from a variety of roles, analysis of documents) to determine if a consistent picture emerges for any given theme of the results. In some ways this is the subjectivist analogy to the objectivist strategy of using multiple, independent measures to estimate the quantitative error in a measurement process.

A useful strategy when trying to ensure that all issues of high relevance to a study have been identified and explored is to seek *closure*, *saturation*, or *convergence*. In very general terms, these three concepts suggest that if the investigators remain properly open-ended throughout their approaches to participants, and no longer hear anything substantially new, it is likely that they have identified the full range of issues as well as the full range of views about each one.

Verification by individuals external to the study and by participants themselves is another important check on the veracity of the findings. When people familiar with the setting of a study read a report or a preliminary document, the message should be meaningful or insightful to them. They should say, perhaps with enthusiasm, "Yes, that's right. You've portrayed it correctly." External verification can be sought by asking an experienced investigator not associated with this particular study to review for logical consistency the data and the derived conclusions. What is sought here is not necessarily agreement with the conclusions themselves but, rather, an affirmation that the conclusions were reached in a scientifically competent and responsible manner, and that the conclusions are consistent with the data on which they are based. Members of a study team routinely audit each other, but the addition of external reviewers reduces the possibility that some perspective affecting the entire team will skew the results.

Comparing Objectivist and Subjectivist Studies: Importance of a Level Playing Field

When all is said and done, how do we know that the findings of a subjectivist study are "correct"? How do we know if the findings carry any truth? What makes a study of this type more than one person's opinion, or the opinion of a study team that may share a certain preexisting perspective on the resource under study? To explore this question fairly, both subjectivist and objectivist studies should be seen as belonging to a more general family of methods for empirical investigation. Neither approach should be placed on the defensive and required to prove itself against a set of standards produced by proponents of the other. When seen in this light, the credibility of both objectivist and subjectivist approaches derives from five sources:

- Belief in the philosophical basis of the approach
- Existence of rules of good practice

- The investigators' adherence to these rules
- Accessibility of the data to others if necessary
- Value of the resulting studies to their respective audiences

We discussed how these factors apply to objectivist studies earlier in the book, and we have discussed them as they apply to subjectivist studies to some extent in this chapter. A more thorough discussion is found in Chapter 10.

Ultimately, each reader of this volume must make a personal judgment about the credibility of any of the evaluation approaches presented. None of the approaches is beyond challenge. We specifically caution the reader against establishing an objectivist approach as a standard, and then assessing subjectivist approaches using the specific characteristics of this standard. This would inequitably frame the competition using the logic, definitions, and assumptions unique to one of the competitors. For example, consider the question of whether subjectivist approaches can establish causality as well as their objectivist counterparts. If cause and effect are defined as proponents of objectivist methods see the world, of course the answer is no. (Objectivist work establishes cause and effect through randomization and experimental control. Since subjectivist work does not employ randomization and control, it cannot therefore establish cause and effect.) The argument changes if cause and effect are defined more generically, however. If both sides accept that one can establish cause and effect by building a logical, believable case, they will conclude that both objectivist and subjectivist approaches can approach such issues. They will just do it differently.

It is also human nature to compare anything relatively new to an idealization of what is familiar. Because objectivist studies may be more familiar, it is tempting to compare subjectivist methods against the perfect objectivist study, which is never realized in practice. Every objectivist study has limitations that are usually articulated at the end of a study report. Many such reports end with a lengthy list of limitations and cautions and a statement that further research is needed. For these reasons, rarely has any one study, objectivist or subjectivist, ended a controversy over an issue of scientific or social importance.

Two Example Abstracts

To convey both the substance and some of the style of subjectivist work in informatics, we include below abstracts of two published studies. The first is Forsythe's[10] 1992 work, which had substantial impact on a project at the design stage. The second is Aydin's[13] 1989 work, which addressed the impact of a deployed information resource.

Forsy the Abstract

The problem of user acceptance of knowledge-based systems is a current concern in medical informatics. User acceptance should increase when system-builders understand both the needs of potential users and the context in which a system will be used. Ethnography is one source of such understanding. This paper describes the contribution of ethnography (and an anthropological perspective) during the first year of a 3-year interdisciplinary project to build a patient education system on migraine. Systematic fieldwork is producing extensive data on the information needs of migraineurs. These data call into question some of the assumptions on which our project was based. Although it is not easy to rethink our assumptions and their implications for design, using ethnography has enabled us to undertake this process relatively early in the project at a time when redesign costs are low. It should greatly improve our chances of building a system that meets the needs of real users, thus avoiding the troublesome problem of user acceptance.[10]

Aydin Abstract

This paper explores the effects of computerized medical information systems on the occupational communities of health care professionals in hospitals. Interviews were conducted with informants from the pharmacy and nursing departments at two hospitals currently using medical information systems for communicating physicians' medication orders from the nursing station to the pharmacy. Results showed changes in tasks for both pharmacy and nursing, resulting in increased interdependence between the two departments. This interdependence was accompanied by improved communication and cooperation, providing an opportunity [to] encourage better working relationships between departments. The use and maintenance of the common computerized data base became a superordinate goal for the two groups, with the computer system itself as the topic of communication.[13]"

Food for Thought

1. Return to Self-Test 2.2. After rereading the case study presented there, consider the following questions:
   a. What specific evaluation issues in this case are better addressed by objectivist methods and which are better addressed by subjectivist methods?
   b. If you were conducting a subjectivist study of the T-HELPER project, consider the various data collection modalities you might employ. Whom would you interview? What events would you observe? What artifacts would you examine?
   c. How would you immerse yourself into the environment of this project?
2. Consider the following about subjectivist' studies:
   a. Are they/can they be credible in the world of biomedicine?
   b. What personal attributes must a subjectivist investigator have?
   c. Which of these attributes do you personally have?

d. Should medical informatics professionals themselves perform these studies, or should they be "farmed out" to anthropologists or other social scientists?

References

1. Winograd T, Flores F. Understanding Computers and Cognition: A New Foundation for Design. Reading, MA: Addison-Wesley, 1987.
2. Norman DA. The Design of Everyday Things. New York: Basic Books, 1996.
3. Davis WS. Business Systems Design and Analysis. Belmont, CA: Wadsworth, 1994.
4. Bansler JP, Bødker K. A reappraisal of structured analysis: design in an organizational context. ACM Transact Inf Syst 1993;11:165–193.
5. Zachary WW, Strong GW, Zaklad A. Information systems ethnography: integrating anthropological methods into system design to insure organizational acceptance. In: Hendrick HW, Brown O, eds. Human Factors in Organizational Design and Management. Amsterdam: North Holland, 1984:223–227.
6. Becker H. Boys in White: Student Culture in Medical School. Chicago: University of Chicago Press, 1963.
7. Bosk CL. Forgive and Remember: Managing Medical Failure. Chicago: University of Chicago Press, 1979.
8. Fafchamps D, Young CY, Tang PC. Modelling work practices: input to the design of the physician's workstation. Symp Comput Applications Med Care 1991;15: 788–792.
9. Osheroff JA, Forsythe DE, Buchanan BG, Bankowitz RA, Blumenfeld BH, Miller R. Analysis of clinical information needs using questions posed in a teaching hospital. Ann Intern Med 1991;14:576–581.
10. Forsythe DE. Using ethnography to build a working system: rethinking basic design assumptions. Symp Comput Applications Med Care 1992;16:505–509.
11. Forsythe DE. New bottles, old wine: hidden cultural assumptions in a computerized explanation system for migraine sufferers. Med Anthropol Q 1996;10: 551–574.
12. Forsythe DE. Using ethnography to investigate life scientists' information needs. Bull Med Libr Assoc 1998;86(3):402–409.
13. Aydin CE. Occupational adaptation to computerized medical information systems. J Health Soc Behav 1989;30:163–179.
14. Kaplan B. Initial impact of a clinical laboratory computer system. J Med Syst 1987;11:137–147.
15. Wilson SR, Starr-Schneidkraut N, Cooper MD. Use of the Critical Incident Technique to Evaluate the Impact of MEDLINE. Palo Alto, CA: American Institutes of Research, 1989. Final Report to the National Library of Medicine under contract N01–LM-83529.
16. Travers DA, Downs SM. Comparing user acceptance of a computer system in two pediatric offices: a qualitative study. Proc AMIA Symp 2000;24:853–857.
17. Ash J, Gorman PN, Lavelle M, et al. A cross-site qualitative study of physician order entry. J Am Med Inform Assoc 2003;10:188–200.
18. Kaplan B, Duchon D. Combining qualitative and quantitative methods in information systems research: a case study. MIS Quarterly 1988;12:571–586.

19. Manning B, Gadd CS. Introducing handheld computing into a residency program: preliminary results from qualitative and quantitative inquiry. Proc AMIA Symp 2001;25:428–432.
20. Hunt DL, Haynes RB, Hanna SE, Smith K. Effects of computer-based clinical decision support systems on physician performance and patient outcomes. JAMA 1998;280:1339–1346.
21. Geertz C. The Interpretation of Cultures. New York: Basic Books, 1973.
22. House ER. Evaluating with Validity. Beverly Hills: Sage, 1980.
23. Stake RE. Evaluating the Arts in Education: A Responsive Approach. Columbus, OH: Merrill, 1975.
24. Scriven M. Objectivity and subjectivity in educational research. In: Thomas LG, ed. Philosophical Redirection of Educational Research. National Society for the Study of Education. Chicago: University of Chicago Press, 1972.
25. Scriven M. Maximizing the power of causal investigations: the modus operandi method. In: Popham WJ, ed. Evaluation in Education. Berkeley, CA: McCutchan, 1974.
26. Parlett M, Hamilton D. Evaluation as illumination. In: Parlett M, Dearden G, eds. Intro duction to Illuminative Evaluation. Cardiff-by-the-Sea, CA: Pacific Soundings, 1977.
27. Fielding NG, Lee RM. Using Computers in Qualitative Research. Newbury Park, CA: Sage, 1991.

10
Performing Subjectivist Studies in the Qualitative Traditions Responsive to Users*

According to the typology of evaluation approaches introduced in Chapter 2 and based on the work of House, four different approaches fall under the subjectivist tradition: quasi-legal, art criticism, professional review, and responsive/illuminative. This chapter focuses on the last of the four approaches: the subjectivist tradition that is responsive to the multiple stakeholders engaged in any evaluation activity. This is a particularly apt approach for evaluating biomedical informatics projects and information resources, since the success of these efforts most often depends on understanding and meeting the needs of the resource developers, the end users, and other important constituencies that inevitably are engaged in these complex undertakings.

The methods discussed in this chapter have many different labels. They are sometimes called "interpretive" to connote that they seek to go beyond simple documentation and description of phenomena. They are sometimes called "qualitative" to connote the predominantly non-numerical nature of the data that are collected and the non-statistical methods of data analysis. They are sometimes called "naturalistic"[1] to connote that studies are performed without purposeful manipulation of the environment under study. Since no single term does full justice to these methods, we use multiple terms in the title of this chapter, and we consider the terms *qualitative, subjectivist, responsive*, and *interpretive* as practically synonymous.

Whereas the previous chapter offered an overview of the subjectivist family of approaches and provided much of the rationale for their value to biomedical informatics, this chapter has more of a "how to do it" character. While there are many schools of thought about how to pursue these kinds of evaluation (discussed in Appendix A of this chapter), we focus on the methods that we have found most relevant to the domain of biomedical informatics. The references cited in the chapter can provide further information on both the methodological issues and the philosophical underpinnings of these approaches. The two appendices provide additional detail.

---

* This chapter was written by Joan S. Ash, Allen C. Smith III, and P. Zoë Stavri.

What Do We Mean by Qualitative Studies?

Strauss and Corbin[2] define qualitative/subjectivist research (and, by extension, evaluation) as "any type of research that produces findings not arrived at by statistical procedures or other means of quantification." Qualitative studies generally gather data in an open-ended way through interviews or observation, and the data are then progressively interpreted by the investigators. These data are usually words and pictures, not numbers. Qualitative studies are usually conducted at the site where the work of interest is actually being done; typically these are sites where an information resource is or will be in actual use. This study setting is called "the field" and the studies themselves are often called field studies.

Qualitative studies are designed so that the topic of interest is considered within a larger context. For example, a clinical researcher's success in using a new protocol management system depends in part on whether the system is consistent with other features of the local research environment such as institutional human subjects procedures and perceptions of the system by colleagues. Qualitative methods might be used to evaluate the system within such a context, and the data collected can be the source of both rich descriptions and explanations. Qualitative methods can illuminate the evolution of important phenomena over time if the study has an historical component; they can indicate what led up to certain consequences; they can lead to new questions and insights; and their results can be presented in particularly vivid ways by using quotes to illustrate points. As discussed in the previous chapter, well-executed qualitative studies are credible, dependable, and replicable. (Readers interested in the variants of qualitative methods that have evolved over time may wish to refer to Appendix A at this point.)

Why Is It Important to Understand the Qualitative Framework?

Qualitative/subjectivist studies have become an accepted alternative or complement to quantitative/objectivist studies in the health care literature because they make it possible to address certain research questions that cannot be investigated any other way. Because they accommodate study of "attitudes, beliefs, and preferences, and the whole question of how evidence is turned into practice,"[3] they are ideal for evaluating information resource implementation processes, for example. Like their objectivist counterparts, subjectivist studies can be done either well or poorly. Examples of both exist in the literature. It is therefore critical that persons knowledgeable in informatics be able to distinguish the useful studies from the flawed ones, as well as be able to do high-quality evaluation studies themselves.

When Are Qualitative Studies Appropriate?

A study design needs to be appropriate for the investigative questions and for the setting. For evaluation of biomedical information resources, knowledge of the context or environment within which the implementation takes place is critical. Diana Forsythe,[4] an anthropologist who was influential in promoting the use of qualitative studies for evaluation of biomedical information systems, has offered strong arguments in favor of studying these resources as they are used in context. Kaplan[5] has outlined four areas for which qualitative evaluations are most useful: when the focus is on communication, care, control, and context or, as she calls them, the 4 C's. If the investigator seeks to evaluate human interactions, the effects on delivery of care, the political aspects of a system, or the importance of the practice setting on the success of an implementation, all of which involve context and the social environment, he should consider using qualitative methods. Qualitative techniques are especially useful, therefore, when studying informatics applications at the organizational level, such as enterprise-level implementation of systems designed for use by health care providers or biomedical researchers.

Case Example

The rest of this chapter proceeds in the context of an example. We present it first here, and then revisit it to illustrate aspects of qualitative methods arising in this discussion.

The Nouveau Clinic has recently selected an electronic medical record (EMR) system for its five community practices. After a year of exploration and consultation, the administration and information technology staff determined they had found the most effective system and, anxious to move forward, decided that after a 6-month transition period, all patient records in the clinics would be in the system. Anticipating some problems with the clinical staff, they asked a consultant to evaluate the new system and the implementation process over a 2-year period. They expect the evaluation to provide the basis for smoothing out the rough spots in the system and to guide the training and ongoing support they provide to staff. Their working assumption is that the clinical staff will grumble at first, but will accept the system after a short period of time.

As we begin to think about what this consultant might do, we can imagine a wide range of possibilities in terms of the focus (workflow and efficiency issues, quality of health care and patient safety, attitudes of personnel, and others), the calendar for the evaluation (a short project to help develop the training to be provided or a longer study to find and address currently unknown issues), and the boundaries of the problem (a narrow look into the new system, or a wider look at the other issues that are inevitably attached to it). Selection among these alternatives would be required at the beginning of the study, particularly in view of the management expectation, whether justified or not, that the clinicians will accept the EMR after a short transition period. It is also critical to realize that the initial answers to these questions might change as new facts are clarified and new questions identified. More fundamentally, it would be essential to clarify the character of the evaluation, and then maintain contact with the client group at the Nouveau Clinic to ensure that the outcomes are understandable and present no major surprises when submitted in a final report. These points, and many others, all imply the need for serious discussion early in the life of the study.

What Distinguishes Qualitative Inquiry?

Qualitative inquiry, when successfully undertaken, answers research and evaluation questions at two levels: descriptive and explanatory. At the descriptive level, the conclusions that emerge offer a "thick description," a term initially used by Geertz[6] in application to ethnography.* Thick description portrays "particular events, rituals, and customs" in detail.[7] At the explanatory level, qualitative inquiry also offers interpretation of the events that are described. If the conclusions of a study are to have utility, they must go beyond the telling of a story, no matter how interesting that story may be. To offer a useful indication of the value inherent in an information resource or service, the study must do more than assemble the apparent facts. Qualitative inquiry, like all other serious inquiry, must combine description with explanation. How this is accomplished is the major focus of this chapter.

Qualitative inquiry both draws upon and builds theory. Many kinds of theory come into play at different stages of a study. Personal theory stems from an investigator's own professional training and background. "Hunches" based on personal experience fall into this category. A second type of theory, somewhat more formal in nature, is based on prior research by others who do work closely related to that of the investigator. Theories of why information resources succeed or fail, derived from the biomedical informatics or general information technology literatures, fall into this category. The third kind of theory is formal theory found in the literature of the organizational, social, behavioral, and other related sciences. Such theories, for example those relating to the communication and adoption of innovations, have applicability to a very broad domain, but certainly can be supportive of studies within biomedical informatics.

---

* Ethnography, which is closely aligned with the qualitative methods emphasized in this chapter, is a methodology used by researchers who observe daily life within a defined cultural group in the field and then describe it.

Qualitative inquiry is distinguished by the organization and sequence of investigative actions within a study. Within objectivist studies the familiar sequence progresses along a linear path from the research problem, through a literature review, the development of a research design, the collection and analysis of data, and finally arrives at a statement of conclusions. Each of these activities is also included in qualitative work, but the sequence is neither linear nor quite so predictable. As discussed in Chapter 9, every element of a qualitative study—the questions, relevant literature, data collection, and interpretation of results—is continually examined and refined. Work proceeds continuously through an iterative loop with frequent adjustments as the data and theory are gradually combined into explanation. We can define a starting place for a study, where a decision is made to invest resources into answering a set of questions. We can also define a stopping place, where a decision is made that an argument has been assembled that adequately captures the significant data and answers the initially posited questions. The path between beginning and end is flexible by design and intention. We use the term "argument" to denote the key findings of the study and the rationale that supports them.

The Four Qualitative Processes

Within a qualitative/subjectivist study, the processes of gathering and interpreting data happen continuously in a cycling or spiraling fashion. There are cycles of data collection in which the deliberate effort is to explore— to find data that suggest new questions as well as answers. This requires an openness to and curiosity about events and details. There are times when the purpose is to seek data that either confirm to or conflict with an emerging explanation. Confirmatory work includes the effort to ensure that the findings from the most recent experience "in the field" are cross-checked against data from other times and places. It also includes a search for other kinds of data that should be evident or absent if current thinking is accurate. Work that explores conflicting data is also necessary so that many perspectives can be understood and the study can be as thorough as possible.

One way to conceptualize the qualitative/subjectivist investigation process, and perhaps set it apart from objectivist work, is to describe four types of thought processes that take place throughout the lifetime of a study. Typically, these are turned on and off by the investigative team, as they are needed.

The Managerial Planning Process

Planning allows the investigator to maintain control over the study process. Starting with imagination about the full range of what might be possible to accomplish in a study and ending with concrete schedules and appointments and tasks, planning is continuous. As part of planning, the investigator needs to reach an agreement with the person, or client, who desires the evaluation. That agreement will outline the purpose of the evaluation, the resources available for conducting the evaluation, and the roles of the client and evaluator. Another major planning decision is whether to conduct the study as a solo investigator or assemble a study team. Involving others can be more expensive and time consuming, but provides more data and different perspectives. If a team is formed, there is a continuing need to keep all members of the team up to date on the plans to ensure that the overall work is coordinated and to allow members to seize appropriate opportunities as they continue with their individual roles.

Maintaining a boundary around the project, which restricted the scope of work, is a continuing challenge to management and planning. Qualitative studies have a remarkable tendency to expand. For example, in Ash et al.'s[8] studies of computerized physician order entry (CPOE), it became evident that CPOE is a subset of a large information system environment at each institution, with fuzzy boundaries between CPOE and results reporting, notes entry, and decision support systems. Since she had grant funding to study the narrowly defined domain of CPOE, she had to remain constantly diligent in keeping CPOE as a focus, yet be flexible enough so that the effects of the other systems could be considered as they inevitably affect and are affected by CPOE.

In qualitative studies there is an inevitable tension between a realistic plan for a study and the emergent possibilities that imply adjustments to that plan. In a study conducted by a team, planning becomes even more important because team members need to communicate continuously about the needs for adjustments.

The Scholarly Theory Review Process

The investigator may turn to the literature during a study, as the investigator's personal theories begin to be confirmed through fieldwork and she seeks a broader theoretical framework to gain a better understanding. The dominant mode of thought in this process is akin to traditional scholarship. Sometimes the analysis and the report require the investigation to venture into unfamiliar literature and theory. When a potential answer lies wholly or partially outside the familiar intellectual ground of the investigator, there is a new challenge in finding useful literature and theory. Assistance from colleagues who have different backgrounds may be fruitful at these points. For example, if the investigator has a hunch that diffusion of innovations theory might be applicable to the project at hand, he may want to ask a colleague in sociology or marketing for advice; if social learning theory seems applicable, he may need to approach a friend with a background in education. A multidisciplinary approach that takes advantage of literature and expertise outside of informatics can expose the team to relevant theories that might otherwise go undiscovered.

The Open-Minded Data Gathering Process

This process entails recognizing, finding, collecting, and recording data according to the emergent design of the study. (Specific data gathering methods will be discussed in detail later in this chapter.) During data gathering, the mode of thinking required of the investigator is best described as "open minded." This thought process is inevitably shaped by personal and formal theories and assumptions that evolve with the study. The data gathering process generally begins with an effort to gain an overview of the issues and context and moves toward more focus later. It might entail initial strategies such as visiting the site, gathering information about the organization using library resources, talking to colleagues who may know something about the organization, or learning more about the information resource that is to be evaluated. Open-mindedness in qualitative/subjectivist studies is critical. In contrast with objectivist work, where data are gathered according to a predetermined plan and deviations are to be minimized, qualitative investigators are actively seeking opportunities to change the plan.

The Analytical Interpretation Process

This process entails capturing and explaining the events through analytical acuity, creativity, and intuition as the data and personal/formal theory are progressively brought together, from the hunches that give the argument initial shape to the interpretation in its final form. The process unfolds such that, over time, the theory explains the data in an integrated, persuasive statement of what the investigator sees as the primary findings of the study. Interpretation is the central intellectual work of the study. Over time, interpretation progresses from small, tentative fragmented possibilities to a coherent, confident answer.

In the more familiar world of quantitative work, these four processes occur in a sequence. Revisiting any one of them is viewed as a problem. In qualitative studies, any process, including those that perhaps had been considered completed, can be revisited at any time. This is considered normal and healthy.

Strategies for Study Rigor

There are a number of important considerations when designing and conducting rigorous qualitative studies. The following sections describe methods for safeguarding the integrity of the work. Safeguards imply a deliberate rigor to achieve a descriptive and explanatory argument that can be used by others with confidence. There are five strategies that should be considered part of every qualitative study: (1) reflexivity, (2) triangulation, (3) member checking, (4) saturation in the field, and (5) an audit trail.

Reflexivity

This concept, also known as "self-reflection,"[9] should operate in the investigator's mind during every phase of the study.

It is natural and perfectly acceptable that the investigators enter any study with their own biases. Reflexivity is the conscious recognition of these biases and the equally conscious design of the study to address them. Recognizing bias from the beginning is essential because other investigators who do not have the same biases may need to be called upon to view the data as well, so that multiple perspectives can be gained.* In qualitative study, the investigator is the tool for data gathering, and must also be aware of personal interests and predilections. For example, it is often difficult for persons with clinical backgrounds to observe patient care. Their tendency is to focus on the validity of diagnostic and management decisions when perhaps, in the interest of the evaluation study, they should be watching work processes and technology usage. Once aware of this bias, however, they can put their attention where it should be, while still exploiting their clinical knowledge by making acute observations that would elude most nonclinicians.

At the Nouveau Clinic, the consultant might feel a sense of surprise on noticing a physician smile when the business manager reminds him that diagnostic labels should be drawn from the codes prespecified on the system. On reflection, she recognizes that she expected the physician to feel angry. When she later asked about this situation, the physician responds that he had helped to create the codes himself and he had suddenly realized that he had been a bit lazy when completing a patient's record, by not following methods of his own creation. The consultant moves from her original sense of surprise to a new curiosity about how the physicians came to accept elements of the computerized system as "their own." Without her self-awareness when she recognized her sense of surprise, the consultant would have missed out on gaining an important new insight.

Triangulation

Triangulation is a term borrowed from surveying and navigation, and represents a process by which the location of a third point is deduced from the

---

* This is of course a major point of departure between subjectivist methods and their objectivist counterparts. In objectivist work, investigators do not acknowledge bias, and if they do, they are typically disqualified from participating in the study.

locations of two known points a fixed distance apart. Triangulation was originally used in the social sciences to describe multiple data collection techniques employed to measure a single concept. The definition of the term has expanded to include the use of multiple theories, multiple researchers, and multiple methods, or combinations of these, to obtain a "fix" on a specific issue. In qualitative studies, triangulation means the weaving together of different data gathering techniques, data elements, or investigators[10] to help ensure that the resulting descriptions and interpretations are as useful as they can be. Comparing and contrasting data from these varying sources verifies and strengthens the results that emerge.

Member Checking

Member checking employs the actual subjects in the study, at various points, to confirm that the investigator's findings are reasonable.[11] This can be based on brief, individual contacts ("Did I get the main point from the meeting yesterday?") or on repeated contact with an intact group within the organization that will serve this function progressively throughout the study. The investigator asks if his/her notes and arguments are logical and to the point. To the extent that these informants confirm that the argument makes sense, this constitutes an important kind of support for it. Member checking can be used both to validate and sharpen preliminary hunches at the early stages of a study, and to confirm an almost-finalized argument toward the end.

Data Saturation

At some point in the life of the study, the next cycle in the field seems like it will be repetitive. During the analysis process, little that is new emerges. The search for confirmation and contradiction only supports the interpretation that has already been done. During interviews, answers given are similar to those offered by prior interviewees. During periods of observation in the field, observers find themselves taking fewer notes because they are seeing nothing new. It is hard to predict how much time a study will take before this point of data saturation is reached. Often the constraints of the resources available and the investigator's other roles limit the project and bring it to an end sooner than the end might come through a natural sense of saturation. However, if saturation is reached first, the fieldwork can stop at that point.

Audit Trail

The audit trail is a record of the study, one sufficiently detailed to allow someone else to follow the study's history and determine if the investigation and the resulting data provided an adequate basis for the argument and conclusions.[12] Such a record would also enable someone external to the study to determine if there were flaws in the investigative process. Most records composing the audit trail emerge as natural by-products of properly executed fieldwork. If a solo investigator has maintained files of her field notes, a chronology of her coding and outlines, notes on her efforts to find contradicting data, and a log of her experiences, the audit trail is essentially complete.

The audit trail becomes more complex in a study conducted by a team. There is a greater amount of data collected, and the audit trail must also capture the interactions among the team members. So a team audit trail might include minutes of analysis and planning meetings involving all or a subset of the team members. Overall, the clarity of the trail and the depth of its detail are indicators of the care with which a study was conducted.

The consultant for the Nouveau Clinic has been told that her job is to evaluate the success of the system over the next 2 years. She might plan initial strategies after first visiting one or two of the clinics. She might observe at the computer stations, at the nurses' stations, in the hallways and exam rooms, or in offices, laboratories, and staff meetings. She might notice the people who make use of the records and the system, the kinds of paper records and notes they produce, the gestures they make, the clutter they leave behind. She might talk with some physicians and nurses casually and then ask a selection of them to give her more detailed information. She might ask to review minutes of staff and committee meetings. She is carefully getting the lay of the land during this initial foray into the field.

The Nouveau Clinic will be undergoing major change as the EMR is implemented, and the consultant decides to try to identify an "insider" to play a key role in the study by becoming a member of a study team. It turns out that one of the primary care physicians is a neighbor who has expressed interest in the evaluation. This physician agrees to collaborate and assist, especially in making introductions and in gaining user involvement.

The consultant must make some early decisions about how to design the evaluation. She meets with the client and together they formulate the overarching question to be "What are the factors that affect the success of this EMR implementation?" Since communication, care, control, and context are all involved, she begins thinking about using qualitative methods. This stage can be problematic, since many evaluators are comfortable in either the quantitative or qualitative school of thought, and will see the question from the beginning in relation to their preferred strategies. It is important to be able to recognize the full range of methods that may be appropriate, and perhaps recommend another consultant or evaluator for the work. Our consultant recognizes this as an appropriate situation for a qualitative study. First, she determines that she wants and needs to do a high-quality, rigorous study, since the Nouveau Clinic has invested heavily in the new system. She then needs to make decisions about how to gather the data and analyze them.

Our consultant, an astute practitioner of reflexivity, knows that she has some bias about her assignment from past experience: she already sympathizes with the users of the yet-to-be-installed EMR. Fortunately, she knows several graduate students at a nearby university who are seeking practical experience in evaluating informatics projects, and have taken a qualitative methods course. She recruits several of them to be part of the study team. The team subsequently meets and outlines its strategy. Each member comes from a different background, so the members discuss their personal biases and how they will provide checks on one another. To facilitate triangulation, they decide that all members of the team will participate in observing clinician workflow, performing interviews, and obtaining forms presently used in patient care—all to try to understand how the EMR will affect the staff. Another focus they articulate is the need to gain a picture of the prevalent attitudes of users toward the forthcoming EMR. They outline a timeline bounded by the 2 years specified by the client, so they will gather data throughout the implementation period and beyond or until they sense they have reached data saturation. They will keep a careful audit trail. To this end, one team member volunteers to gather, disseminate, and archive files as field notes and transcripts become available. Another agrees to keep records of analysis meetings and enter into the qualitative data analysis software the themes identified in team discussions. They outline a schedule for delivering reports to the client, and once each report is in draft form, they will do a member check by meeting with as many of the staff as they can to go over the preliminary results.

Specifics of Conducting Qualitative Studies

The preceding sections have provided strategic background information on qualitative/subjectivist approaches to evaluation. This section provides an overview of some of the specific decisions about techniques and procedures that need to be made while planning and executing a qualitative study. In this section we are emphasizing what has worked for the authors of this chapter in their studies of information system implementations in hospitals and outpatient settings. While what follows may seem overly prescriptive and formulaic in light of the numerous options available within the qualitative framework, we would like in this section to remove some of the mystery that is often attached to qualitative research. Once familiar with the basics, readers can refer to the references for more detail and other methodological options.

The basic steps are as follows: Once the research questions have been articulated and it is clear that qualitative methods are appropriate for answering them, it is necessary to select the sites for fieldwork if these are not constrained, select the study team members and the individuals to be interviewed or observed, determine the techniques for gathering the data, outline a time frame for data collection, and decide what resources and budget are needed.

Site and Informant Selection

In many evaluations, the sites for field investigation are predetermined, but this is not always the case. When there is flexibility in site selection, the choices are invariably driven by the study goals or research questions. For example, if the goal is to understand how house staff (interns and residents) view a new EMR, teaching hospitals should be the focus. On the other hand, to compare views of clinicians at teaching and nonteaching hospitals, it would be necessary to do fieldwork at at least one site of each type. Even if the evaluation site is predetermined, the investigators still need to decide, for example, which unit(s) of the organization might be the focal points for fieldwork.

Whether selecting a study site or selecting the individuals to interview or observe, the logic of the selection procedure is similar. Qualitative methods usually entail a "purposive" selection, meaning that deliberate selection is based on the purpose of the study, and the selection strategy can evolve as the progress of the study reveals initially unanticipated needs for subjects who bring potentially novel viewpoints. Investigators use their judgment to select appropriate sites and subjects. They may begin selecting individual study subjects, customarily known as "informants," by finding the most knowledgeable people, those who know something about the focus of the evaluation (the EMR, for example) and who also know other people in the organization. These important contacts can then identify others in the organization who may be productively included in the study, and these subjects can in turn recommend others, creating a "snowball" effect.

This approach contrasts with convenience sampling, which is less deliberate, and based purely on availability and happenstance. For example, an investigator studying the utilization of a new bioinformatics consulting service based in a health sciences library might engage as an informant anyone who happens to use the service on the days the investigator is on site. Because measurement and estimation, as discussed in Chapters 4 to 8, are typically not performed in qualitative studies, random sampling does not enjoy in qualitative work the preeminent role it plays in quantitative/objectivist studies.

Careful purposive selection of informants is almost always the preferred method for qualitative investigation. This is especially the case when choosing subjects for interviews that are very expensive to conduct when the costs of transcription and analysis are added to the very real costs of the time of the interviewer and interviewees. Informants should be selected based on the information or expertise that they can share.[13] As a general rule, both expert and nonexpert users of an information resource should be included. It is useful to seek out the outlier and the skeptic in addition to those who are known to be heavy system users. Generally, investigators will not have a complete list of informants at first; the list will be constantly expanded and adjusted. Skeptics and other new informants with special viewpoints will be identified by the informants previously identified.

When considering the numbers of informants to interview or observe over an extended period, Crabtree and Miller[14] suggest five to eight informants if most people are like-minded, or 12 to 20 if there is a good deal of variation. Obviously, these numbers may increase as additional issues emerge, bringing with them requirements for additional points of view. For observation, the number of people will depend on the focus of the study and the context. If one were evaluating a large-scale information resource implementation in a large, complex environment, such as a medical school with 1500 faculty members, a larger number of informants would be needed than would be the case for a study set in a small rural clinic.

The Team

Informatics evaluation studies are applied research projects and "it is in applied research that ethnographers most often find themselves members of teams, usually multidisciplinary ones."[15] As a rule, a team approach to qualitative study is almost always desirable. Whatever the focus of the evaluation, it should be viewed through different lenses so that the most complete picture has the opportunity to emerge. Teamwork can sometimes be frustrating and seem slow; nonetheless, it provides a higher level of trustworthiness to the study. A team study needs an overall leader. The leader must recognize that he or she will need to spend considerable time managing the team and performing administrative duties such as writing interim reports for the client(s) and tracking expenses.

In addition to expertise in data collection techniques, team members need to be effective collaborators in every sense of the word, but above all in producing what they have promised to do on time. Effective teams often include individuals with different backgrounds, and roles in the study. For example, clinicians and nonclinicians can be deliberately paired during observations in the field so that they can offer different perspectives on the same activity. If resources permit, it is helpful to have an experienced qualitative researcher employed to scan all of the data and provide judgment about the reasonableness of the interpretations made by team members.

Team planning includes extended periods of time for meetings to develop strategies and timelines. Early in the life of the project, the team might gather for a half-day or full day in a retreat setting, using flip charts or project management software to plan tasks, timelines, and resource use. During regular team meetings once a study is underway, it is important to set time aside to track progress and do further planning. Dividing the meeting agenda into two major segments, separating study planning from data interpretation and assigning fixed amounts of time to each, helps assure that all tasks will be achieved.

Selection of Data Gathering Techniques

For qualitative studies largely conducted in the field, the selection of data gathering techniques depends on the purpose of the evaluation, the questions being asked, and the resources available. As described below, plans for entering the field must be carefully formulated and executed.

Entering the Field

Entering the field as an investigator can be a daunting experience, even for team members who are clinicians or researchers, to whom the environment is familiar. Gathering some background information about the sites—by looking at routine organizational publications, Web sites, or perhaps vendor information about the information resource under study—is invariably helpful. One central contact person within the organization who can act as a "key informant," someone who knows the people involved and the resources being studied, can provide names of other possible informants. It is a good idea to do a "lay of the land" visit first so the investigators not only know their way around the physical space, but also feel comfortable when the real work starts. Each informant with whom the study team will spend considerable time should be given a fact sheet outlining the purpose of the study, and a consent form if it is required by the local human subjects committee. While both necessary and important, the consent process can make for awkward introductions, so it is helpful to have an informative verbal statement ready that outlines the purposes of the study, the data collection methods to be employed, safeguards of confidentiality, and something perhaps a bit personal about members of the study team to build rapport.

The evaluation team, which has named itself the Nouveau Evaluation Team (NET), now includes the original consultant, graduate students, and an "insider" who is an employee of the organization. The consultant discusses the project with an additional person, a colleague who has qualitative analysis experience and asks if the person would serve as the objective outsider who would provide an overview of the data and audit trail later in the project to make sure bias has not crept into the study. This person agrees and the client approves the additional expense.

The insider gives the NET a tour and makes brief introductions. She recommends that the NET members provide a pizza lunch and several coffee breaks and be in the staff room to chat with everyone so that their faces are known and they can distribute fact sheets and explain about informed consent. They do this and find that a large number of staff members, including busy clinicians, agree to participate in these activities.

Techniques for Data Collection

This section discusses in some detail procedures that help generate data useful to building a cohesive argument by the end of the study. We focus on interviews, observation, and document analysis because they are the techniques most commonly used in biomedical informatics studies.

Interviews

There is a continuum of interview structure ranging from very structured to very open-ended. Scripted, highly structured interviews are basically quantitative surveys or questionnaires administered face to face. Highly open-ended interviews are often like conversations, with the interviewer suggesting a subject but providing little guidance. Semi-structured interviews occupy the middle position. They provide guidance and focus while allowing flexibility in the topics addressed. The ability of the interviewer to offer gentle guidance, without interrupting the continuity of the interviewee's thoughts, constitutes the art of interviewing. There are numerous variations of qualitative semi-structured interviews, including cultural interviews to find out what shared meanings group members hold; oral histories, which gather reminiscences about a focus or theme; life histories, which gather memories about one's life; and so-called evaluation interviews, which discover whether new efforts are meeting expectations. With evaluation interviews, "the researcher learns in depth and detail how those involved view the successes and failures of a program or project."[16]

When studying biomedical information resources, it can be useful to use elements of each of these four kinds of interviews. For example, a comprehensive interview can begin with a few life-history questions, because it is always helpful to understand people's background and learn the roots of their involvement in the project. Life history questions are also good rapport builders. One then builds questions into the interview that can elicit descriptions of organizational culture, such as "From your viewpoint, what group or groups were influential in shaping the plans to implement the EMR?" An oral history technique can be used with great success to explore recollections, for example, of different phases of informatics system implementations. Oral history is a technique "for obtaining first person accounts of how modern society has been shaped by causative factors of historical significance."[17] Oral history questions might be designed to elicit memories about the history of an information resource implementation. (Often, one major goal of a qualitative study is to establish "what really happened.") The goal of semi-structured interviews is to generate perspectives on a specific topic by asking questions that open the door to informants' beliefs. Oral history questions that evoke memories and stories are ideal for generating these narratives.

Although it is not always possible or practical, interviews should ideally be tape recorded so that the interviewer does not need to take detailed notes and eye contact can be retained. Human subjects committees often have special requirements for interviews that are to be recorded. For example, these committees will usually require that the consent form specify where the actual tapes will be stored and for how long. As part of further preparation, the interviewer should gather information about the interviewee ahead of time and develop an interview guide listing several main questions and many subquestions that can probe for answers if the interviewee does not spontaneously respond. Some questions may be asked of everyone who is interviewed, while other questions will be reserved for specific types of individuals. It is absolutely critical that the interviewer be a good listener and avoid making any value judgments during the interview. Judicious use of silence can often stimulate responses. Interrupting is to be avoided. Many investigators prefer to allocate a full hour to conduct an interview of this type; however, shorter interviews can be useful if they have a well-defined focus or if the informant is being contacted on multiple occasions. After the interview, the tapes should be transcribed by someone with experience in capturing nuances such as laughter and sighs; it usually takes 3 hours or longer to transcribe 1 hour of tape. Further details about conducting semi-structured interviews are provided in Appendix B.

Group interviews, or focus groups, differ fundamentally from the one-on-one interviews discussed above. They should not be viewed as a way to gather more interview information in less time. Focus groups are not easy to do well and, if several participants speak at the same time, audiotapes of focus groups can be hard to transcribe. When run properly, however, focus groups have distinct advantages. In particular, useful synergy among the participants can develop. When this happens, participants build on the thoughts of one another to generate new insights or more accurate recollections of past events. (It is interesting to listen to members of a focus group correct one another's personal recollections of a past event, until a more accurate consensus develops.) Focus groups can employ many of the same types of questions as those used in one-to-one interviews. Gathering a group of up to 10 informants over pizza at lunchtime can generate lively narratives. The moderator needs an interview guide and must set some fairly strict ground rules to discourage participants from interrupting or monopolizing the discussion. An assistant moderator can take general notes that specify who is speaking (which will help the transcriptionist), and can also manage the audiotaping.[18]

Consensus or expert panels can also be treated like group interviews. The advantage here is that informants may be together for extended periods of time, perhaps for days, so rapport and synergy can build over time and settled opinions of the full group can be generated. Audiotaped transcripts of these discussions can be formally analyzed as qualitative data sources. Often the conversation leading up to an agreement is filled with vivid stories and examples, and worthy of capture and analysis.[19]

Back at Nouveau, our insider has urged us to interview at least 12 of the 150 primary care providers because there are several one would call champions who are always at the cutting edge of information technology; there are three who are skeptical; and there are many others who are neutral. The team agrees, but also asks for names of nurses, pharmacists, and laboratory staff who will be affected by the EMR. They also ask for names of hospital administrators and information technology personnel, and for vendor contacts.

Observations

Ethnographic observation, in which a investigator is immersed in the daily life and culture of a group for extended periods of time, is an excellent way to confirm what is discovered through other data-gathering methods such as interviews, and to generate new hypotheses and explanations. There are times when informants will say one thing during interviews, but will act differently when observed. This occurs not because informants are disingenuous, but rather because they may not be conscious of the differences between what they state and what they actually do.

Data collection by observation grew out of anthropological research methods employed initially to understand unfamiliar cultures. For our purposes in evaluation within biomedical informatics, those original methods have been significantly modified. In this respect, Berg[20] offers a useful distinction between *macroethnography*, which strives to describe a way of life in general terms, such as the work of nurses in a hospital, and *microethnography*, which focuses on specific activities within a culture, such as use of an electronic information resource. The original work of anthropologists falls largely in the first category, and what we do in informatics falls largely in the second. When evaluating biomedical information resources, a short but intense period of observation, ideally conducted by a multidisciplinary team, can be of enormous value, whereas traditional macroethnography requires one individual or a very small team to observe a social unit over a long period. An "insider" team member, someone who works within the organization, can make arrangements and introductions to lay the groundwork for observation of ongoing health care, research, or educational activities. Practitioners of these activities vary in the degree to which they are accustomed to being observed as they work, so care must be taken at the outset. Insiders, at first, may have to accompany the observers, but after the first day or two, the other study team members may be able to routinely observe on their own.

There is a spectrum of roles for observers, ranging from passive following of informants to full participant observation, during which the investigator, if qualified, contributes to the work being done in the study setting. For informatics studies, participant observation can be problematic in active clinical and biomedical research settings, because the primary focus of the observation needs to be the information resource under study and not the health care or research being practiced. Full participant observation is not often used. More typically, members of the team who are practicing clinicians or researchers function in a more passive observer role, following the practitioners and quietly watching. Since consent to be observed must usually be obtained from each informant, it is more efficient to observe fewer people for longer periods, or to follow intact groups of workers, such as a research lab or a ward team. There may be opportunities, during a break in the work routine, to perform brief informal interviews of one or more informants to ask questions about what has been observed. This can be particularly useful if an important event in the work of the group (e.g., analysis of clinical trial data that reveals a positive result) has just occurred. Focused follow-up interviews can capture informants' immediate reactions to the event before these are forgotten. For this reason, observers should routinely carry small tape recorders. The possible occurrence of spontaneous interviews should be reflected in the general consent form, so informants do not have to be "reconsented" before such an interview can occur.

So-called field notes are handwritten notes, sometimes called "jottings," about the setting or physical layout of the facility, activities, and events under observation. Field notes can be taken unobtrusively in a health care setting since many people are routinely taking notes. Pocket-sized notebooks are recommended for these jottings. Clipboards should be avoided because, in professional cultures, these evoke images of surveillance by accrediting agencies or managers.*

Jottings or initial notes taken in the field are meant to capture key ideas, for later expansion into full field notes. Just as with interviews, there is a spectrum of structure to field notes. If the notes are completely structured, akin to checklists, they are not actually qualitative field notes because they do not allow recording of interpretations and unanticipated events. Some level of structure—for example, five to 10 foci identified from prior investigation—can help organize initial field notes and facilitate recording of new observations. Completely unstructured initial field notes are compatible with, and indeed recommended for, forays into the field that occur at the beginning stages of a study.

Field notes from an episode of observation often begin with the observer's assumptions, which are preconceived notions about what the observer expects. Writing such pieces ahead of time is a form of reflexivity. These notes can be followed by a diagram of the observed physical space, and can move on to a description of the events actually observed. Investigators often record thoughts that come to mind regarding theory and future plans for investigation. It is best to write these down immediately, for

---

* For the same reasons, the observers should not dress too formally. They should dress as comparably as possible to the workers being observed in the field.

otherwise they are frequently forgotten. Personal notes, thoughts about the investigator's own feelings about the events as they are being observed, should also be jotted down to enhance reflexivity.

As soon as possible after a session in the field, the observer should type out or dictate more complete "full" field notes. At the beginning of a study, if a very open approach is being taken, it could take 3 or 4 hours to think through and produce full field notes based on jottings from 1 hour of observation,[20] so time should be set aside for this task. This time can be decreased later in the study when observations become more focused and if the jottings are written in a somewhat structured format, because the researcher does not need to labor over how to organize the full field notes. Debriefings of team members, during which each shares impressions of the field experience and a description of accomplishments, should take place often. For more information about observational techniques, refer to Appendix B.

Video recording can be an enhancement to both interviews and observation, but the use of video presents special challenges related to confidentiality and analysis. It is fairly easy to de-identify transcripts and audiotapes by deleting headers or introductory information. Something analogous can be done with videotapes, but confidentiality is a much greater problem with this medium. Anyone acquainted with an informant can identify him/her from a segment of video. Researchers need to be sensitive to these considerations.[21] Also, in order to take full advantage of the medium, analysis of video requires explicit attention to the nonverbal aspects of the subjects' behavior.[22] While this can provide especially useful and rich data, the analysis process is time intensive and expensive.

Document or Artifact Gathering

Another extremely important data source is artifacts: documents or physical objects that are natural products of the work ongoing in the field. Organization charts of a hospital, e-mail correspondence of a team of researchers about their research, notes taken in class by students, and paper hospital forms are all examples of artifacts that can be used as data sources. Note that the artifact must be naturally occurring, and not induced by the study. In this sense, an e-mail message from an informant in response to a question posed by a member of the study team is "data" but not an artifact. Informants will often offer artifacts to the investigators. For example, even if a hospital has an electronic medical record, some of the care process may still be documented on paper forms. A nurse may reach into a drawer while you are informally interviewing him and give you a blank form as an example. If the observer sees something he would like to keep or copy as an artifact, he should, of course, ask permission. Investigators need to be careful about artifacts that are offered by well-meaning informants but in fact represent a breach of confidentiality—for example, a completed paper form with patient data already written on it.

To use documents appropriately, the original motivation for the creation of the artifact must be understood. During interviews, the researcher can refer to an artifact he may have available and ask questions about it. How was the text recorded in the document collected? Who collected it? How was it generated? Why was it generated? Was the artifact creation mandated or spontaneous? Such questions must be addressed in order to interpret the meaning of a document.

The NET meets several times to map out strategies for this study. They have already decided to use observation and interviews, but they need to outline interview questions and foci for observations, along with a format for field notes. Although the consultant has agreed to interview a core set of informants herself to maximize consistency, and although she will vary the questions for each interviewee, she spends considerable time with the team outlining six main questions to ask each person. The team agrees that field notes will include personal, theory, observational, and methods sections when they are in their final form. The team also agrees that the focus will be on describing the attitudes and actions of physicians as they use computers in general, and the EMR in particular, and also on the impact of physician use of the EMR on other staff. In addition, the research team asks the insider for a copy of the contract with the vendor and copies of various paper forms as artifacts. The contract contains privileged information and the request is denied, but paper copies of provider order forms and order sets, used only when the system is unavailable, are provided.

Building the Argument: "Measurement" and Analysis

The end product of a qualitative/subjectivist study is a set of conclusions—the "argument"—built on the data and rooted in relevant theory. Qualitative investigators seek for their conclusions trustworthiness, confirmability, credibility, and transferability. While objectivist studies also strive for these characteristics, they are conceptualized, approached, and attained in qualitative/subjectivist work in distinctive ways that are not dependent on statistical constructs such as confidence intervals and inference. In qualitative studies, trustworthiness implies total authenticity of findings. Confirmability denotes objectivity or freedom from bias. Credibility is akin to internal validity or gaining a true and believable picture. Transferability is an analog to generalizability—the degree to which the results are applicable to other contexts. Dependability, like reliability, is the extent to which the process of the study has been undertaken with consistency and care.[23]

In general, approaches to qualitative data analysis employ progressive abstracting or "progressive focusing" as described in the previous chapter. Meaning is assigned, through categorization and coding, initially to segments of raw textual data taken directly from field notes. Initially, the number of categories is large. Then the categories themselves are analyzed, aggregated, and reanalyzed to develop a relatively small number of themes.

Subsequently, the themes are assembled into a coherent argument addressing the goals or questions of the study.

There is a spectrum of specific approaches to qualitative data analysis, just as there is for data collection. Also, just as in data collection, different approaches are chosen and interwoven by investigators in building their argument. At one extreme of the analytical spectrum is a quasi-statistical style, such as word counting, to find how often a particular term occurs in interview or field notes.* At the other extreme is completely unstructured data analysis, in which the investigator reads and considers the data and reaches conclusions without formal intermediate steps.

Crabtree and Miller[24] describe three points on the data analysis spectrum. They categorize the chief organizing styles used in qualitative data analysis as template, editing, and immersion/crystallization. The template style is the most structured. It uses a code manual and is similar to indexing in librarianship. The investigators develop a code list at the outset of the data analysis process, and use it to count occurrences of a particular word or phrase representing a concept, and to index text. Although the template style permits the creation of new codes throughout the analysis process, this is considered exceptional. The editing style generates codes in a different way. Investigators develop codes as they review the data, making notes as they read and reread the various texts they have assembled. The resulting code list is continuously modified as new data are collected and reviewed. The editing style requires frequent recoding of textual items, as the codes themselves evolve, and for this process qualitative data analysis software can be very helpful. The immersion/crystallization style is the least structured, with investigators spending extended periods of time reading and interpreting the text and gaining an intuitive sense of the data prior to writing an interpretation. The coding process, in this style, is much less formal and systematic.

The different approaches contribute in different ways to the attributes of sound qualitative argument. The template and editing styles work to improve the credibility of a study. These impart a natural internal consistency to the analysis, and they allow analysis to be conducted collaboratively. In the beginning stages of fieldwork, the editing approach can be used in an open ended way to produce themes, and later these themes can be used in a template style as new data enter the study. One begins coding by underlining words or phrases of importance in the transcript and writing them in the margin. As the researcher reads more transcripts, phrases will reoccur, some of which are exact synonyms, and others that are more or less specific but clearly related. At this point, there are several techniques for beginning to "chunk," or aggregate, synonyms into patterns and then to chunk patterns into larger themes.

---

* Some researchers use the term *content analysis* to refer to word counting, but others broaden the idea of content analysis to include both counting/quantitative analysis and interpretation/qualitative analysis.[20]

Qualitative analysis software is one method for supporting this analytical process, but some researchers find handwritten lists or spreadsheets more workable at early stages of a study because they are more compatible with the personal style of the investigator. (Even the most flexible software imposes a process or structure that the investigator may not find congenial.) The investigative team needs to come to agreement on patterns and themes that emerge from the data; this is best done face to face. Tracking these discussions is critical because the records of them become a highly distilled form of data. As larger themes emerge from the data, it is possible to revisit the older data with new insight. The discussion of themes often generates new research questions or new foci for future fieldwork. As soon as some themes seem to be coalescing, it may be time to introduce member checking, taking the results back to the informants and asking if they seem right. As the study progresses, the themes might become codes for a code manual or a template for further data collection. At this point, an "outsider" who has not been involved in collecting the data can review both the data and the ultimate themes as a further confirmatory step.

Another way of analyzing the data is to use narrative analysis. This kind of analysis examines both the content of the text and its structure. For example, the structure of informants' stories can be analyzed for their plot development. Stories are narrative descriptions that generally follow a standard format: the stage is set; something happens; there is an ending. The stories of different informants can also be compared with one another. For example, Stavri and Ash[25] analyzed stories told by informatics experts using this comparative approach. Analyzing the structure as well as the content of the stories, they found that stories about successful implementations of computerized physician order entry usually began with descriptions of prior failures. This finding was important because it raised a new research question (how might failure of CPOE systems breed future success?) and it provided insight into the thinking of the storytellers (their memories focus on the failures first, perhaps because those are more vivid than memories of success).

Computer Software

Software can be helpful during both the data analysis and result reporting processes, especially when there is a large amount of data to be analyzed by multiple researchers. Such software may be highly compatible with the working style of persons aligned with the field of informatics, who may prefer reading and coding using a laptop over marking up paper documents. The software must be able to easily import text documents in a standard word processing format since undoubtedly transcripts and field notes will be in such a standard format. It is up to the investigator to determine the granularity of the coding: by line, sentence, paragraph, or section. During coding, the investigator reads each segment and assigns terms just as he would do manually, but the software keeps track of the assignments so that later the segments assigned to each code can be retrieved using keyword searches. This feature is especially helpful when writing study results. By reviewing all of the text pieces associated with a particular code, it is easier to find relevant material to quote.

Programs that provide code-and-retrieve capabilities include HyperQual, NUD*IST, QUALPRO, and Ethnograph. For example, one interviewee in Ash's CPOE studies said of an EMR: "It's timely, legible, accurate, comprehensive information then, so I think it beats the heck out of the paper chart, and the one big drawback then and still to this day is that it takes longer for the doctors I think to go back and type it." This one sentence could be coded "benefits," "drawbacks," and "time issues." If the researcher later wanted to find all text that related to perceptions of the time it takes to use an EMR and used the software to search on the word *time*, this snippet would be found.

As coding progresses, terms can be grouped into higher level patterns and examined for relationships to build themes and develop theory. Programs that are especially useful for looking at relations among themes are NUD*IST, ATLAS, HyperRESEARCH, QCA, and AQUAD. The products that allow sharing of codes among different researchers are most desirable for team research. Within this class of software, graphics capabilities for building conceptual networks are helpful, though not essential. Programs with these graphics capabilities include Inspiration, Decision Maker, ATLAS, MECA, and NVIVO. This family of software is also useful for version control, so members of the team do not chaotically edit each other's work. For a more complete discussion, see Crabtree and Miller.[26]

The NET members decide to analyze data using the "editing style" described by Crabtree and Miller, and to manage the large amount of data to be collected by multiple researchers, they select an appropriate software package. They hold regular analysis meetings to review the coding that each individual has done and then they agree on "team" codes, patterns, and themes by consensus. The patterns and themes evolve until all of the data have been analyzed and a final consensus is reached about what should be reported.

Presenting Evaluation Results and Criteria for Evaluating the Quality of Qualitative Inquiry

As a rule, at least at the present time, most people who read evaluation and research reports in biomedical informatics are more familiar with objectivist methods than with subjectivist, qualitative methods. For this reason, the presentation of qualitative reports must be undertaken with special care, clarity, and explanation.

Presenting Evaluation Results

Presenting results of qualitative studies poses a challenge. After analyzing masses of textual data, skills unique to qualitative inquiry are required to reduce to a few pages the argument that needs to be presented. The necessary clarity and completeness of description can be difficult to attain when the evaluation report is intended for a busy administrative team, as might be the case for an in-house technology implementation. Similar difficulties can arise when the report is intended for publication, because of page limitations. At the same time, much of the power of qualitative/subjectivist studies lies in the appeal the report can have to a wide audience, whose members do not have to be proficient in statistical methods to understand it. So time taken to write a report that communicates well to the intended audience is time well spent. Detailed verbal description about data gathering and analysis is necessary to lend credibility to the findings. This process cannot be reported as concisely as often is the case for a quantitative study, where the symbolic language of mathematics can convey a great deal of information in relatively few pages. Also, in presenting qualitative study results, it is always effective to offer representative quotations to support each component of the argument. These quotations, in their totality, are often quite lengthy. This requires a balancing act between the inclination to include more quotations to empower the argument, and the inclination toward fewer quotations to make the report more concise.

The reporting process for qualitative studies is supported by several techniques. First, the conceptual framework can be described with the help of a diagram. For example, Ash et al.[27] used a simple diagram to illustrate how a multiple perspectives framework was employed to analyze the views of clinicians, information technology, and administrative staff about computerized physician order entry. Information about sites or informants can be illustrated in a table or matrix. For example, the matrix may list types of people across the top (administrators, nurses, physicians, information technology personnel), and their locations along the left side. The cells of the matrix would include numbers of people in each cross-categorization who were observed. Diagrams of various kinds, tables of quotations, flowcharts, and timelines are all useful.[28] The format for these more concise representations cannot be prescribed, and is specific to the study methods and results being reported. While a team approach to data collection and analysis is almost always fruitful, preparation of the actual report usually falls to one or a small number of study team members. Nonetheless, a team discussion is ideal for reaching consensus about how to best communicate in a succinct, artful, and easily grasped manner.

A final study report or manuscript can be organized into standard sections: introduction, background, methods, findings or results, discussion, and conclusions. This is a conservative approach that almost always communicates effectively as long as each section itself is well written. Most often, the results section of a qualitative study is organized by theme or concept, but such reports can also be arranged in more creative ways, depending on the purpose or the requirements of the report. For example, May and Ellis[29] present a study of a telemedicine project as a narrative story written in a dramatic tone, complete with a plot and actors. These authors have also used a chronological approach in the results section of another paper,[30] tracing informants viewpoints at different points in the evaluation process through representative quotes. Patton[31] suggests that a formal qualitative evaluation report might include the purpose of the evaluation; the methods; presentation of the data (describe the information resource, describe the findings, and offer interpretations); validation and verification of the findings; and conclusions and recommendations.

After member checking and writing several drafts, the NET members prepare a final report for the Nouveau Clinic following Patton's outline. However, they also ask for and receive permission from their sponsor to prepare several papers for publication. They mask the identity of the clinic and, of course, the informants. They write a case study paper for publication in an informatics journal and a paper about their methods for a social science and medicine journal. The NET story is a success story: they have helped smooth the transition to the EMR by providing ongoing feedback and a summary report, the students have gained valuable fieldwork experience and the team has both of its papers published in peer reviewed journals.

Evaluating the Quality of Qualitative Research

When study reports and manuscripts for publication are reviewed, those employing primarily qualitative methods should be evaluated using somewhat different criteria from those employing quantitative methods. The criteria for appraising qualitative work are somewhat less formulaic and perhaps best described in a series of questions. First, were qualitative methods appropriate for answering the study questions and, if so, were the specified methods (interviews with more or less structure, observation, etc.) appropriate? Was there a theoretical framework guiding the work and was that framework well developed? Was the study context clearly described? Were sites and subjects carefully selected and described? Was the method used for analysis appropriate for both the study questions and the type of data gathering selected and was it well described? Were divergent points of view deliberately integrated (were skeptics as well as champions interviewed, for example)? Did more than one investigator review the data and analysis? Were the reported results considered insightful and helpful? When new qualitative studies are proposed in grant applications, these same criteria can be applied to the plans for the proposed work.

Special Ethical Considerations in Qualitative Studies

Informants must provide formal consent to be observed or interviewed if a study is being performed for research purposes. If the study is strictly an internal evaluation for administrative or quality improvement purposes, informed consent may not be required, but the human subjects review board of the organization should make that determination—not the study team. It may in fact be necessary to approach two or more such boards: that of the institution sponsoring the evaluation and that of the institutions where fieldwork will be conducted. For example, a university team may be conducting a study of advanced information technology in the military. In that case, it is necessary to consult the university's review board as well as the military review boards with jurisdiction over the data collection sites. There is an extremely fine line between "research" studies and studies conducted for internal purposes.

Whether or not informed consent procedures are required, informants should be made aware of the purpose of the study, that their help is voluntary, and that confidentiality will be completely respected. Unlike survey respondents in quantitative studies, these informants will be studied in detail over time. They will be observed while doing their jobs. Obtaining useful data requires gaining their trust, and identities should be protected as much as possible. This is somewhat harder to do with audiotapes than it is with field notes, and even harder with videotapes. Names should be coded and, after analysis, tapes kept under lock and key or destroyed. Special issues need consideration if the investigators are members of the organization where data are collected. Team members need access to the data, but sensitive issues can arise if the investigators and informants are colleagues. For example, a mistake, criticism, or embarrassing incident may be recorded in field notes. If the team is collectively certain that the incident has no bearing on the evaluation or can add nothing new to the study, the outside members on the team should consider deleting the description of it. If, however, the information is deemed critical to the study, the entire team, including the insider, will need to decide what to do. There is always tension between the research benefits, the organizational benefits, and the informant benefits of qualitative studies. If the only product of the study is an academic paper written by the investigator, then the informants may feel they were exploited—perhaps with significant justification.

There are special considerations related to participant observation in health care settings. We discussed earlier the need for investigators to focus on the subject of the evaluation, usually information resources, and not basic issues of medical or nursing management. If a clinically trained field researcher encounters an extreme situation of suboptimal care where patients may be harmed, there is a professional obligation to take action.

This can be done with subtlety by suggesting a different course of action to the informant. For example, if an observer who is a pharmacist encounters a situation where a nurse is about to administer the wrong medication, he could suggest that she might take a second look at the order. While conducting fieldwork in informatics, it is likely that researchers will be in patient care settings. If the focus of the study is the actions of clinicians, the patient is not a direct informant and general consent from the patient for investigators being in the area may suffice. (Some academic institutions may routinely ask patients to consent to this level of observation when they are admitted to the hospital.) If patients are being directly observed, in a study of patient–physician–computer interactions, for example, patients' formal informed consent will be needed. Again, an organization's human subjects research committee should make the final decisions about the consent process. Investigators should anticipate that the pertinent issues are often not trivial to resolve and may require significant time. Timelines for studies should be designed accordingly.

The Future of Qualitative Inquiry

Qualitative, interpretive methods are receiving more respect in health care disciplines, as evidenced by the increasing number of research reports based on these methods that can be found when one searches the medical or nursing literature. This is partly because objectivist quantitative methods cannot address some of the research questions now being raised, particularly when the focus of the question is "why" or "how" instead of "what" or "how much." Qualitative methods are also receiving more attention because the standards of scientific rigor for qualitative work have become increasingly well established. At the same time, many believe that even more effective use of these methods in the future will require several open issues to be resolved. Miles and Huberman[28] state:

We should be mindful of some pervasive issues that have not gone away. These issues include the labor-intensiveness (and extensiveness over months or years) of data collection, frequent data overload, the distinct possibility of researcher bias, the time demands of processing and coding data, the adequacy of sampling when only a few cases can be managed, the generalizability of findings, the credibility and quality of conclusions, and their utility in the world of policy and action.

As qualitative inquiry receives greater acceptance and investigators gain more experience with these methods in informatics, a number of the above issues will be addressed. For example, as more knowledge is gained about combining qualitative and quantitative methods (a form of triangulation), it will be possible to perform more efficient and therefore less resource-intensive inquiry to address the full range of research and evaluation questions that continually arise in biomedical informatics.

References

1. Lincoln YS, Guba EG. Naturalistic Inquiry. Newbury Park, CA: Sage, 1985.
2. Strauss A, Corbin J. Basics of Qualitative Research: Grounded Theory Procedures and Techniques. Newbury Park, CA: Sage, 1990.
3. Green J, Britten N. Qualitative research and evidence-based medicine. BMJ 1998;316:1230–1233.
4. Forsythe DE. Studying Those Who Study Us: An Anthropologist in the World of Artificial Intelligence. Stanford, CA: Stanford University Press, 2001.
5. Kaplan B. Addressing organizational issues into the evaluation of medical systems. J Am Med Inform Assoc 1997;4:94–101.
6. Geertz C. Interpretation of Cultures. New York: Basic Books, 1973.
7. Denzin NK, Lincoln YS. Handbook of Qualitative Research, 2nd ed. Thousand Oaks, CA: Sage, 2000:15.
8. Ash JS, Gorman PN, Lavelle M, et al. Perceptions of physician order entry: Results of a cross-site qualitative study. Meth Inf Med 2003;42:313–323.
9. Crabtree BF, Miller WL, eds. Doing Qualitative Research, 2nd ed. Thousand Oaks, CA: Sage, 1999:14.
10. Patton MQ. Qualitative Evaluation Methods. Beverly Hills, CA: Sage, 1980:329.
11. Crabtree BF, Miller WL, eds. Doing Qualitative Research, 2nd ed. Thousand Oaks, CA: Sage, 1999:308–309.
12. Lincoln YS, Guba EG. Naturalistic Inquiry. Newbury Park, CA: Sage, 1985: 319–320.
13. Johnson JC. Selecting Ethnographic Informants. Newbury Park, CA: Sage, 1990.
14. Crabtree BF, Miller WL, eds. Doing Qualitative Research, 2nd ed. Thousand Oaks, CA: Sage, 1999:42.
15. Erickson K, Stull D. Doing Team Ethnography: Warnings and Advice. Thousand Oaks, CA: Sage, 1998.
16. Rubin HJ, Rubin IS. Qualitative Interviewing: The Art of Hearing Data. Thousand Oaks, CA: Sage, 1995:6.
17. Brunet LW, Morrissey CY, Gorry GA. Oral history and information technology: Human voices of assessment. J Org Computing 1991;1:251–274.
18. Morgan DL, Krueger RA. The Focus Group Kit. Thousand Oaks, CA: Sage, 1998.
19. Ash JS, Stavri PZ, Kuperman GJ. A consensus statement on considerations for a successful CPOE implementation. J Am Med Inform Assoc 2003;10:229–234.
20. Berg BL. Qualitative Research Methods for the Social Sciences, 5th ed. Boston: Pearson, 2004.
21. Crabtree BF, Miller WL, eds. Doing Qualitative Research, 2nd ed. Thousand Oaks, CA: Sage, 1999:239.
22. Pink S. Doing Visual Ethnography: Images, Media, and Representation in Research. Thousand Oaks, CA: Sage, 2001.
23. Miles MB, Huberman AM. Qualitative Data Analysis, 2nd ed. Thousand Oaks, CA: Sage, 1994:277–278.

24. Crabtree BF, Miller WL, eds. Doing Qualitative Research, 2nd ed. Thousand Oaks, CA: Sage, 1999:135.
25. Stavri PZ, Ash JS. Does failure breed success: narrative analysis of stories about computerized physician order entry. Int J Med Inform 2003;72:9–15.
26. Crabtree BF, Miller WL, eds. Doing Qualitative Research, 2nd ed. Thousand Oaks, CA: Sage, 1999:195–218.
27. Ash JS, Gorman PN, Lavelle M, Lyman J. Multiple perspectives on physician order entry. J Am Med Inform Assoc Suppl AMIA Proceedings 2000:27–31.
28. Miles MB, Huberman AM. Qualitative Data Analysis, 2nd ed. Thousand Oaks, CA: Sage, 1994.
29. May C, Ellis NT. When protocols fail: technical evaluation, biomedical knowledge, and the social production of 'facts' about a telemedicine clinic. Soc Sci Med 2001;53:989–1002.
30. May C, Gask L, Atkinson T, Ellis N, Mair F, Esmail A. Resisting and promoting new technologies in clinical practice: the case of telepsychiatry. Soc Sci Med 2001;52:1889–1901.
31. Patton MQ. Qualitative Evaluation Methods. Beverly Hills, CA: Sage, 1980: 31–32.

Appendix A: Schools of Thought About Qualitative Studies

There are nearly as many philosophical approaches to qualitative inquiry as there are research teams. These philosophical stances strongly influence the researchers' selection of methods, which is why these approaches are introduced here. The positivist approach to qualitative research tries to apply the criteria of validity and reliability, and is basically a deductive approach such as that used in biomedical studies.[1] Post-positivist approaches argue that a new set of criteria needs to be developed, and that there are multiple views of reality. Along similar lines, the constructivist approach, or naturalistic inquiry, maintains that truth is relative and is a result of perspective. It considers the social construction of reality and uses the criterion of trustworthiness. Our primary focus has been the constructivist tradition throughout the preceding chapter.

The grounded theory approach in its purest form is the most inductive and constructivist. First Glaser and Strauss[2] and then Strauss and Corbin[3] described this approach that is becoming more widely used in biomedical informatics research. It is an approach that is firmly based or grounded in the data. This means that few preconceived notions are allowed to structure the outcomes of the study. For example, when Crabtree did his early work studying what it is like becoming a physician, he gathered observational and interview data, and did his coding by selecting the residents' own words as a beginning coding scheme. He saw patterns as codes were grouped together, but the larger theme became clear in what he calls a "thunderbolt" moment.[4] The central organizing theme describing the lives of residents, he realized, was "surviving." He then revisited his data and became more and more confident that this was the central issue. His subjects did not talk directly about survival, so it was not until he reached the highest level of interpretation that in the investigator's view, full understanding emerged. The insight emerged directly from the data and is an excellent example of the outcome of a grounded theory approach.

Another approach, one that grew out of the organizational development movement, is participatory action research (PAR). It is receiving increasing attention in medicine. A recent Institute of Medicine workshop explored the role of the public in the design, review, and setting of the research agenda for clinical research. The workshop built upon Green's definition of PAR, reported as "systematic inquiry, with the collaboration of those affected by the issue being studied, for purposes of education and taking action or effecting change."[5] *Participatory action research, participatory inquiry*, and *action science* are all terms that refer to the cooperative efforts of researchers and those who work inside an organization to improve the situation. Qualitative evaluation studies that involve the stakeholders in the design, execution, analysis, and determination of what will be done with the results fit this definition.

Another approach is to conduct the evaluation as a case study. Case studies are detailed descriptions of real situations in which the context and decision-making processes are explored. Case studies are an ideal way of summarizing the results of an evaluation study by combining what has been learned using different methods. They can include one or more sites and can be either quantitative or qualitative, but are generally a blending of both. They can be used for evaluation purposes or as teaching aids, but would be written differently for those different purposes. Evaluation or research case studies must be accurate and rigorous; teaching cases need not be, as long as they stimulate dialogue. We will limit our discussion to evaluation cases.

Case studies can be descriptive or explanatory and, like the qualitative methods described above, they can help to answer research or evaluation questions that ask why or how something happened. Also as outlined above, there must be a clear strategy for selecting sites and informants and specific foci or measures appropriate for the research questions. Cases can be either representative of the norm or unique. Evidence for the study can come from any of the qualitative methods described and from any documents, including those presenting facts and figures from quantitative data. The goal is to gather enough information in different ways so that the multiple sources of evidence help the investigator paint an accurate picture. Analysis consists of gaining a broad view of the data as well as finding patterns and themes. Again, it is recommended that multiple researchers partake in analysis in order to have more perspectives on interpretation. The final report might be prepared in different versions, depending on the audience. Usually, a case is written in traditional narrative form that describes and explains the situation. If multiple cases are to be described, they can be reported separately and followed by a cross-case analysis, or the cross-case analysis can stand alone. Another possible format is to organize the report by issue and describe the individual cases to illustrate each issue. Either the cross-case analysis or issues-based description can help keep the study sites anonymous, if that is a goal. Above all, the case study report must be well written and engaging.[6]

References

1. Denzin NK, Lincoln YS. Handbook of Qualitative Research, 2nd ed. Thousand Oaks, CA: Sage, 2000:276–277.
2. Glaser B, Strauss A. The Discover of Grounded Theory. New York: Aldine, 1967.
3. Strauss A, Corbin J. Basics of Qualitative Research: Grounded Theory Procedures and Techniques. Newbury Park, CA: Sage, 1990.
4. Crabtree BF, Miller WL, eds. Doing Qualitative Research, 2nd edition. Thousand Oaks, CA: Sage, 1999:155.
5. Institute of Medicine Board on Health Sciences Policy. Exploring Challenges, Progress, and New Methods for Engaging the Public in the Clinical Research Enterprise: Clinical Research Roundtable Workshop Summary. Washington, DC: National Academies Press, 2003.
6. Yin RK. Case Study Research: Design and Methods, 3rd ed. Thousand Oaks, CA: Sage, 2003.

Appendix B: Interviewing and Observation Tips

Interviewing

Note: these tips are for a semistructured interview format.

Preparation

- Prepare an interview guide prior to each interview. This should outline five or six main areas you would like to explore and should also list more detailed subquestions that you can ask if the interviewee does not spontaneously cover them. These will guide your probing questions.
- Organize what you need to have with you: the interview guide, background information on the interviewee, a notebook for writing or recorder for taping, a consent form, an information sheet outlining the project, and a token thank you gift (if appropriate).

Getting Started

- Review the information sheet and consent form and briefly outline verbally what is on the interview guide. Make it clear that although you have a set of issues you wish to address, you are interested in hearing everything the interviewee thinks is important to the subject. If the study plan calls for sending a summary back to the interviewee for approval or if you will be making a copy of the consent form to give him later, state that at the beginning. Give appropriate reassurance about anonymity and confidentiality.
- Tell the interviewee that you will make every effort to end the interview on time, where "on time" means whatever time has been negotiated. That gives the interviewee a chance to say that it is all right to run overtime—or not.
- Begin the interview with an open-ended, easy question about the person's background and what led up to his involvement in the project being evaluated. Then ask about his role in the project and move on to more specific questions. It is easier to go from more general to more specific questions and, if asked early on, specific questions may constrain the person's thinking too much.
- Glance down at your interview guide as necessary and jot a note or two to remind you to follow up on something later, but keep eye contact most of the time. Taping is recommended so that eye contact is not broken by your having to write notes. If you must rely on notes, keep them brief or have a human recorder in the room. You can minimize the awkwardness of having a third person involved in the interview by introducing him or her and by explaining that person's role.

Topic Flow and Question Format

- You have provided some structure to the interview by this point, so you can now allow and invite the interviewee to dictate the flow of topics. However, if time is running out and you still have not covered some important topics, you need to take more control of the agenda. Do it with an apology. Make a note on your interview guide to remind you to return to this interesting subject if there is time or if a second interview is possible.
- Before making any major shift in subject, ask the interviewee if she has anything else to add on this issue.
- Always avoid leading questions, questions that tell the interviewee the answer you want, questions like "You don't approve of the way this is being done, do you?"
- Do not be drawn into a conversation with the interviewee. You are there to listen, not to talk. You can offer encouragement as the interviewee talks, but not a value judgment.
- Ask for clarification if you do not understand what the interviewee is saying or if you would like him to expand on a point.

Ending the Interview

- When time is up, say so and make it clear that the interview can end now. Many interviewees want to keep on talking and some save their most insightful remarks until the end. For this reason, do not schedule back-to-back interviews and be flexible with your time.
- Thank the interviewee, ask if he or she has any questions, present a token gift, and explain the next steps.
- Always send a formal thank you note afterward.

Observation

Preparation

- Negotiate entry into the site by making contacts with people within the organization who can grant you access, give you information, and make arrangements such as getting identification badges, space for your personal items, access to schedules, etc.
- Put aside the time for observation; there should be no other demands on your time. Also put aside time for writing field notes after the observation is complete.
- Have some initial research questions in mind so that you can focus your attention in a general way.
- Dress so that you blend into your surroundings, and dress comfortably, since you will probably be doing a lot of walking.

Getting Started

- If you have an appointment to observe someone, have your contact person introduce you, be prepared to give a two-sentence summary of the study's purpose, have information sheets available in case the informant wants to know more, and go over and sign the consent form if it is needed.
- If you are doing a "lay-of-the-land" visit, pick a place in the flow of activity and simply watch for a while and pay particular attention during transitions in the activities, such as shift changes.

Data Recording

- Take notes briefly and occasionally and step out of the situation often to work on your jottings in more detail.
- If you want to dictate notes into a small tape recorder, do this outside the situation; if you do a short informal interview with the recorder, step away so no one is disturbed.
- Include jottings about personal, theory, observational, and methods issues in your notes.

Ending the Session

- Express your thanks and describe the next steps; offer a token gift if appropriate.
- Review your trigger notes soon after leaving the site. Keep adding to them.
- Put ample time aside for transforming jottings into full field notes.

11
Economic Aspects of Evaluation*

In this chapter we return to a primarily objectivist mode of thinking as we embark on a discussion of costs, and particularly how issues of cost and various conceptions of outcome can be figured conjointly into the logic of an evaluation. Although largely linked to objectivist evaluation approaches, we have elected to put this chapter toward the end of this volume because economic issues seem to span all evaluation approaches. Studies that are otherwise subjectivist in approach could incorporate a formal cost analysis selected from the methods described below. While the focus and examples in this chapter address clinical issues, the methods introduced apply across all of the application domains of biomedical information resources.

Motivation for Economic Analysis

The dramatic rise of health care expenditure over the past several decades has focused attention on resource allocation in health care at several levels. For example, the United States spends close to 14% of its gross domestic product (GDP) on health care, which totals just over $1.4 trillion *or* $1,400 billion.[1] Other nations spend from 5% to 11% of their GDP on health care, and in all countries, the percentage of GDP directed toward health care expenditure continues to rise. The rising costs have prompted substantial efforts to reduce the ever-increasing component that health care represents in national budgets. However, technology and medical advances continue, and at a time when federal, state, and private insurance payers are cutting back reimbursement, there are continuing expansions in new pharmacological agents, diagnostic tests, and other procedures. At a more local level, hospitals, health care providers, and caregivers are faced with increasing costs and rising demand for new services and treatments, but have limited (and sometimes shrinking) budgets with which to meet those demands. Finally, there has been an increase in the desire of patients to have a role

---

* This chapter was written by Mark S. Roberts.

in health care decisions, which may require a more detailed understanding of costs and benefits and the response of consumers to changes in prices.

Therefore, at several levels there has been increasing interest in understanding the economic impact of decisions that administrators, clinicians, and health care systems make regarding which programs to institute, what services to offer, etc. The overall goal of these investigations is to ensure that the resources that are expended at a national, regional, or local level are spent wisely, and that the decision maker is maximizing the benefit of the resources spent to provide health care services. All financial resource expenditure decisions involve choices: monies spent in one area cannot be spent in another, and putting financial resources into a particular program implies that the program has more value for the resources spent than other potential programs that were not implemented.

For example, a·hospital must decide how to distribute limited financial resources between several competing demands for new services or programs. Should the hospital purchase a new clinical information system that contains an electronic health record in hopes of improving information flow, reducing error, and improving quality—or should it place those financial resources into purchasing more modern radiological imaging equipment that will improve the diagnosis of particular diseases and improve efficiency in the emergency departments? At a finer level of detail, departments within the hospital face similar decisions. Should the information systems division purchase hardware upgrades to its file servers because of increasing complaints of long wait times for laboratory results in busy clinical areas, or spend its resources on implementing physician order entry?

The motivation for all economic analyses is to place decisions such as these in a rigorous, analytic framework. This will include all the relevant components important to the particular decision makers, to allow a pre-decision estimate of the effects (in both resources and other outcomes) of the consequences of the decision. This chapter briefly introduces the principles of economic analysis as applied in health care, focusing on the components that are unique to biomedical informatics and clinical information systems.

Principles of Economic Analysis

Figure 11.1 illustrates the generic description of the choices facing a decision maker and describes the outcomes that must be simultaneously evaluated in the economic analysis of health care programs. A decision maker is faced with a choice regarding whether to institute an innovation, perhaps in the context of a clinical information system: each choice implies a different stream of costs and outcomes. The purpose of any economic analysis is to make a quantitative comparison between the stream of costs and benefits that arise from each of the possible options being compared. The idea is to highlight the tension between costs and outcomes by calculating

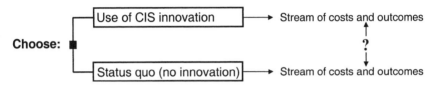

FIGURE 11.1. Basic structure of an economic analysis. In general, all types of economic analyses follow this structure. A new program or strategy that can be introduced to replace an existing strategy produces a stream of costs and outcomes that are different from the stream of costs and outcomes produced by the alternative. CIS, clinical information system.

the costs required to achieve a given change in outcomes. It is important to emphasize that economic analyses can rarely if ever indicate the "correct" choice; they can only provide estimates of the likely economic and clinical consequences of various choices. Whether a particular outcome gain is worth the costs involves political, ethical, and other concerns that are specific to the situation.

There has been recent increasing interest, both in the United States and abroad, in the development of formal, consistent standards for the conduct of economic analyses in health care. In the United States, prompted by the realization that economic analyses were quite variable and had differing adherence to even minimal standards of analysis and reporting,[2] the Public Health Service commissioned the Panel on Cost Effectiveness in Health and Medicine, which consisted of experts who developed a series of recommendations regarding the conduct of cost-effectiveness analyses in health care.[3] Their recommendations, although not entirely complete, have become the de facto standards for conducting, analyzing, and reporting cost-effectiveness analyses in the United States. In the United Kingdom, a similar effort and structure has been put forward by the National Institute for Clinical Excellence (NICE), which carries out cost-effectiveness studies on novel medical technologies using a procedures manual published on its Web site: www.nice.org.uk. Over the past 5 years the NICE organization has completed dozens of effectiveness and cost-effectiveness analysis of medical procedures, which are used in coverage and reimbursement decisions by the U.K. National Health Service and other services around the world.

Types of Cost Studies

There are several types of economic evaluation that are used to compare the effects of different choices and options in a health care setting. Table 11.1 provides a brief description of the various types of analysis and how they differ in terms of the measure of outcomes. The characteristic that differentiates most economic analyses is the metric used to evaluate the ben-

TABLE 11.1. Types of economic evaluation in health care.

Type of analysis	Description	Measurement of cost	Measurement of outcome
Cost minimizing	Assumes outcomes are equivalent	Dollars	None
Cost consequence	Lists the costs and outcomes (even if multiple endpoints are used) of each option	Dollars	Variable, possibly multiple
Cost-effectiveness	Measures outcomes in clinical terms (lives, life expectancy, number of infections averted)	Dollars	Clinical outcome
Cost utility	Measures outcomes in utilities: measures of the preferences for the outcome state	Dollars	Quality-adjusted life years (QALYs)
Cost-benefit	Requires that outcomes (lives, quality of life) be given a monetary value	Dollars	Dollars

efits.[4] In the simplest case, an analysis of the benefits goes no further than to assume the clinical effect of the possible strategies is the same; the only difference arises from difference in costs. This type of analysis is termed a cost-minimizing study, because with outcomes assumed equal, the only relevant goal would be to minimize costs. The most common clinical example of a cost-minimizing study would be an evaluation of a therapeutic drug substitution program in which the efficacy of the two drugs was equivalent and the analysis looks only at the costs of the drug, its administration, and monitoring. Cost-consequence studies are only slightly more complicated, as they list the costs in dollars and outcome in whatever units are appropriate for the particular situation being evaluated. For example, suppose new upgrades are being proposed for network hardware to try to improve both network performance (perhaps measured in loading time for an electronic record of a standard size) and reliability (measured in expected number of minutes of unscheduled downtime per month). A cost-consequence study would simply generate lists, such as option A will cost $238/workstation, will require 6.8 milliseconds to load a chart, and will have 35 minutes of unscheduled downtime per month; whereas option B will cost $312/workstation, will require 3.2 milliseconds to load a chart, and will have 41 minutes of unscheduled downtime each month. No attempt is made to equate the value of downtime and speed; the results are presented to allow the decision makers to place their own value on the relative worth of the various outcomes and the trade-off between them.

Cost-effectiveness analysis (CEA) is defined by the use of a clinically relevant outcome to quantify the benefits, and is consequently the most common type of economic analysis used in health care. The clinical effectiveness measure may span a wide range, from global outcomes such as lives saved to limited outcomes such as number of infections avoided. The critical aspect is that the alternatives being evaluated be measured using the same outcome and the same metric. For example, a new component of a clinical information system may reduce the number of duplicate laboratory tests and x-rays ordered, but may cost resources to install and maintain. Assuming one believes the actual quality of care is unchanged, an appropriate metric might be the cost per number of duplicate tests avoided. For a clinical reminder system that warns clinicians when they are prescribing a drug to which a patient is allergic, the appropriate outcome might be cost per medication error avoided or even anaphylactic reaction avoided. For interventions that affect the quality of care and have the potential to affect mortality, the appropriate outcome may be cost per life saved, or perhaps life-years saved, which would also incorporate the remaining life expectancy of a patient who benefited from the program.

Cost utility analysis (CUA) is an extension of CEA that differs by measuring the outcome as a "utility." This is a measure of the strength of preference for the particular clinical outcome state, and is a measure of the quality of life attributable to living in a particular health state. It is intuitively obvious that people do not place the same value on various outcome states: a year of life after a stroke is worth less than a year of life without a stroke. There are multiple methods, such as SF-36 and EuroQOL, for measuring these preferences, as reviewed by Lara-Munoz and Feinstein.[5] There are several examples of scales throughout the literature.[6,7] The debate about appropriate utility measures began three decades ago. The unique attribute of utilities is that they provide a quantitative assessment of the magnitude of difference between the values of various health states. This allows the various outcome states to be measured in quality-adjusted life years (QALYs).

Cost-benefit analysis (CBA) is a form of economic evaluation that requires that both costs and benefits be valued in monetary terms. Therefore, to use CBA in health care, it is usually necessary to determine the value of the clinical outcome in dollars. Because this means placing a value on the cost of human life, it is often avoided as a mechanism for analysis in health care settings.

Each of the above analysis types is appropriate in a particular setting. For example, if outcomes are truly known to be equivalent between two different options, then ignoring outcomes and only analyzing costs (cost-minimizing study) may very well be an appropriate analysis. However, whichever analysis type is chosen, the costs (and benefits if included) need to be measured accurately, and in a manner comparable to other, similar studies. This chapter describes the techniques for conducting economic analysis, including the measurement of costs and outcomes; concentrates on their use in cost-effectiveness; and provides examples of cost-benefit analysis that has been used by health systems and hospital administrations to make various financial resource decisions in health care.

Conducting an Economic Analysis

When conducting an economic analyses, several decisions need to be made initially that set the stage for the type of costs and outcome data that will be used, the level of detail required in that data, and the sources and type of analysis that will be carried out. First, the investigator must decide the perspective from which the analysis will be carried out: The patient? The hospital? The insurance company? Society? Second, the overall time frame of the analysis needs to be decided: does the investigator care only about short-term effects, or will the technology choices alter the stream of resource use and benefits for many years to come?

The Perspective of the Analysis

The perspective of an analysis specifies from whose point of view the decision is being evaluated. The perspective of the analysis is important, because different types of costs and benefits accrue to different components of the health care system, and therefore different costs and outcomes should be included in an analysis depending on who is making the decision and who accrues benefits. For example, consider a clinical decision rule in an information system that allows a nurse to triage symptomatic urinary tract infections and treat a portion of these women over the telephone rather than have everyone be seen and evaluated. Although this may reduce overall costs and improve the quality of care, whether or not it makes sense to a particular provider group depends on the reimbursement mechanism. Under a capitated system where the health care provider is paid a monthly amount for all services provided, the benefit will accrue to the health care provider. Conversely, if providers operate under a fee-for-service insurance system where they are paid only for people they see or tests they perform, they may lose resources that the insurance company gains.

The preceding example illustrates the critical importance of choosing an appropriate perspective from which the analysis is completed. Different perspectives will include different types of costs and outcomes, depending on who bears the costs and who accrues the benefits. We consider below four specific perspectives.

Societal Perspective

The societal perspective is by definition the broadest perspective, and therefore should include all costs and benefits, regardless of who pays the costs or to whom benefits accrue. Furthermore, in addition to a global inclusion of all monetary costs and clinical outcomes, a societal perspective should include many of the costs and benefits that an individual payer or insurance company might not choose to include, such as out-of-pocket expenses of the patients, or the time spent by family members in the care of an ill relative.

Health Care Payer or Insurance Company Perspective

The perspective of a large health care provider, system, or insurer makes substantial sense for many economic analyses because they are often making resource allocation decisions regarding what type of services to cover, and what resources to expend in the production and provision of those services.

Hospital Perspective

The hospital perspective is commonly used to evaluate the effects of information systems, as it is often the hospital that is expending resources. The hospital perspective is also usually straightforward: the cost structure of the institution is generally known, and the costs that the hospital must include in national cost reports are published. Furthermore, the financial responsibility of the hospital is generally straightforward, with nonprofit or government hospitals responsible for working within a global budget, while in private or for-profit hospitals there is the financial oversight of a board of directors or investors. The costs and benefits included are those that directly accrue to the bottom line of the hospital.

Patient Perspective

Although arguably one of the most important perspectives from the individual patient's point-of-view, the patient's perspective is rarely used in comprehensive analyses. Part of the difficulty with the patient's perspective is that it does not include many costs simply because the patient doesn't pay them, the most obvious being costs paid by an insurance company.

Time Frame of the Analysis

Most decisions to implement a new program or introduce a new device or treatment set into motion a series of events (in terms of costs and benefits) that occur over time. It is not uncommon for these costs and benefits to occur at different times. When a hospital decides to implement a clinical information system, the majority of the expenses may be required at the beginning (capital expenses to purchase hardware, software, and installation costs, resources required for training), whereas many of the benefits do not occur for several years, when clinical processes have been changed. The important concept is that the time frame used in an economic analysis must match the actual duration of time required to encompass all of the important costs and benefits of the program. The classic example of this is the evaluation of the cost-effectiveness of a preventive intervention (lowering cholesterol) with a therapeutic intervention (coronary artery bypass surgery). Unless the data collection is carried out for a sufficient time for the cholesterol lowering strategy to have realized a benefit, the analysis will be biased in favor of the surgical intervention. On the other hand, since the treatment of acute urinary tract infection in otherwise healthy women carries no real risk of long-term events, a time frame of only a matter of days could be appropriate when comparing two different treatments for acute dysuria in women.

Self-Test 11.1

1. For the following types of information technology innovations, indicate which study methodology would be most appropriate for an economic analysis: cost minimizing, cost consequence, cost effectiveness, cost utility, or cost benefit.
   a. You are a vendor of an electronic medical record, and you want to show that installation of your product improves health care of hospitalized patients by decreasing length-of-stay, and improving quality of care.
   b. Your pharmacy department has proposed purchasing a new inventory control mechanism that will eliminate the need to carry large stocks of inventory on some items and decrease the number of pharmacy technicians that you need to hire. No changes in therapeutic outcome are expected.
   c. A large employer wants to assess the impact of an electronic algorithm for detecting high-risk employees so that preventive healthcare measures can be offered that will decrease future illness burden, absenteeism, and improve the efficiency and quality of life of its employee base.
   d. A pathology department is considering two different electronic pathology slide reviewing machines that allow the remote viewing of slides by an off-site pathologist. The resolution quality is equivalent, but the hardware, software, and personnel costs appear different.
2. For the following proposed economic analysis, list the most appropriate perspective (payer, hospital, society):
   a. A study of the economic effects of instituting a therapeutic substitution program in a pharmacy.
   b. A study that investigates the overall impact of the electronic transfer of clinical information between hospitals, home health agencies, nursing homes, private practitioners, and rehabilitation facilities of the overall quality of care of patients with orthopedic surgery in a region.

Definition and Measurement of Costs

For all types of economic analyses, the costs of each option must be clearly delineated and appropriately measured. There is tremendous variability in the methods with which health care providers, hospitals, and insurance companies calculate costs. In addition, there are differences between certain definitions traditionally used by accountants from those used by health care economists. In this section, the differences between costs and charges are discussed, the various types of costs included in economic analyses in health care defined, and a general overview of the types of cost accounting systems typically used in hospitals provided. Finally, more generalized national or regional measures of costs that can be used in economic analyses are described.

How Costs Do Not Equal Charges

One of the most important realizations over the past few decades with respect to health care costs is that there is little relationship between charges (the price that a hospital or provider asks the insurer or patient for payment) and the actual costs of that particular item or service to the provider.[9] There are many reasons for this, from the market strength of many insurance companies that negotiate lower charges from providers to desires on the part of certain institutions to magnify the appearance of donated free care by having high prices for self-pay patients.

Direct Costs

Direct costs are those costs that are an immediate consequence of the choice or decision being made. They typically include the costs of medical services (hospitalizations, medications, physician and other health care professional fees, durable medical equipment, etc).

Time Costs

The amount of time required by patients to participate in a treatment should be included as a real cost to any program. If two health programs are equally effective and have equal monetary costs, the program that required less patient time would be preferred. Details for measuring and evaluating different types of time expended in health care activities can be found in Gold et al.[3] The fundamental concept is that time is a valuable commodity that should be included in the overall costs of a particular intervention. It is often true, however, that when considering clinical information system interventions, patient time considerations are ignored, often because the patient is in the hospital the entire time under either program, and the time-costs would likely cancel out. On the other hand, if a particular information system intervention had the effect of decreasing length-of-stay, the differential times of the patients could be included in the analysis (and should be, if the analysis is being conducted from the societal point of view).

Indirect Costs (Productivity Costs)

There are differences in the definition of indirect costs used by health care economists and accountants; many authors choose the term *productivity costs* to more directly describe the types of costs being considered. Indirect costs or productivity costs are the monetary values of lost productivity that occurs as a consequence of the intervention and the disease being treated. For example, if a patient treated under one particular strategy can return to work but a patient treated under an alternative strategy cannot, the values of the lost productivity should be charged to the first program. As noted above, this type of cost would be appropriately included only if the analysis were being conducted from a patient or societal perspective.

Intangible Costs (Pain and Suffering)

There is no question that patients place a value on pain and suffering, as evidenced by the fact that patients spend resources (purchase pain relievers, accept operations that palliate symptoms) to eliminate or alleviate symptoms even if the intervention has no effect on the length of life or survival. However, finding an appropriate value may be extremely difficult, and most investigators do not include pain and suffering as a cost; rather, they include the values of that pain and suffering in the estimate of the quality of life of the particular health state. This is most commonly accomplished by using QALYs as the outcome measure, where the value of living in a state that includes pain and suffering is less than living in a state from which the pain and suffering are absent.

Mechanics of Cost Determinations

Once the perspective and time frame of the analysis is chosen, one must develop a method to assess and measure the costs that accrue from a particular intervention. There are, in general, two basic methods of determining costs: micro-costing methods and macro-costing methods. Each has benefits and difficulties, but can be used to develop accurate, robust cost analyses.

Micro-costing methods make use of detailed accounting principles to develop measures of what each product, service, or option costs by breaking it down into individual parts and determining the cost of each component. For example, the cost of a chest x-ray includes the cost of the film, a small portion of the amortized cost of the equipment, staff time to take and process the x-ray, radiologist time to read it, some small amount of power to run the equipment, a small part of the cost of housekeeping to clean the radiology areas, etc. The process can be extremely complicated, but many cost-accounting systems keep track of inputs to the various products that they produce at that level of detail. Often, the calculation is accomplished at a slightly higher level of detail, in which the costs of an entire department (say radiology) are calculated based on what portion of the overall hospital budget is attributable to the department (salaries, capital equipment costs, overhead, etc.), and these costs compared to the total charges for the product produced (billed) by that department. This global *cost-to-charge ratio* is then applied to the charge for each individual product or service produced by that department to estimate the cost of that item. More detail regarding costing methodology is found in Drummond et al.,[10] Chapter 4.

Macro-costing techniques use truly global measures of the costs (or payments) for services. For example, in the United States, the Centers for Medicare and Medicaid Services (CMS) has calculated (through a very complicated resource-based analysis) the estimated average cost for every physician service from office visits to various procedures to the costs of hospitalization for all categories of diagnoses. For hospitals, these are called diagnostic related groups (DRGs). They not only represent what the federal government will pay for particular services, but also are designed to represent the average true cost of that service or procedure. In the U.S., for individual providers, CMS pays practitioners according to the Resource-Based Relative Value Scale (RBRVS), which represents a complex calculation of the education, training, difficulty, and risk of various services and procedures. More information on cost analyses are available in Drummond et al.,[10] Chapter 4, Gold et al.,[3] and at the NICE Web site.

Often, cost analyses do not need to be conducted at a level of detail that requires knowledge of the costs of every component of a health care provider or hospital's cost structure. This is especially true in determining the costs of information systems, when the costs may be dictated by market forces (a particular vendor sells a system for a particular price). Costs savings (in terms of decreased need for personnel, changes in pharmaceutical costs, changes in maintenance fees) can also often be calculated from data derived from vendors, personnel files, and current hospital contracts. However, if a portion of the costs or benefits are measured in changes in the quantity of services, procedures, or clinical outcomes, a rigorous analysis of the true cost of those components needs to be accomplished.

Definition and Measurement of Outcomes and Benefits

With the exception of studies in which the clinically important outcomes are assumed to be equivalent, economic analyses in health care must have a mechanism for measuring and quantifying the outcome of interest. One of the most difficult aspects of this task is making sure that the various outcomes are measured using the same metric, that is, that the units of measurement for all possible choices or strategies are the same. The simplest cases are those in which the mortality and morbidity outcomes of a particular set of choices can legitimately be assumed to be the same; then the outcome measure such as changes in length-of-stay or numbers of duplicate tests avoided can be appropriate. It is even possible to ignore the long-term beneficial effects of a strategy if it has already been decided that the intermediate outcome that leads to a mortality benefit is desired. Consider a decision between different strategies to increase mammography screening in an outpatient setting. There might be a paper-based alert system placed on charts, a reminder and tracking system instantiated into an electronic medical record, a postcard reminder to patients incorporated into the scheduling software, or the development of a publicity campaign within the physical confines of the practice. Each one of these would have different costs and different impacts on the mammography rate for the practice. Provided information was known (e.g., from literature reports from other practices that had tried particular methods), estimates of the success rates could be determined, and estimates of the costs of each strategy could be derived as well. In this example, it would be appropriate to consider the cost-effectiveness outcome as costs per extra mammogram obtained, even though the long-run effect of the increasing mammography rate is to lower breast cancer incidence and mortality.

Matching the Correct Outcome Measure to the Problem

The choice of the appropriate outcome measure is dependent on the intended purpose of the economic analysis. If the analysis is designed to be used in global resource allocation decisions across many different possible uses of the financial resources, it is necessary to measure outcomes in a quantity such as lives saved or QALYs that can be compared across the various different options. However, economic analyses restricted to a much narrower outcome measure can be appropriate and valuable if their intended use is more local and restricted. For example, when considering the decision to purchase a new pharmacy module for a clinical information system to prevent medication errors and interaction checking, a hospital administration may be satisfied with simple cost-consequence analyses, such as reporting the cost per medication error avoided by implementing a particular system. Again, this ignores the long-term health benefits of error reduction, but considers "error reduction" as an outcome in its own right.

Adjusting for Quality of Life

It is intuitively obvious and supported by innumerable quality-of-life studies that patients do not value all health outcomes similarly: a year of life after a stroke is not valued as highly as a year of life in full health. Therefore, if the analysis is being conducted from society's perspective, the appropriate outcome is QALYs. However, the actual measurement of QALYs is not always straightforward: different assessment methods may arrive at different values, the assessed values may change over time, and the values may vary systematically with characteristics of the individuals responding to questionnaires. For these reasons, one should include an expert in utility or quality of life assessment if the analysis is intended to be done with QALYs as the outcome measure.

Cost-Minimizing Analysis

As noted above, the fundamental assumption in cost-minimizing analyses is that the clinical outcomes expected under each possible option are the same. The best example of such studies in health care are therapeutic substitution policies, where less expensive (usually generic) drugs are substituted for more expensive brand name drugs if the more expensive drug is ordered. Such therapeutic substitution policies are commonly embedded in clinical information systems that have pharmacy components. As an example, we will examine a simple case of an antibiotic substitution program.

Example 1: Antibiotic Substitution

The chair of the hospital formulary committee has requested that the pharmacy system institute an automatic therapeutic substitution program of a less expensive antibiotic (Cheapocillin) for the commonly ordered new antibiotic Cephokillumall. This program is to be built directly into the pharmacy component of the hospital's clinical information system (CIS). The argument is that Cheapocillin is substantially less expensive and by all reports equally effective for the treatment of infections. The infectious disease service agrees, and does not object to the therapeutic substitution on clinical grounds. Therefore, the most important prerequisite for conducting a cost-minimization study has been met: there is good evidence and agreement that the two strategies have equivalent outcomes. This allows the economic analysis of the new information system to concentrate entirely on costs.

The most important concept in cost-minimizing studies is the appropriate identification and enumeration of the costs of the various strategies. Table 11.2 outlines the costs of the various therapeutic strategies. Cheapocillin has very low pharmaceutical costs per dose ($0.50), but comes as a powder that must be reconstituted with saline by the pharmacist. This procedure is calculated to cost $11.00 per dose. Because of its short half-life, Cheapocillin must be administered four times a day, resulting in a daily cost of $46.00. Cephokillumall is substantially more expensive for each dose ($22.00) but comes in a ready-to-administer vial, so preparation and administration costs for the pharmacy are reduced ($8.50). The recommended regimen is one dose per day, producing a daily cost of $30.50. However,

TABLE 11.2. Example of a cost minimizing study of therapeutic substitution.

Cost	Cheapocillin	Cephokillumall
Cost per dose	$0.50	$22.00
Administration costs/dose	$11.00	$8.50
Doses per day	4	1
Total daily costs:	$46.00	$30.50
Cost of 5-day course	$230.00	$152.50
Laboratory costs (day 3)	$0.00	$28.00
Total costs	$230.00	$180.50

Note: This type of analysis assumes that the effectiveness of the two strategies (drugs) is the same, and only examines the costs of each alternative.

because of potential side effects of this drug on the kidney, laboratory tests need to be obtained to assess kidney function, which cost $28.00. Since both drugs are given for 5 days, the total cost of Cheapocillin is $230.00, and the total cost of Cephokillumall is $152.50 plus $28.00 for the laboratory test, or $180.50.

The point of the example is that even cost-minimizing studies may be more complicated than initial impressions, and the intuitive answer (Cheapocillin is obviously cheaper) may not hold up after an appropriate accounting of all costs related to a particular strategy.

The analysis can be relatively straightforward as described or it can be more complicated, in several possible ways. For example, the costs of implementing a therapeutic substitution program will be substantially less in an information system that already has a pharmacy module with decision support functions built-in than would be the case if it had to be developed from a CIS system that did not already have the pharmacy module. The costs of developing, implementing, and maintaining a particular function may also need to be included in the analysis, but the exact form and magnitude will be very dependent on the specific characteristics of the local information systems components that are available.

Cost-Effectiveness Analysis

The defining characteristic of cost-effectiveness is that the outcomes for each strategy are measured in the same, clinically meaningful outcome. The most general of these outcomes would be life expectancy (or its quality-adjusted companion, QALY). The purpose of this uniform measurement is that it allows various strategies (even if they are in different diseases) to be compared to each other and decisions about the efficient distribution of resources across various choices to be made. The economic principle that forms the foundation of CEA is that resources should be spent on the most cost-effective options first, and strategies or programs added or funded in order of their cost-effectiveness. In theory, this ensures that the resources expended are purchasing the most "health" possible. So, when faced with a series of choices between possible health-improving programs and a limited budget, economic principle would dictate that you rank the possible options in order of cost-effectiveness ratio (from the most cost-effective to the least cost-effective) and purchase programs in decreasing cost-effectiveness order until the budget limit is reached. In practice, this rank ordering of options followed by spending the available health care resources is rarely explicitly done. Often resources directed in one area (e.g., information services) cannot be redirected to another area of public service (e.g., social work). This is true at all levels of decision making, with each level containing a series of political, social, and organizational barriers to the strict application of CEA. However, it remains useful to understand this as the underlying concept in the intended use of CEA, which is designed to achieve the highest quantity of the outcome (chosen and valued by the investigator) for the least cost.

Graphically, the comparisons used in cost-effectiveness analysis are illustrated in Figure 11.2, which represents the cost-effectiveness plane. For any new therapy or choice that is being made, the costs and benefits need to be compared to the current strategy. For any new option, the new strategy can be more effective, less effective, or equivalent to the current strategy, and can be more expensive, less expensive, or equal in costs to the current strategy. This divides the cost-effectiveness plane into four quadrants that have useful interpretations. The lower right quadrant would represent strategies that are both *cheaper* and *more effective* than the existing strategy: these programs should simply be implemented. Similarly, those strategies that fall in the upper left quadrant are both *more expensive* and *less effective* than the current strategy: these should be avoided. It is only in the two remaining quadrants (the upper right quadrant, where strategies are *more expensive* and *more effective*, and the lower left, where strategies are *less expensive* but *not as effective*) that the use of CEA is appropriate. It is in these areas, where there is a *trade-off* between costs and benefits, that CEA is most useful.

The Incremental Cost-Effectiveness Ratio

A crucial aspect of a CEA is that something cannot be cost-effective in and of itself; it is only cost-effective (or not) compared to another alternative. Consequently, the statement "This clinical information system is cost-effective" is nonsensical; it must be accompanied by a description of what the system is being compared to. In fact, CEA is most useful when the strategies being examined represent a range of possibilities, each with different costs and effectiveness. Typical CEA studies provide the results of each possible strategy, and compare each to the next least effective or expensive.

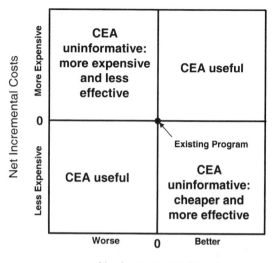

FIGURE 11.2. The cost-effectiveness (CE) plane. Compared to the costs and effects of a baseline program, a new strategy can be either more or less expensive or more or less effective that the current strategy. This divides the CE plane into four quadrants. The upper left quadrant represents those strategies that are both less effective and more expensive that the existing program; these programs require no choice and are clearly dominated by the current strategy. Similarly, no analysis is required for strategies that fall in the right lower quadrant. Projects in this quadrant are cheaper and better than the existing strategy, and should simply be adopted. The real benefit of cost-effectiveness analysis (CEA) is in the right upper quadrant (where strategies are more expensive but produce better outcomes) and in the left lower quadrant (where strategies are cheaper, but do not produce equivalent outcomes). It is in these areas that a trade-off exists between cost and effectiveness, the condition required for a CEA.

The global outcome measure that defines cost-effectiveness analysis is the incremental cost-effectiveness ratio (ICER). It represents the ratio of the net costs that will be expended by implementing a particular program divided by the net benefit, measured as an appropriate clinical outcome. It is defined as

$$\frac{Cost_B - Cost_A}{Effectiveness_B - Effectiveness_A}$$

or the net costs of moving to strategy B from strategy A divided by the net benefits (measured as a clinical outcome) of choosing strategy B over A. The units of the ICER are dollars per unit outcome, which represents the cost of an additional unit of the particular outcome measure. For example, if the outcome of an intervention is measured in lives saved, the ICER would be in units of dollars per life saved.

TABLE 11.3. Example of cost-effectiveness (CE) analysis of several lifesaving interventions.

Strategy	Cost	Outcome (year of life)	Net cost	Net effect	Incremental CE ratio
Strategy A	$10,000	3.5	n/a	n/a	n/a
Strategy B	$20,000	4.5	$10,000	1 year	$10,000/yr
Strategy C	$35,000	5.0	$15,000	0.5 years	$30,000/yr

Note: For each strategy, the table provides the cost of the strategy and the outcome in life-years gained. The net costs are calculated as the difference in costs from the previous strategy, and the net effects are the difference in outcomes for a strategy compared to the next least effective. The incremental cost-effectiveness ratio (ICER) is simply the net cost divided by the net effects.

To illustrate, we first examine a completely generic example, with hypothetical programs that both cost resources and save lives. Although this may not be the most common outcome measure used in CEA studies in biomedical informatics, it represents the most common application of CEA in health care, and is a reasonable starting point to develop an understanding of the technique.

Example 2: A Series of Lifesaving Therapies

A simple CEA is illustrated in Table 11.3 and displayed graphically in Figure 11.3. In the figure, only the upper right quadrant of Figure 11.2 is

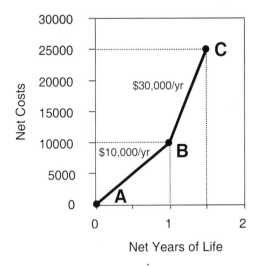

FIGURE 11.3. The cost-effectiveness plane. Assume the baseline strategy is A; the graph depicts the net (incremental) costs required to purchase the next best strategies B and then C, as well as the net or incremental gains that the strategy would provide.

represented for simplicity; all three strategies evaluated are more expensive and better than the current strategy. Assume that there are three possible strategies for treating a particular disease, and they have different costs and effects, as shown in the table. Current therapy is described by strategy A, which costs $10,000 and produces a mean of 3.5 years of survival. Two new therapies have been devised: strategy B costs $20,000 (an additional $10,000 compared to strategy A) but produces a longer survival of 4.5 years (an additional year compared to strategy A). A third treatment (strategy C) is even more expensive at $35,000, but does produce improved results, with patients living 5.0 years after receiving that therapy.

To calculate the ICER, the first step is to calculate the net costs and effects of moving from the base strategy to the next best strategy. From strategy A to B, the net cost is $10,000, the net effectiveness is 1 year: the ICER is therefore $10,000/life year gained. Then, the use of strategy C instead of strategy B costs an additional $15,000 ($35,000–$20,000), and gains another 0.5 life years (5.0–4.5): the ICER of moving from strategy B to strategy C is $30,000/life year. The calculations are illustrated graphically in Figure 11.3. The net costs and effects (in terms of life years) are plotted in the cost-effectiveness plane. The slope of the line between each possible strategy is the ICER of that strategy.

It is left to health policy makers to decide how they will use such figures. For example, if controlling health expenditure is important, they may decide to sanction widespread use of strategy B but reserve strategy C for those patients most likely to benefit, in view of its much higher ICER.

Cost-Benefit Analyses: The Cost-Benefit Ratio

As noted in the section on types of cost analyses, cost-benefit analyses (CBAs) are distinguished by the valuation of both the costs and outcomes of a strategy in monetary terms. The cost-benefit ratio then simply measures the ratio between the incremental costs of choosing a strategy over the benefits (measured in monetary units) of each strategy:

$$\frac{Cost_B - Cost_A}{Monetary\ Benefit_B - Monetary\ Benefit_A}$$

The advantage of CBA, and one of the reasons for its use in many fields other than health care, is that the interpretation of the cost-benefit (CB) ratio is straightforward: any strategy with a CB ratio less than 1 means that the benefits are valued more than the costs, and instituting that strategy produced a net benefit. Cost-benefit ratios of greater than 1 indicate that the costs are greater than the benefits: such projects should not usually be undertaken. This applies even for projects undertaken for the public good since if something has a value, for the purpose of CBA it is necessary to quantify that value in dollars. The value of the public good is then contained in the benefit side of the equation. The problem often is trying to agree on

TABLE 11.4. Simple cost-benefit analysis.

	System A	System B
Costs		
Cost of system	$16,000	$12,500
Cost of personnel training	$2,850	$1,000
Maintenance contract	$1,850	$1,250
Total cost:	$20,700	$14,750
Benefits		
Increased billing revenue	$32,000	$22,000
Decreased staffing requirements	$14,000	$0
Decreased debt service	$1,340	$1,340
Total benefit:	$47,340	$23,340
Cost-benefit ratio	0.44	0.63

Note: In this analysis, two replacement billing systems are compared with respect to their system and maintenance costs, as well as the effects they have on personnel needs and their effect on billing revenue and debt service from decreased time in accounts receivable.

a monetary value for commodities like health status or increased security resulting from police protection, military strength, etc.

Example 3: Cost-Benefit Analysis

A hospital needs to upgrade its billing and patient accounts system because the current version of the system is no longer supported by the vendor. There are two options, A and B, which differ in their startup and maintenance costs. These options also have different effects on the ability to produce accurate bills, their personnel staffing requirements, and the speed with which bills are submitted (which decreases the financial resources caught up in accounts receivable). Table 11.4 details the costs and benefits (both measured in dollars) for each option. For example, system A is more expensive to purchase than system B, and has higher costs of personnel training and higher maintenance fees. However, it also is a more accurate system, leading to increased billing revenue, as well as requiring fewer personnel to operate and maintain, which may save the salary of a part time data-entry clerk ($14,000). Assume that all these costs have been properly spread over the expected life of the product. Although system A is more expensive, it returns more benefit for every dollar spent. The CB ratio indicates that it costs only 44 cents for each dollar it saves, whereas system B costs 63 cents for each dollar it returns. Although any project with a CB ratio of less than 1 produces more benefit than it costs, choices can also be ranked, based on which options produces the highest return. It is important to note that some authors report the *benefit-cost ratio* (which is benefits divided by costs), which inverts the ratio. If reported in this manner, ratios over 1 are favored, and ratios under 1 are not.

Self-Test 11.2

1. Consider the following costs of alternative components of a information systems deployment and the number of lives each component is expected to save. If the particular group making this decision feels that it can spend no more than $75,000 per life year saved, which components strategy should it pursue? (Calculate the ICER of each strategy, ranked by effectiveness.)

Strategy	Cost	Outcome (life years gained)
Strategy A	$80,000	3.5
Strategy B	$50,000	3
Strategy C	$30,000	2.5
Strategy D	$90,000	3.6

2. Currently, a health plan is spending $150,000 on a health prevention program that the plan feels increases the life expectancy of the patient population by 10 life-years (averaged over the entire population). A proposal has been made for a new program that costs $130,000, and is known elsewhere to save 15 life years. Is a formal CEA of this program necessary?

Discounting Future Costs and Benefits

It is clear from basic economic analysis (and common sense) that dollars spent today are not directly equivalent to those spent in the past or in the future. The changing value of a dollar over time has two components: inflation and the real rate of return. Inflation represents the change in prices in an economy, and requires that prices (and therefore costs) be standardized to a common base year if expenditures from multiple different years are to be added, compared, or analyzed. Dollars spent in different years can be adjusted to a base year through the consumer price index (CPI).[11] There is also a health care specific price index, the Medical Price Index (MPI), which is used to adjust the prices of medical and health care goods and services.[11] In addition, however, even after adjusting for inflation, there is a need to account for the fact that dollars can be invested and produce greater value in the future. Even if the inflation rate were zero, the real rate of return (interest rate) in society would return more dollars next year to an investment made today; therefore, a dollar spent today is not worth the same as a dollar spent tomorrow.

The *present value* (PV) of an expenditure of X dollars t years in the future with an interest rate of r is

$$PV = \frac{X}{(1+r)^t}$$

So if a particular strategy incurs a cost of $100 next year, and the interest rate is 5%, the value today of that $100 expenditure next year is only $95.23

[100/(1 + 0.05)^1] This is because $95.23 invested today at 5% interest produces the $100 needed for the program a year from now. For a stream of costs $(X_1, X_2, \ldots, X_n)$ made over time under an interest rate of r, the present value is

$$PV = \frac{X_1}{(1+r)^1} + \frac{X_2}{(1+r)^2} + \frac{X_3}{(1+r)^3} + \frac{X_4}{(1+r)^4} \ldots + \frac{X_n}{(1+r)^n}$$

For all resource use that occurs generally more than a year in the future, it is both reasonable and appropriate to discount those costs to their present value equivalents.

Discounting Benefits

There is a natural intuition about the reasons we must discount costs: it is clear that a dollar today is not worth the same as a dollar tomorrow. Although the same intuition regarding benefits does not exist, there are equally persuasive reasons why an appropriate analysis must discount the value of benefits (years and/or quality of life) as well. One of the consequences of discounting costs but not discounting benefits is that the analysis would produces a change in the relative valuation of outcomes with respect to resources over time. In other words, by discounting costs but not benefits, the amount of monetary value attached to a particular outcome would change over time, even if the societal value for those outcomes were constant. If a life-year is worth $50,000 today, discounting costs, but not benefits, implies that the optimal ICER next year is less than $50,000/life year. The problem of discounting benefits is described in more detail in Gold et al.,[3] Drummond et al.,[10] and in a landmark technical paper by Keeler and Cretin.[12] However, virtually all methodology groups that have examined the problem agree that costs and benefits should be discounted at the same rate.

Choosing a Discount Rate

The choosing of an appropriate discount rate is not trivial, however. It is important to remember that the discount rate is quite different from the inflation rate, which represents the "price" of money. In economic analyses, the discount rate refers to the real growth rate of money, after the effects of inflation have been removed. There are several recommendations for choosing a discount rate; they differ by country and are sometimes dependent on what type of resource (public or private) is being used. Most recommendations are between 3% and 5%, and discussions regarding these choices can be found in Drummond et al.,[10] Chapter 4.

Sensitivity Analysis

It is virtually impossible to conduct an economic analysis without making assumptions regarding a particular component of the costs or benefits. One of the most powerful attributes of placing an analysis in a quantitative analytic framework is the ability to test the effect of different assumptions on the outcome. However, such "sensitivity analyses" have many other uses. During the design and development of an economic analysis, the investigator can use sensitivity analysis to ensure that the components of the analysis represent the situation as designed. For example, it is often possible to know ahead of an analysis what the expected effect of a particular change in a particular parameter will have on the answer. If one of the inputs in a CEA is the effectiveness of a particular therapy, then the cost-effectiveness (CE) of an option should increase as the predicted effectiveness of that particular treatment increases. To make sure an analytic model is working as expected, a series of these analyses should be conducted: an option's CE ratio should increase as the cost of that option increases, and should decline as the cost decreases. Although it seems obvious, when the analytic model that has been constructed to evaluate a problem is complex, this is the easiest mechanism for checking that the model represents the actual problem well.

There two major types of sensitivity analysis: structural sensitivity analysis, in which the actual components of the analysis are varied to understand the effects of various different assumptions regarding the structure of the model, and parameter sensitivity analysis, in which the values of the variables in the model (costs, probabilities of various outcomes, etc.) are varied over reasonable ranges to understand the effect of variability in the parameter estimates.

Structural Sensitivity Analyses

The goal of structural sensitivity analysis is to help ensure that the important and correct components of the problem have been included and are related in an appropriate manner. For example, an analysis of an antibiotic interaction and allergy-checking program in a pharmacy system might be analyzed only considering the effect on error reduction (number of allergic reactions, number of medication side effects). However, the new procedures may have an unpredictable effect on pharmacists' time, and a complete analysis would generally include what happens to the work loads of the pharmacists. Although a common assumption is that it would save pharmacist time, it is possible that a whole new set of activities (responding to complaints from clinicians regarding the medication interactions checker) may actually increase pharmacist time. Also, it is possible that the interaction program would teach the clinicians, and actually affect the accuracy and efficiency of their prescribing behavior over time. Therefore, a simple analysis would not include pharmacist time or the effect on long-term clinical behavior, and there is no direct way of including that in a simple model by just changing a probability or value in the analysis. Including pharmacist time and long-term effects on behavior would require a model with entirely new components in it, and would represent a structural sensitivity analysis in that the actual structure of the model representing the strategies is extended to include a different level of detail concerning the potential outcomes of each strategy.

Parameter Estimate Sensitivity Analyses

Virtually every number involved in an economic analysis is at best a point estimate of a quantity that could, in reality, be different from the specific number estimated in that particular instance. For example, even in the situation in which the estimate of a particular cost is the result of an economic analysis conducted alongside a randomized controlled trial, the cost estimate is only accurate within some confidence limits; had the trial been conducted in a different set of patients or a different setting, undoubtedly the estimated costs would be (at least slightly) different. More commonly, the estimate may come from the literature, and is accompanied by a measure of its accuracy given by confidence limits or standard deviation. Although the accuracy with which parameters for a particular analysis are known may vary, it is rarely (if ever) the case that a parameter is known exactly. Therefore an analysis of the model outputs using slightly different estimates for each parameter is necessary.

One of the most common methods of describing the variability of results in an economic analysis is to provide *baseline*, *best-case*, and *worst-case* calculations. This is illustrated in Figures 11.4 and 11.5. Assume that a CEA has been done as described in Figure 11.4. There are two strategies, A and B, each with different costs in several categories (hospital costs, ambulatory costs, pharmacy costs, and time costs) and strategy B is both more expensive and more effective (it adds 5 years of life expectancy for this particular disease). The straightforward calculation of the ICER is to

Strategy A			Strategy B	
Variable	Baseline		Variable	Baseline
Hospital costs	$60,000		Hospital costs	$102,000
Ambulatory costs	$4,600		Ambulatory costs	$9,400
Drug costs	$900		Drug costs	$2,000
Time costs	$2,800		Time costs	$8,000
Total costs:	$68,300		Total costs:	$121,400
Outcomes:	5.0 years		Outcomes:	10.5 years

$$\frac{\text{NET Costs: Strategy B} - \text{Strategy A}}{\text{NET Benefits: Strategy B} - \text{Strategy A}} = \frac{\$121,400 - 68,300 = \$53,100}{10.5 \text{ years} - 5.0 \text{ years} = 5.5 \text{ years}} = \$9.655/\text{year}$$

FIGURE 11.4. Sample cost-effectiveness analysis, describing the comparison between two strategies, A and B, in which B is both more expensive and more effective than A, and calculating a cost-effectiveness (CE) ratio.

Net Difference in costs

Variable	lowest	baseline	highest
Hospital costs	$30,000	$42,000	$85,000
Ambulatory costs	$3,900	$4,800	$6,800
Drug costs	$,900	$1,100	$1,300
Time costs	$4,000	$5,200	$6,400
Total costs:	$38,800	$53,100	$99,500

Net Difference in Benefits

Life expectancy	4.8 years	5.5 years	8.2 years

Best Case:	**Baseline Case:**	**Worst Case:**
Least Expensive	Best estimate of	Most Expensive
Most Effective	Costs and effects	Least Effective

$$\frac{\$38,800}{8.2 \text{ years}} = \$4732/\text{year} \qquad \frac{\$53,100}{5.5 \text{ years}} = \$9655/\text{year} \qquad \frac{\$99,500}{4.8 \text{ years}} = \$20729/\text{year}$$

FIGURE 11.5. Best-case/worst-case sensitivity analysis. A common method to evaluate the sensitivity of a result is to combine all of the worst (least favorable) assumptions and calculate a worst-case CE ratio, and repeat the analysis with all of the best (most favorable) assumptions and calculate a best-case CE ratio.

calculate the net change in costs incurred by moving from the standard therapy A to strategy B, and the net change in benefits. As shown, strategy B produces 5.5 additional years of life for a cost of $53,000, for an ICER of $9,655/year.

However, it is extremely unlikely that all of the estimates of costs and benefits are exact. In fact, they are all only estimates, and there are likely high and low limits of those estimates. For example, the extra life expectancy gained may be 5.5 years at baseline, but the confidence limits surrounding that gain could be wide. For the sake of this example, assume that the net benefit ranges from a low of 4.8 years to a high of 8.2 years. Similarly, each of the cost estimates has some inherent variability. Figure 11.5 provides the ranges of each component cost that goes into the estimates of the costs of strategy A and strategy B, producing low, baseline and high estimates of the difference in costs. Coupled with the best, baseline, and worst estimates of the benefits, these can be used to create best-case, baseline, and worst-case scenarios, shown in the bottom of Figure 11.5. The worst-case scenario would be produced if the most pessimistic estimates of costs were correct and the least optimistic estimates of benefit were also correct, which would produce an ICER of about $20,700 per year of life gained. The best case (which would represent the least expensive, most effective combination) would result in an ICER of only $4,700/year of life gained, and the baseline estimate (representing our best estimate of the difference in costs and difference in effects) would estimate an ICER of around $9,700/year of life gained.

Although the best case/worst case scenario is a common method for presenting the variability in results, it is crucially dependent on the accuracy of the estimates of the high and low values for component costs and effects.

One-Way Sensitivity Analysis

Although the best-case/worst-case method provides an estimate of the spread of possible results from an overall analysis, it does not provide an estimate of the effect of individual variables on the ICER. One-way sensitivity analysis examines the effect of a single variable on the outcome. This is calculated by varying the values of that single variable while holding all others constant, and examining the effect on the ICER implied by changes in that one variable. A simple one-way sensitivity analysis is shown in Figure 11.6, in which the hospital costs portion of strategy B in the example in Figures 11.4 and 11.5 is systematically varied from $100,000 to $200,000 while all of the other costs and benefits are held constant at their baseline values. The resulting graph indicates the effect of changes in that one parameter (hospital costs in strategy B) on the outcome measure, the ICER. It is common practice to conduct multiple one-way sensitivity analyses to check the effect of all the primary variables in a cost model and

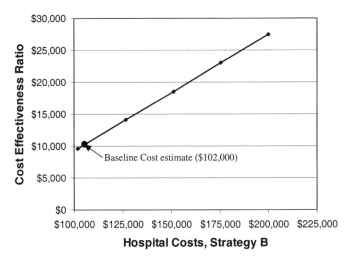

FIGURE 11.6. One-way sensitivity analysis. The x-axis represents the values of the hospital costs component for strategy B of the cost analysis example shown in Figures 11.5 and 11.6, the y-axis depicts the incremental cost effectiveness ratio (ICER) implied by those values of hospital costs, holding all other costs and benefits constant. As the costs of strategy B increase, the ICER worsens.

understand which estimates have the potential to have a large impact on the answer.

Multiway Sensitivity Analysis

A direct extension of the one-way concept, two-, three-, and multiway sensitivity analysis calculates the effect of simultaneously varying two, three, or more variables at once, again holding all others constant. Because multiple dimensions are difficult to graph, multiway sensitivity analyses rarely plot the ICER by the various combinations of component variable; rather, they plot whether the ICER passes some threshold ICER or not. For example, a two-way sensitivity analysis might plot the ranges of hospital costs and expected outcomes for which the ICER is over $50,000/year.

Monte Carlo Sensitivity Analysis

Sensitivity analysis is really more a statement about how the model is constructed than a measure of how the world represented by the model behaves. The reason is that sensitivity analyses are deterministic; they simply state that, if the values of the component parts of an analysis are W, X, and Y, then the calculated answer (the ICER) is Z. However, the analysis makes no statement concerning which of those values is the most likely, or how often a particular combination of values is believed to occur. This is a problem for the best-case/worst-case scenario methods as well; how likely is it that the least expensive estimates will coincide with the most effective estimates to produce the best-case scenario?

This problem can be addressed through the use of Monte Carlo or probabilistic sensitivity analysis. In this method, instead of representing each variable as a single number, it is replaced by a probability distribution that represents the inherent variability in that particular parameter. These distributions can be empirical (derived from real data from which the estimates have been made), or hypothetical. For example, many of the data used in economic analyses come from hospital discharge costs; over a large number of patients these data will have a mean and a standard deviation. The data resemble some distribution (normal, log-normal, etc.), and a distribution with the appropriate parameters can represent the variability in the input data. Then, the analysis is duplicated by running the model thousands of times, and in each iteration a different number is pulled from each distribution representing a variable in the analysis. This produces thousands of answers to the analysis, and these can be plotted in the cost-effectiveness plane. Figure 11.7 illustrates the results of a hypothetical Monte Carlo sensitivity analysis of a new strategy. The center of the graph represents the status quo; the large circle labeled "baseline estimate" represents the best estimate of the difference in costs and effects of the new program. Each dot represents one replication of the analysis with a specific set of values for

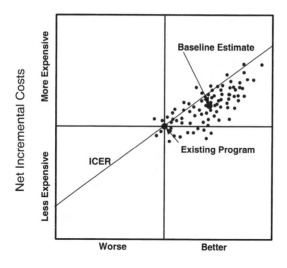

FIGURE 11.7. Monte Carlo sensitivity analysis. In this technique, individual variables in the analysis are replaced with probability distributions, and the analysis is recalculated hundreds or thousands of times: for each iteration a different set of data randomly drawn from the distributions describing the variables is used. The resulting plot indicates the various possible cost and effectiveness answers for each iteration. In this figure, most of the iterations result in points lying in the right upper quadrant, where CEA is appropriate. On only very few iterations does the analysis indicate the new strategy is worse than the existing strategy. Note that in the CE plane, the acceptable ICER is represented by the slope of a line through the existing program. Points below the line represent areas where the intervention is cost-effective in that the ICER is less than the acceptable range; points above that line represent combinations of variables in which the ICER is above the acceptable level.

the input variables drawn from the distributions. The analysis is repeated many times, represented by the multiple dots. In this analysis, most of the dots cluster around the baseline, and the majority are found below a line that represents the acceptable cost-effectiveness threshold, indicating that there is a high likelihood that this strategy is economically preferred to the existing strategy.

Self-Test 11.3

1. The implementation of a particular information technology in your health system will produce the following streams of costs and benefits (all defined in terms of dollars).

New information technology (IT) installation projected
costs and benefits

	Year 1	Year 2	Year 3	Year 4	Year 5
Costs	$100,000	$40,000	$10,000	$10,000	$10,000
Benefits	0	$30,000	$40,000	$50,000	$60,000

a. Without considering discounting, is investing in this project a good strategy?
b. Also without discounting future revenue and cost streams, what is the cost-benefit ratio of this project?
c. Assume a discount rate of 5%, and assume the hospital considers all costs and benefits as occurring at the end of the year. What are the present values of the cost and benefit streams?
d. What is the cost benefit ratio of this project with the inclusion of discounting at 5%?

Confidence Limits on Cost-Effectiveness Ratios

(This more advanced material can be skipped without loss of continuity.)

As with any analysis that involves a decision, decision makers must have methods for assessing how sure they are of the particular results. In traditional biomedical studies, this takes the form of the p value, which indicates how likely it is that the result was found by chance alone. Small p values provide high confidence that the particular result is real and not simply an effect of chance. In economic studies, it is difficult to estimate a quantity equivalent to a p value, primarily because many of the parameters may be estimates that have ranges but do not come from a specific distribution. For example, the estimated cost of installing a new component of an electronic medical record may be estimated at between $15,000 and $25,000, but there is no specific, statistical estimate of the mean and spread of the possible costs for that particular component.

The analysis of the variability of the ICER is further complicated by the fact that it is a *ratio*. Ratios do not have the stable statistical properties of sums. For example, although the variance of a sum of random, independent variables is the sum of the variance of each variable, the variance of a ratio is *not* the ratio of the variances. Therefore, it is extremely difficult to develop statistical confidence limits surrounding the ICER. Most commonly, graphical or simulation methods are used to estimate these confidence limits.

Box Method

The most straightforward method is a graphical one, illustrated in Figures 11.8 and 11.9. In Figure 11.8, imagine there is a cost-effectiveness study for which the net difference in effects is known for sure, but there is some uncertainty concerning the net difference in costs. Specifically, assume that

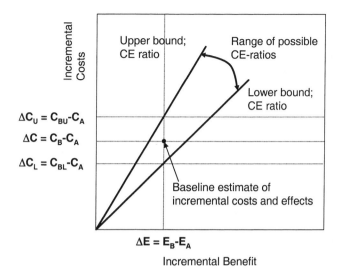

FIGURE 11.8. Box method for evaluating the confidence limits of a CE ratio. This figure assumes that the net difference in effectiveness is known for sure, but that the net change in costs is known with uncertainty, indicated by the upper and lower limits on the change in costs (ΔC_u, ΔC_L). Since the slope of the line from the origin to the intersection of the incremental costs and benefits represents the CE ratio, the two lines shown indicate the upper and lower bound of the ratio in this case.

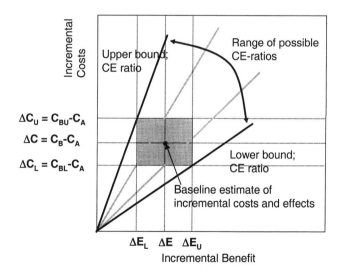

FIGURE 11.9. Box method for confidence in CE ratios when both parameters contain uncertainty. This figure is identical to Figure 11.8 except it is assumed that there is uncertainty in both the net benefit and the net costs, and each has a range of possibilities. As you can see, the possible range of CE ratios increases when there is unknown variability in both parameters.

there is an upper and lower bound of the estimates on the difference in costs, indicated by the point ΔC_U and ΔC_L in the figure. Because a line from the existing program to the estimate of the net costs and effects of the other strategy represents that program's ICER, the upper and lower bounds of the cost-effectiveness ratio for the program can be represented by the two lines indicated in the figure. Of course, the more realistic situation is that there will be uncertainty in both estimates of the net costs and net effects, as represented in Figure 11.9. Here, there are upper and lower bounds for both the net costs and effects, and the upper and lower bounds of the cost-effectiveness ratio are even larger, touching the edges of the box (hence the name "box" method) that represents the set of possible points that could contain the true ICER.

Special Characteristics of Cost-Effectiveness Studies in Biomedical Informatics

Although the principles of economic analysis are the same regardless of the content area of the problem being addressed, there are special circumstances surrounding the specific nature of a particular health care problem that an investigator needs to incorporate in economic analyses of that particular area. There are several such special circumstances in informatics that need to be understood in order to conduct accurate and appropriate economic analyses.

System Start Up

The deployment of a particular feature or use of a clinical information system may appear very different depending on what components of the system are already in place. For example, the decision to introduce order entry into a clinical information system will appear very different if the existing clinical information system already has components that can accept orders and relay them to the pharmacy, radiology system, etc. Similarly, consider the decision to introduce an allergy-checking and medication interaction system after a high-profile error has occurred in a hospitalized patient. The costs of such a system could look very different if it required purchasing an entire pharmacy system, as compared to the situation where adding a new module to an existing system will accomplish the task.

Similarly, costs that have already been expended (whether the decision was appropriate or not) should not be included in the costs of a new strategy, even if that strategy uses those components. This makes use of the incremental concepts that we have stressed. For example, in the decision to implement computerized physician order entry in a clinical record system that is scheduled for deployment already, the cost of the record system installation, development, maintenance, etc., is not appropriately charged to the physician order entry component; the decision to install those components had already been made for other reasons. The only reasonable costs to include in the decision regarding physician order entry are the additional costs that will now be incurred to install, manage, and update the order entry component.

Sharing Clinical Information System Costs

This applies because the costs of systems are often distributed across many departments. The hospital can't exist without billing, so if the billing is used system for an additional purpose, how much of the cost should be attributed to the new program? Certainly, any additional costs required to modify or interface with the CIS should be included, as should some component of the maintenance contracts, upgrades, and other ongoing costs. However, it is sometimes very difficult to understand how to distribute those costs across various components that use them.

Information systems may have life cycles running on a different time scale than the process they are used for. For example, a particular clinical system that is installed to improve patient safety and decrease fatal drug errors may have a system life of 5 to 8 years, and require multiple upgrades. At the end of the life span of the product, a new system or comprehensive upgrade may have to be purchased. If the benefits of this medication interaction system have long-term effects, the evaluation from a societal point-of-view would require including the continuing costs of system replacement, etc. However, these distant future costs are often not included in individual hospital analyses.

Examples of Cost-Effectiveness Studies in Biomedical Informatics

This section provides examples of two cost studies in which the effects of a clinical information system were economically evaluated. The guides to the evaluation of economic analyses by Drummond et al.[13] and O'Brien et al.[14] provide a useful template for the critique of published studies. There are four important components in the analysis of the validity of economic study results (from Drummond et al.):

1. Did the analysis provide a full economic comparison of health care strategies?
2. Were the costs and outcomes properly measured and valued?
3. Was an appropriate allowance made for uncertainties in the analysis?
4. Are estimates of the costs and outcomes related to the baseline risk in the treatment population?

The two articles are reviewed using these questions. We would recommend having a copy of the full article available while reading the critiques.

The study by Wang et al.[15] examines the financial costs and benefits of instituting a hypothetical electronic medical record. No attempt is made to associate the effects with clinical outcomes; the study is only concerned with financial results such as increased charge capture, decreased drug utilization, and decreased costs in maintaining and pulling paper charts. The article uses data from the published literature, the authors' own electronic medical record system, and expert opinion to make assumptions regarding the costs and benefits of system implementation. The setting of the study is a U.S. practice in which some of the patients are fully capitated (the practice only receives a set amount per month to care for these individuals, and must pay for health care expenditures out of that pool) and some of the patients have fee-for-service insurance, in which the practice is paid according to a bill that is generated by the practice. The practice, therefore, accrues benefit if it reduces expensive medication use and laboratory tests in the capitated group, and accrues benefit if it can improve and enhance billing practices in the fee-for-service group. The analysis is carried out for 5 years, with setup and initialization costs only accruing in year 1, and maintenance costs, license fees, and other recurring costs charged in the years that they occur. The costs and expected changes in expenditure for various laboratory tests and the increase in billing accuracy for patients and other benefits are listed, with ranges placed on those estimates. The authors calculate that, on average, the net benefit from instituting an electronic medical record was over $86,000 per provider over a 5-year period of time, or $13,000 per provider per year.

With respect to the first question posed by Drummond et al., the answer is mixed: the authors provide only a single alternative (electronic medical record, EMR). However, this is the relevant comparison, and multiple possible EMRs could be evaluated through the extensive sensitivity analyses. With respect to the second point, although extensive analysis was completed regarding the various costs and benefits, all the values represent only the financial gains: no clinical gains are included, making the analysis undervalue the EMR. The analysis clearly incorporated uncertainties in the estimates of input parameters and conducted multiple one-way and several multiway sensitivity analysis of critical estimates to determine how robust the analysis was to variability in assumptions. Finally, the last criterion regarding validation asks whether the outcomes and costs are related to the baseline risks of the population: this requirement relates much more directly to the economic analysis of a particular disease process, and is not particularly relevant in this study. On the whole, this study adheres to formal methodological recommendations quite well.

The second study by Evans et al.[16] details the effects of the implementation of a computerized program to help clinicians choose the proper antibiotic regimen for seriously ill individuals in the intensive care unit at a large academic hospital, using a pre–post design where the outcomes are measured for a year before implementation and then for a year after implementation. The program has multiple clinical algorithms that evaluate the type of infection, the current, local resistance patterns of bacterial strains at that hospital, and the level of illness of the individual, as well as many other clinical factors. The program not only recommends whether or not a particular patient needs an antibiotic, but also makes recommendations on the particular drug to use, the dose, and the interval. Over the course of the hospitalization, as clinical conditions and laboratory results change, the program makes recommendations for the modification of the patient's antibiotic regimen. Benefits of the program are measured in terms of the number of antibiotics ordered, the duration of dose, the number of days of excess antibiotics provided, and the length and costs of hospital and intensive care unit stays.

The analysis clearly does not provide a comprehensive analysis of the economic outcomes of the program. Many of the outcomes are clinical, and there is no attempt to include evidence that the program improved life expectancy, etc.; length of stay and avoidance of allergic reactions are the only two clinical outcomes. Furthermore, with respect to whether costs and outcomes were correctly valued, again the answer (for a comprehensive analysis) must be no. There are no costs of developing and implementing the program included in the analysis, yet the authors indicate that they have been working on the program for over a decade, which must represent a large amount of resources. As noted, clinical outcomes are not valued, and benefits are essentially only calculated as a pre–post change in these outcome variables; long-term effects (survival, etc.) are not included. There is very little attention to sensitivity analysis, although ranges for the outcomes found in the trial are provided. Finally, since the analysis takes place in an environment identical to the expected use, the incidence of various infections, antibiotic uses, etc., are exactly what would be expected to be seen in clinical practice at a similar facility.

From an economic point of view, this study is clearly more a cost-consequence than a true cost-effectiveness or cost-benefit analysis. Because there was no attempt to include the costs of development and implementation, it is not possible to evaluate the benefits of duplicating this effort elsewhere. However, the study provides a remarkable amount of useful information, indicating that, if well conducted, any type of economic analysis may be useful. It provides an excellent estimate of the amount of wasted and inappropriate care that can be removed from the use of antibiotics in seriously ill hospitalized patients through the use of computer-based treatment algorithms.

References

1. Centers for Disease Control and Prevention. Total health expenditures as a percent of gross domestic product and per capita health expenditures in dollars: Selected countries and years 1960–2000 in Health, United States, 2003, Table 111 on the CDC Web site: http://www.cdc.gov/nchs/hus.htm.

2. Udvarhelyi IS, Colditz GA, Rai A, Epstein AM. Cost-effectiveness and cost-benefit analyses in the medical literature. Are the methods being used correctly? Ann Intern Med 1992;116(3):238–244.

3. Gold MR, Siegel JE, Russel LB, Weinstein MC. Cost Effectiveness in Health and Medicine. New York: Oxford University Press, 1996.

4. Doubilet P, Weinstein MC, McNeil BJ. Use and misuse of the term "cost-effective" in medicine. N Engl J Med 1986;314(4):253–256.

5. Lara-Munoz C, Feinstein AR. How should quality of life be measured? J Invest Med 1999;47(1):17–24.

6. Feeny D, Furlong W, Torrance GW, et al. Multiattribute and single-attribute utility functions for the health utilities index Mark 3 system. Med Care 2002;40(2):113–128.

7. Torrance GW, Feeny D. Utilities and quality-adjusted life years. Int J Technol Assess Health Care 1989;5(4):559–575.

8. Rosser R, Kind P. A scale of valuations of states of illness: is there a social consensus? Int J Epidemiol 1978;7(4):347–358.

9. Finkler S. The distinction between costs and charges. Ann Intern Med 1982;96:102–109.

10. Drummond ME, O'Brien B, Stoddart GL, Torrance GW. Methods for the Evaluation of Health Care Programmes, 2nd ed. Oxford: Oxford Medical Publications, 1997.

11. United States Department of Labor. Consumer price Index. http://www.bls.gov/news.release/cpi.toc.htm.

12. Keeler EB, Cretin S. Discounting of life-saving and other nonmonetary effects. Management Sci 1983;29:300–306.

13. Drummond MF, Richardson WS, O'Brien BJ, Levine M, Heyland D. Users' guides to the medical literature. XIII. How to use an article on economic analysis of clinical practice. A. Are the results of the study valid? Evidence-Based Medicine Working Group. JAMA 1997;277(19):1552–1557.

14. O'Brien BJ, Heyland D, Richardson WS, Levine M, Drummond MF. Users' guides to the medical literature. XIII. How to use an article on economic analysis of clinical practice. B. What are the results and will they help me in caring for my patients? Evidence-Based Medicine Working Group. JAMA 1997; 277(22):1802–1806.

15. Wang SJ, Middleton B, Prosser LA, et al. A cost-benefit analysis of electronic medical records in primary care. Am J Med 2003;114(5):397–403.

16. Evans RS, Pestotnik SL, Classen DC, et al. A computer-assisted management program for antibiotics and other antiinfective agents. N Engl J Med 1998; 338(4):232–238.

Annotated Bibliography

Books

Drummond ME, O'Brien B, Stoddart GL, Torrance GW. Methods for the Evaluation of Health Care Programmes, 2nd ed. Oxford: Oxford Medical Publications, 1997.
  This text presents a comprehensive, easy-to-follow description of the various components that go into an economic analysis. After an introduction and description

of methods to critiques economic analyses, the chapters are organized by type of cost study: studies that just consider costs, cost-effectiveness studies, cost-utility studies, and cost-benefit studies. Practical chapters regarding data collection and analysis, as well as recommendations on the presentation of economic analyses are provided.

Gold MR, Siegel JE, Russel LB, Weinstein MC. Cost Effectiveness in Health and Medicine. New York: Oxford University Press, 1996.

This book reports the findings, conclusions, and recommendations of the U.S. Public Health Service Panel on the Cost-Effectiveness in Health and Medicine. Not designed as a text, it covers the economic foundations of CEA, presents the rationale for and implications of choosing a particular perspective for the analysis, and provides summaries of the determination of costs and benefits. The book also describes many of the current controversies that exist surrounding the determination of confidence surrounding the results, and which costs and benefits to include.

Articles

Detsky A, Naglie IG. A clinician's guide to cost-effectiveness analysis. Ann Intern Med 1990;113:147–154.

Primarily directed toward physicians, this article provides an overview of CEA in the context of simple medically related examples.

Doubilet P, Weinstein MC, McNeil BJ. Use and misuse of the term "cost-effectiveness" in medicine. N Engl J Med 1986;314:253–256.

This article catalogs the poor state of published economic analyses in the 1970s and 1980s, and provides a set of criteria that all economic analyses should adhere to. The authors reviewed years of published economic analyses from multiple high profile journals, and found that only one quarter of these papers contained sufficient information to fully interpret or critique the work.

Drummond MF, Richardson WS, O'Brien BJ, Levine M, Heyland D. Users' guides to the medical literature. XIII. How to use an article on economic analysis of clinical practice. A. Are the results of the study valid? Evidence-Based Medicine Working Group. JAMA 1997;277(19):1552–1557.

O'Brien, Heyland D, Richardson WS, Levine M, Drummond MF, Users' guides to the medical literature. XIII. How to use an article on economic analysis of clinical practice. B. What are the results and will they help me in caring for my patients? Evidence-Based Medicine Working Group. JAMA 1997;277(22):1802–1806.

This pair of articles provides an excellent synopsis of the important aspects of a well-designed economic analysis, and provides mechanisms to aid the reader in interpreting and using the results of a published economic study.

Eisenberg J. Clinical economics: a guide to the economic analysis of clinical practice. JAMA 1989;262(20):2879–2886.

This is an excellent review of the application of economic principles to health care problems, written from a clinician's point of view.

Finkler S. The distinction between costs and charges. Ann Intern Med 1982;96: 102–109.

This seminal article outlines the multiple market forces and other characteristics of fees for health care services that render charges almost unusable as a measure of actual costs.

Kuperman GJ, Gibson RF. Computer physician order entry: benefits, costs, and issues. Ann Intern Med 2003;139(1):31–39.

This is an excellent review of the pros and cons of the implementation of a particular clinical system: physician order entry. It reviews the types of costs and benefits that should be included, and reviews the existing literature on studies that examine the clinical and cost-effectiveness of physician order entry.

Weinstein MC, Stason WB. Foundations of cost-effectiveness analysis for health and medical practices. N Engl J Med 1977;296:716–721.

A classic introductory article that describes the rationale and fundamental methods of economic evaluation in health care.

Answers to Self-Tests

Self Test 11.1

1.
  a. Cost-effectiveness (if quality of life were included, could be cost-utility as well).
  b. Cost-minimizing (or could be cost-consequence).
  c. Cost-utility.
  d. Cost-minimizing.

2.
  a. Hospital.
  b. Society.

Self Test 11.2

1. First, rank the strategies by effectiveness (C, B, A, D), and calculate the incremental costs and benefits of moving to the next best strategy. Then calculate the ICER by dividing the incremental costs by the incremental effectiveness for each strategy:

	Cost	Incremental costs	Life-years	Incremental effectiveness	ICER
Strategy C	$30,000		2.5		
Strategy B	$50,000	$20,000	3	0.5	$40,000
Strategy A	$80,000	$30,000	3.5	0.5	$60,000
Strategy D	$90,000	$10,000	3.6	0.1	$100,000

Since the decision makers feel that they can only spend up to $75,000 year, the optimal decision is strategy A as it yields the greatest gain in life years white remaining within the spending limit; strategy D is too expensive for the small extra benefit it provides.

2. No, this is a program that falls into the "cheaper and better" quadrant of the CEA plane. No further analysis is necessary.

Self-Test 11.3

a. Undiscounted, the value of the streams simple $170,000 in costs and $180,000 in benefits, so it is a good investment.

	Year 1	Year 2	Year 3	Year 4	Year 5	Present value
Costs	$100,000	$40,000	$10,000	$10,000	$10,000	$170,000
Benefits	0	$30,000	$40,000	$50,000	$60,000	$180,000

b. The undiscounted cost-benefit ratio is $170,000/$180,000 or 0.94, indicating that it costs you 94 cents for each dollar of return.

c. To calculate the present value of a discounted stream, each year's costs and benefits must be discounted by

$$PV = \frac{X}{(1+r)^t}$$

which produces the following table (for the first entry, $0.9524 \times 100,000 = \$95,239$, excluding rounding error.

	Year 1	Year 2	Year 3	Year 4	Year 5	Present value
Discount multiplier	0.9524	0.9070	0.8638	0.8227	0.7835	
Costs	$95,238	$36,281	$8,638	$8,227	$7,835	$156,220
Benefits	$0	$27,211	$34,554	$41,135	$47,012	$149,911

d. The cost-benefit ratio is now $156,220/$149,911, or 1.04, indicating an unfavorable CB ratio.

This example shows that, when the majority of costs occur early and benefits occur late in a project, discounting can change the conclusion about cost benefit.

12
Proposing and Communicating the Results of Evaluation Studies: Ethical, Legal, and Regulatory Issues

This final chapter addresses a set of critical issues for evaluation. These are the often "hidden" but important considerations that can determine if a study receives the financial support that make its conduct possible, if a study in progress encounters procedural difficulties, or if a completed study leads to settled decisions that might involve the improvement or adoption of an information resource. Whether a study is funded depends on how well the study plan is represented in a proposal; whether a study encounters procedural difficulties depends on the investigator's adherence to general ethical standards as well as more specific stipulations built into an evaluation contract; whether a study leads to settled decisions depends on how well the study findings are represented in various reports.

We will see in this chapter that studies can succeed or fail to make an impact for reasons other than the technical soundness of the evaluation design—the considerations that have occupied so much of this volume. Conducting an evaluation study is a complex and time-consuming effort, requiring negotiation skills and the ability to compromise between conflicting interests. The investigator conducting an evaluation must be a communicator, manager, and politician, in addition to a technician.

This chapter provides a glimpse into this nontechnical set of issues. We focus on proposals that express study plans, the process of refereeing other people's proposals and reports, how to communicate the study results in reports and other formats, and a set of ethical and legal considerations pertinent to evaluation. We are aware that the treatment of each of these issues here includes just the rudiments of what a fully accomplished investigator must know and be able to do. We encourage the reader to access additional resources to amplify what is presented here, including the references and additional readings listed at the end of the chapter.

Writing Evaluation Proposals

Why Proposals Are Necessary and Difficult

A proposal is a plan for a study that has not yet been performed. A proposal usually also makes a case that a study should be performed and, often, that the recipient of the proposal should make available the financial resources needed to conduct the study. In most situations, evaluation studies must be represented in formal proposals before a study is undertaken. This is required for several reasons. First, the negotiations about the scope and conduct of a study require a formal representation of the study plan. Second, if the investigator is seeking resources from an external agency to conduct the study, funding agencies almost always require a proposal. Third, students conducting evaluation studies as part of their thesis or dissertation research must propose this research to their committees, with formal approval required before the work can begin. Fourth, human subjects committees—also called ethics committees or institutional review boards (IRBs)—require written advance plans of studies to ensure that these plans comply with ethical standards for the conduct of research. Field studies of clinical information resources usually involve patient data, which requires that they carry IRB approval. Laboratory studies of information resources supporting clinical work, research, or education may also require human subjects review if data are collected directly from practitioners, researchers, or students who are participants in these studies. Even for laboratory studies, we advise anyone planning an evaluation to assume human subjects review of the study will be required, unless notified otherwise or unless the evaluation scope is absolutely restricted to study of information resource structure or performance with no involvement of human users.

When evaluations are nested within information resource development projects that are funded by the organization developing the resource, a formal proposal for the study may not technically be required. Nonetheless, a written description of the study plan is still a good idea. Sound evaluation practice, as first discussed in Chapters 1 and 2, includes a process of negotiation with important members of the client group for whom the study is conducted. These negotiations cannot occur properly without some written representation of the study plan. An evaluation contract based on an unwritten understanding of how a study will be conducted, absent a written proposal, is bad practice. With no anchor in writing for the conduct of the study, misunderstandings that are difficult to resolve can, and often do, arise. A written evaluation plan, even when not required to secure funding, is also an important resource to support study planning and execution. Conducting a study without a written plan is like building a house without a blueprint. The investigator is always feeling her way along. Changes in a plan are always possible, but it is helpful for the study team to be keenly aware about what changes are being made in the originally conceived plan. Although they are described differently, subjectivist studies can be reflected in a written study plan just as readily as objectivist studies. There is nothing ineffable about the subjectivist approaches that defies clear description.

Evaluation studies in informatics are difficult to describe on paper.[1] Writing a study proposal is difficult largely because it requires the author to describe events and activities that have not yet occurred. For most investigators, writing a plan is intrinsically more difficult than describing, in retrospect, events that have occurred and have been experienced by the people who would describe them. Writers of proposals must portray their plans in ways that are logical and comprehensible. Uncertainty about what ultimately will happen when the study is undertaken must be acknowledged but constrained. In addition to having a clear idea of what they want to do, proposal writers must know what constitutes the complete description of a plan (what readers of the plan expect will be included), the format these descriptions are expected to take, and the style of expression considered appropriate.

Writing a persuasive proposal is part science and part art. Although this assertion is impossible to confirm, it is likely that many potentially valuable studies are never performed because of the prospective investigators' inability to describe them satisfactorily in proposals. Finally, evaluation as a relatively young field has fewer models for good proposals, leaving authors somewhat more in the dark than they would be in mature fields where it would be relatively easy to locate a successful model proposal for a project addressing virtually any topic.

Format of a Study Proposal

To describe evaluation studies, we recommend use of the proposal format embodied in the U.S. Public Health Service Form 398 (PHS 398), even if the investigator is not planning to apply to the U.S. government for funds.[2] This recommendation has several bases. Most important, this format provides a sound, proven generic structure for articulating a study plan. (Writing a proposal is difficult enough; having to invent a format is yet one more challenging thing for the investigator to do.) Even though it was developed by a research agency in one specific country, the format is almost universally applicable. Another reason to use the format of PHS 398 is that many, perhaps most, readers have grown accustomed to reading study plans in this format and writing their own proposals using it. They then tacitly or overtly expect the plan to unfold in a particular sequence. When the plan develops in the expected sequence, it is easier for referees and other readers to understand. Copies of PHS 398 can be

TABLE 12.1. Components of the Research Plan for PHS
Form 398.

Revised applications (3 pages)
Supplemental applications (1 page)
a. Specific aims (1 page)
b. Background and significance (2–3 pages)
c. Preliminary studies/progress report (6–8 pages)
d. Research design and methods (a–d, 25 pages maximum)
e. Human subjects
f. Vertebrate animals
g. Literature cited
h. Consortium/contractual arrangements
i. Resource sharing
j. Consultants

obtained from any university research or grants office, by download
(http://grants.nih.gov/grants/forms.htm).

A complete proposal using PHS 398 has 12 major parts; the proper completion of all of them is important if one is applying to a U.S. government
agency for research funding. We focus here on the one part of the form that
expresses the investigative or research plan itself. The format for expression of the research plan consists of up to 11 sections, as shown in Table
12.1. The discussion here focuses primarily on sections a to d, in which the
investigator represents the core of what she plans to do. In proposals submitted for U.S. federal funding, the total length of these sections is strictly
limited, usually to 25 pages, with recommended lengths for each section.
The specific page limit depends on the type of grant being sought. Investigators preparing evaluation proposals for purposes other than obtaining a
federal grant may not need 25 pages to express their ideas—or, if they
require more space, they have the luxury of doing so.

For proposals that are submitted for funding, investigators usually find
themselves challenged to make their proposals terse enough to comply with
the page length restriction. Writing proposals is thus usually an exercise in
editing and selective omission. Rarely are investigators groping for things
to say about their proposed study. We recognize that in many cases a single
proposal is written to describe a large development project of which evaluation is one component. We explore in a later section (see Evaluations
Nested in Larger Projects) how that situation can be managed.

Suggestions for Expressing Study Designs

Here we provide specific guidance for expressing study designs using the
format of PHS 398, and emphasizing the key sections a to d. A checklist for
assessing compliance with these guidelines is found in Appendix A.

Specific Aims

In this section of the proposal the investigator describes what she hopes to achieve in the proposed work. The format of this section should consist of a preamble, which provides a general rationale for the study, followed by an expression of the specific aims as discrete entities. It is best to number the discrete aims (e.g., Aim 1, Aim 2), so that later in the proposal the aims can be referenced by number. As a general rule of thumb, a study should have three to six specific aims. If the investigator finds herself expressing the study with one or two aims, the aims may be too general; if so, they can be subdivided. Correspondingly, if a study is expressed with seven or more aims, the study itself may be too broad or the aims may be stated too specifically. Even though specific investigative questions might change in an emergent, subjectivist study, the general purposes or "orienting" questions that guide the study from the outset can be stated here.

Background and Significance

This section should establish the need for this particular study/project, not a general need for studies of this type. After finishing this section, the reader should be able to answer this question: "How will we be better off if the aims of this study are accomplished?" Although it is not solely a literature review, this section makes its points with appropriate citations to the literature. For evaluation studies, the need to cite the literature may be less than for more traditional research studies. However, the investigator must think creatively about what is included in the literature. For evaluations, the pertinent literature might include unpublished documents or technical reports about the information resource under study. In general, it is not a good idea for the investigator to cite too much of her own work in this section.

Progress Report/Preliminary Studies

This section describes previous relevant work undertaken by the investigators and their collaborators. When the proposal describes a new line of investigation, this section is called "preliminary studies." When the proposal describes a continuation or extension of a line of work already begun, the section is called "progress report." This section emphasizes results of this previous work and how the proposed study builds on these results. If measurement studies have been performed previously, for example, this section describes the methods and results of these studies. Any pilot data and their implications are included here. Although it is tempting to do so in this section, it is not the place for the investigator to paraphrase her curriculum vitae or describe her awards and accomplishments. In PHS 398, this is accomplished in a separate part of the proposal where the investigators include their biographical sketches.

Design and Methods

This section contains a description of the study being proposed. It includes the following:

- Restatement of the study aims: Even though the study aims were expressed earlier in section a, this repetition helps the reader bring the study back into focus.
- Overview of the study design: To give the reader the "big picture," this should establish the overall evaluation approach being employed as described in Chapter 2 of this book and the type of study as discussed in Chapter 3. If a field study is proposed, it is important to explain how the study will fit into its patient care, research, or educational environment. If the study is objectivist, explain whether the design is descriptive, comparative, or correlational—and why this choice was made. Provide an overview of the study groups and the timing of the intervention. If the study is subjectivist, include an overview of the data collection strategies and procedures that will be employed.
- Study details: For objectivist studies, this part must include specific information about participants and their sampling/selection/recruitment; investigative procedures with a clear description of the intervention (the information resource and who will use it, in what forms); description of the independent and dependent variables; how each of the variables will be measured (the instrumentation, with reliability/validity data if not previously reported); a data analysis plan (what statistical tests in what sequence); and a discussion of sample size, which in many cases will include a formal power analysis. Samples of any data collection forms, or other instruments, should be provided in an appendix to the proposal. For subjectivist studies, the study details include the kinds of data that will be collected (who is anticipated to be interviewed, the types of documents that will be examined, the types of activities that will be observed); how will study documents be maintained and by whom; and the plan for consolidating and extracting patterns and themes from the data. The reader of the proposal, if conversant with subjectivist methods, will understand that many of the ideas expressed in this section may change as the study unfolds.
- Project management plan: For evaluations, it is important to describe the study team and its relation to the resource development team and how decisions to modify the study, should that be necessary, will be made. The "playing field" figure, and related concepts introduced in Chapter 2 of this volume, may be instructive in determining the content of this section.
- Communication/reporting plan: For evaluations, it is important to explain the report(s) to be developed, by whom, and with whom they will be shared in draft and final form. The techniques of reporting are discussed later in this chapter.

- Timeline: The proposal should include, preferably in chart form, a timeline for the study. The timeline should be as detailed as possible.

Special Issues in Proposing Evaluations

Evaluations Nested in Larger Projects

Many evaluations are proposed not in a free-standing manner but rather as part of a larger development project. In this case the evaluation is best expressed as one specific aim of the larger study. The background and significance of the evaluation is then discussed as part of the "Background and Significance" section of the proposal; the same would be true for the "Preliminary Studies" section of the proposal. The evaluation methods would be described in detail as a major part of the "Design and Methods" section. Under these circumstances, the specific evaluation plans must be described in a highly condensed form. Depending on the scope of the evaluation, this may not be a problem. If sufficient space to describe the evaluation is unavailable in the main body of the proposal, the investigator might consider including one or more technical appendices to provide further detail about the evaluation.*

Irresolvable Design Issues

At the time they write a proposal, investigators often find themselves with a design issue that is so complex it is not clear how to resolve it. In this case, the best strategy is not to try to hide the problem. An expert, careful reader will probably detect the unmentioned problem and consider the investigator naive for not being aware of it. Hence, the investigator should admit she has an unsolved problem, show she is aware of the issues involved, and, above all, how others in comparable situations have addressed issues of this type. This strategy often succeeds in convincing the reader/reviewer of the proposal that although the investigator does not know what to do now, she will make a good decision when the time comes during the execution of the study.

The "Cascade" Problem

A related issue is the so-called cascade problem, which occurs when the plan for stage N of a study depends critically on the outcome of stage

---

* Some caution is required here if the proposal is to be submitted for U.S. federal funding. The guidelines for Form 398 specifically state that the appendix should not be used "to circumvent the page limitations of the research plan." It is, for example, acceptable to include specimen data collection forms in the appendix and also to provide in the appendix more technical information about the forms. However, if the main body of the proposal says that "the evaluation design is described in Appendix A" and the appendix in fact contains the entire description of the design, the proposal will likely be considered unacceptable by the funding agency and will be returned for modification.

$N-1$. There is no simple solution to this problem when writing a proposal. The best approach is to describe the dependencies, how the decision about how to proceed will be made, and possibly describe in some detail the plan for stage N under what the investigator considers the most likely outcome of stage $N-1$. Some proposal writers consider the existence of a cascade problem to indicate the boundaries of what they will define as one study. If the outcome of stage N depends critically on stage $N-1$, stage N is considered to be a different study and is described in a separate proposal that is written later, after the work on the previous stage has started and progressed.

Refereeing Evaluation Studies

After a study proposal is submitted to a funding body, it is usually refereed—that is, reviewed for merit by one or more individuals experienced in evaluation design and methods. It is therefore useful for those writing a proposal for an evaluation study also to understand the refereeing process. In addition, once an investigator has succeeded in obtaining funding for several research and evaluation projects, funding organizations are quite likely to send that individual study proposals to a referee. We therefore discuss here briefly how one goes about reviewing a proposed study submitted for funding. Many of these concepts also apply in general to a completed study that has been submitted for formal presentation or publication. Many funding organizations or journals provide referees with a checklist of review criteria they would like addressed, which obviously take precedence over the generic advice that follows. Some generic criteria from the U.S. National Institutes of Health are listed in Table 12.2.

In general, the questions that referees can ask themselves, when refereeing an evaluation proposal, include the following:

- Is there a study question and specific aims, and are they clearly formulated? Often there is more than one question per study.

TABLE 12.2. Some generic review criteria for study proposals, from the U.S. National Institutes of Health.

Criterion	Questions for referee/reviewer
Significance	Does it address an important problem? How will science or clinical practice be advanced?
Approach	Is the conceptual or clinical framework sound? Are potential problems discussed?
Innovation	Are the aims, concepts, methods, and outcomes novel? Do they challenge paradigms?
Investigator	Does the principal investigator or team have appropriate training and experience?
Environment	Does the study benefit from this scientific/clinical environment?

- Is the study question important and worth answering, or is the answer banal or already well-established from other studies?
- Are the investigative methods described in sufficient detail to determine what is being proposed or what was already done?
- Are these methods appropriate to answer the study question, given the potential biases and confounding factors; that is, is the study design likely to result in work that is internally valid?
- Is the study setting sufficiently typical to allow useful conclusions to be drawn for those working elsewhere; that is, is the study externally valid? (This point may not always be crucial for an evaluation done to satisfy a "local" need.)
- Is it feasible for the investigators to carry out the methods described within the resources requested?
- Does the proposal address the standards given in Appendix A?

For completed studies submitted as a report, or for more formal presentation or publication, the following criteria may apply:

- Does the interpretation of the data reflect the sources of the data, the data themselves, and the methods of analysis used?
- Are the results reported in sufficient detail? In objectivist studies, do all summary statistics, tables, or graphs faithfully reflect the conclusions that are drawn? In subjectivist studies, is there a clear and convincing argument? Is the writing sufficiently crisp and evocative to lend both credence and impact to the portrayal of the results?
- Are the conclusions valid, given the study design, setting and results, and other relevant literature?

Some ethical issues related to refereeing are worth mentioning here. If you are asked to referee a proposal and believe that you have a conflict of interest that might skew your judgment about the proposed work, you should of course decline the assignment. In some cases, you might believe that there exists the potential of appearance of a conflict, but you might believe you can be unbiased in your assessment. In such cases, it is wise still to decline the assignment, as the appearance of a potential bias can be as erosive as the bias itself. You should also decline the assignment if you do not have direct experience in the evaluative methods being proposed. For example, persons experienced only with objectivist evaluations should not referee proposals of largely subjectivist work, and vice versa.

Communicating the Results of Completed Studies

What Are the Options for Communicating Study Results?

Once a study is complete, the results need to be communicated to the stakeholders and others who might be interested. In many ways, *communi-*

TABLE 12.3. Reporting as a communication process.

Elements of communication	Equivalent in evaluation studies
A sender of the message	The investigator or investigative team
A message	The results of the study
A communication channel	A report, conversation, meeting, Web site, journal, newspaper or newsletter article, broadcast radio or television, etc.
Recipient(s) of the message	The stakeholders and other audiences for the study results

cation of evaluation results, a term we prefer over *reporting*, is the most challenging aspect of evaluation.

Elementary theory tells us that, in general, successful communication requires a sender, one or more recipients, and a channel linking them, along with a message that travels along this channel (Table 12.3). Seen from this perspective, successful communication is challenging in several respects. It requires that the recipient of the message actually receive it. That is, for evaluations, the recipient must read the written report or attend the meeting intended to convey evaluation results, so the investigator is challenged to create a report the stakeholders will want to read or to choreograph a meeting they will be motivated to attend. Successful communication also requires that the recipient understand the message, which challenges investigators to draft written documents at the right reading level, with audience-appropriate technical detail. Sometimes there must be several different forms of the written report to match several different audiences. Overall, we encourage investigators to recognize that their obligation to communicate does not end with the submission of a written document comprising their technical evaluation report. The report is one means or channel for communication, not an end in itself.

Depending on the nature, number, and location of the recipients, there is a large number of options for communicating the results of a study:

- Written reports
  - Document(s) prepared for specific audience(s)
  - Internal newsletter article
  - Published journal article, with appropriate permissions
  - Monograph, picture album, or book
- One-to-one or small group meetings
  - With stakeholders or specific stakeholder groups
  - With general public, if appropriate
- Formal oral presentations
  - To groups of project stakeholders
  - Conference presentation with poster or published paper in proceedings
  - To external meetings or seminars

- Internet
  - Project Web site
  - Online preprint
  - Internet based journal
- Other
  - Video describing the study and information resource
  - Interview with journalist on newspaper, TV, radio

A written, textual report is not the sole medium for communicating evaluation results. Verbal, graphical, or "multimedia" approaches can be helpful as ways to enhance communication with specific audiences. Another useful strategy is to hold a "town meeting" to discuss a written report after it has been released. Photographs or videotapes can be taken of the work setting for a study, the people in the setting, and the people using the resource. If appropriate permissions are obtained, these images—whether included as part of a written report, shown at a town meeting, or placed on a Web site—can be worth many thousands of words. The same may be true for recorded statements of resource users. If made available, with permission, as part of a multimedia report, the voices of the participants can convey a feeling behind the words that can enhance the credibility of the investigator's conclusions.

What Is the Role of the Evaluator—Reporter or Change Agent?

In addition to the varying formats for communication described above, investigators have other decisions to make after the data collection and analysis phases of a study are complete. One key decision is what personal role they will adopt after the formal investigative aspects of the work are complete. They may elect only to communicate the results, or they may also choose to persuade stakeholders to take specific actions in response to the study results, and perhaps even assist in the implementation of these actions. This raises a key question: Is the role of an evaluator to simply record and communicate study findings and then move on to the next study, or is it to engage with the study stakeholders and help them change how they work as a result of the study?

To answer this question about the role of an evaluator, we need to understand that an evaluation study, particularly a successful one, has the potential to trigger a series of events, starting with the analysis of study results through communication to interpretation, recommendation, and even implementation. The investigator's potential role in this cascade is depicted below.

Conduct study
↳ Analyze study data to yield results
  ↳ Communicate the results as a neutral report to all stakeholders
    ↳ Interpret the results and communicate the meaning of these to stakeholders
      ↳ Recommend actions for stakeholders to take
        ↳ Suggest *to stakeholders* how to implement the recommend*ed* actions
          ↳ Participate *as a change agent* in the implementation process

Viewing the aftermath of a study in this way is most important when a study is conducted for a specific audience that needs to make decisions and then take specific actions requiring careful planning, but it also can assist the investigator when the intended consequences of the evaluation are less clear.

Some evaluators—perhaps enthused by the clarity of their results and an opportunity to use them to improve health care, biomedical research, or education—prefer to go beyond reporting the results and conclusions to making recommendations, and then helping the stakeholders to implement them. Figure 12.1 illustrates the dilemma often faced by evaluators about whether to retain their scientific detachment and merely report the study results—metaphorically leaving the "train" at the first or second "stations"—or stay engaged somewhat longer. Evaluators who choose to remain may become engaged in helping the stakeholders interpret what the results mean, guiding them in reaching decisions and perhaps even in implementing the actions decided upon. The longer they stay on the train, the greater the extent to which evaluators must leave behind their scientific detachment and take on a role more commonly associated with change agents. Some confounding of these roles is inevitable when the evaluation is performed by individuals within the organization developing the infor-

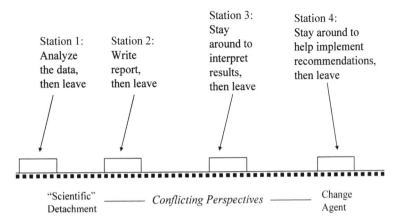

FIGURE 12.1. Scientific detachment or change agent: when to get off the train?

mation resource under study. There is no hard-and-fast rule for deciding when to leave the train; the most important realization for investigators is that the different stations exist and that a decision about where to exit must eventually be made.

Role of the Evaluation Contract

In all evaluations, the evaluation contract assumes a central role in shaping what will happen after the data collection and analysis phases of the study are completed. A possible dilemma arises if an audience member, perhaps the director of the resource development project under study, disagrees with the conclusions of a draft evaluation report. The contract, if properly written, protects the investigator and the integrity of the study, often, but not always, by making the investigator the final authority on the content of the report. A contract typically stipulates that reactions to draft evaluation reports have the status of advice. The investigator is under no obligation to modify the report in accord with these reactions. In practice, the reactions to draft evaluation reports usually do not raise ethical/legal dilemmas but rather provide crucial information to the investigator that improves the report.

The evaluation contract should also help evaluators trying to decide whether they should "pass judgment" on the information resource or leave judgment to the reader. If the role of the investigator does include passing judgment, these judgments should be specific, justified by reference to study results, and not unduly generalized beyond the settings and information resource studied. The readers are left to satisfy themselves about whether the resource is likely to benefit them. In general, the investigator should remain available to the various audiences of the evaluation at least to clarify issues and provide information beyond that included in the formal report, should it be requested.

Specific Issues of Report Writing

As a practical matter, almost all evaluations result in a written report, irrespective of whatever other communication modes may be employed. Deciding what to include in a written evaluation report is often difficult. As a study is nearing completion, whether the study is objectivist or subjectivist in primary orientation, much data will have been collected and many possible interpretations discussed. These alternative interpretations of the data usually have been fueled by reports of other studies in the literature or the investigator's previous personal experiences. As a result, those responsible for writing up the study usually have access to a mass of raw and interpreted data and to comparisons between their results and those of other studies. The key question for reporting, as it is when deciding what to study,[3] lies in distinguishing what is necessary, in contrast to what might be interesting, to include for the audience or audiences who are the "targets" of each version of the report.

Because evaluations are carried out for specific groups with specific interests, the task of report writing can be clarified through attention to what these groups need to know. If the report is for a single person with a specific decision to make, that individual's interests guide the contents of the report. More typically, however, the investigator is writing for a range of audiences, perhaps including resource users, the lay public, biomedical informaticians, policy makers, and others. Each of these audiences expects more detail in the areas of most interest to them, potentially making for a lengthy report. If the investigator plans to prepare a single written report, there is inevitable tension between making the report brief enough to be read by a wide audience, often by publication in a widely read journal, and describing the information resource, clinical problem and setting, the participants studied, origin of tasks/cases, and study methods in enough detail to allow other investigators to reproduce them.

There are at least two dimensions here: how much detail to include and how many audiences to write for in a single document.

One strategy in any sizable evaluation study is to produce modular reports. The investigator could describe in an initial document the details of the information resource, the problem it is addressing, and the setting where it has been deployed, and then refer to this document in subsequent evaluation reports. One problem that may arise, if the investigator plans on publishing reports in academic journals, is the reluctance of many journals to accept publications that merely describe an information resource and its potential application. Once measurement studies are complete, these aspects too can be separately reported, especially if they describe methods and instruments that measure attributes of general interest, such as the dilemmas faced by users,[4] the quality of professional practice, or user attitudes to information resources. The report of the demonstration study can then focus on the details of the study methods, the results, and the conclusions drawn in context. Often publication of measurement studies in the general academic literature is more acceptable than publication of demonstration study results, since the results of demonstration studies may be considered by various stakeholders to be privileged information.

As time goes on and the field of informatics becomes more mature, we expect that evaluation resources such as libraries of standardized problems and cases with which to test information resources, as well as published, validated measurement instruments, will accumulate. Once they are published, citation of these published or otherwise documented resources and methods, used in a particular evaluation study, will provide sufficient detail for most evaluation reports—as is seen in the biological sciences literature for standard assays and preparation methods. Such references make evaluation study reports briefer; the detail that some readers may expect is accessible elsewhere.

Writing Objectivist Study Reports

The format of objectivist study reporting has evolved over the last century into a well-known structure represented by the IMRAD acronym. This format is primarily useful for communicating evaluation study results to technical/scientific audiences. Such a report includes the following components:

1. Introduction to the problem, review of relevant literature, and statement of study goals.

2. Methods employed, including details of statistical tests used, ideally described in enough detail (or by reference to published papers) to allow another investigator to replicate the study.

3. Results, often summarized in tables or graphs. Some audiences, including some professional journals, now ask for full data to be sent with the article for the purposes of refereeing and public access. With the authors' agreement, these data can be made available to other interested parties.

4. Analysis or interpretation of the data.

5. Discussion of the results and potential limitations of the study, and conclusions drawn in the context of other studies.

This formula implies a linear flow in execution of the study, from aims to methods, results, and conclusions—completely in keeping with the objectivist approach to evaluation. Reporting an evaluation study using this model encourages authors to be clear about the evaluation questions that were addressed and the data that were used or collected to answer the questions—helping the reader determine if the inferences drawn from the data are justified.

Authors of papers describing studies of information resources should be guided by the above structure, but may wish to add further sections or detail within sections where necessary. For example, where novel statistical or computational methods have been used, it is useful to include a paragraph describing them in the methods section. In the case of measurement studies, it is wise to include copies of the relevant instruments for publication as figures or an appendix.

The above structure applies equally to reports of evaluation studies that use the methods of randomized clinical trials. Because of the importance of trials in providing the most credible objectivist evidence about the efficacy of clinical interventions,[5] additional guidelines about reporting trials have been published, including the work of the Consolidated Standards of Reporting Trials group.[6] Some journals now require that all clinical trials be reported according to these standards. This practice will aid groups such as the Cochrane Collaboration, who are writing systematic reviews or meta-analyses of the literature, by putting this literature into a more uniform and directly comparable format.[7] Equally, because bibliographic systems increasingly store the abstract along with the citation, many journals are now requesting that authors structure the abstract of an article into sections resembling the IMRAD structure of the article and keep the length of abstracts to a strict word limit.

Writing Subjectivist Study Reports

The goals of reporting a subjectivist study may include describing the resource; how it is used; how it is "seen" by various groups; and its effects on people, their relationships, and organizations. To these ends, the subjectivist investigator will typically include direct quotations, interesting anecdotes, revealing statements, lessons learned, and examples of the insights, prejudices, fears, and aspirations that study subjects expressed—all with due regard to confidentiality and the contract or memorandum of understanding negotiated at the study outset.

Reporting of subjectivist/qualitative studies raises a number of special issues:

- In comparison with an objectivist study, writing a subjectivist report is less formulaic and often more challenging to the written communication skills of the investigator. Conveying the feelings and beliefs, and often the hopes and dreams, of people in their work environment in relatively few words can require talents resembling those of a poet. Reports typically require numerous drafts before they communicate as intended.
- As in all evaluation studies, it is essential to respect the confidentiality of study subjects. In subjectivist studies, fieldwork directly exposes the study subjects to the investigator, and the use of quotations and images in reports can readily reveal identities. Measures to be taken to protect subjects should be laid out in the evaluation contract, also recognizing that the stipulations may need to be altered to address difficult problems or conflicts as they emerge. Before distributing an evaluation report, the investigator must show each subject any relevant passages that might allow them to be identified and allow the subject to delete or modify the passage, if the subject is concerned about his/her identity being revealed.
- The study report is typically an evolving document, written in consultation with the client group. Version control is important, and it is often unclear when the report is "finished." Here again, the evaluation contract may be helpful for determining when "enough" work on the report has been done.
- The report can itself change the environment being studied by formalizing and disseminating insights about the information resource. Thus evaluators must adopt a responsible, professional approach to its writing and distribution.
- It can be difficult when writing journal articles to summarize a subjectivist study in 10 to 20 manuscript pages without losing the richness of the personal experiences that subjectivist studies strive to convey. There is a danger that journal articles describing such studies can be unpersuasive or come across as more equivocal than the underlying data really

are. To counteract this problem, authors can use extracts from typical statements by subjects or brief accounts of revealing moments to illustrate and justify their conclusions in the same way objectivist researchers summarize a mass of patient data in a set of tables or statistical metrics. If there exists a more lengthy report, investigators can make such longer reports available to interested third parties on their Web sites, analogous to the way in which data from objectivist studies are often available.

• Few articles describing subjectivist studies are published in clinical journals, but this is now changing, with a landmark *British Medical Journal* series describing subjectivist methods.[8] As a result, subjectivist studies relevant to medical informatics are increasingly being reported.[9–11] We believe there is no intrinsic or insurmountable reason why subjectivist studies should be not be published in the traditional archival literature. If one is writing an evaluation report for a journal, it is important to be brief but describe comprehensively the data collection and interpretation methods used, give illustrative examples of results (data collected and analyzed) to support the conclusions, and avoid any implication that the subjectivist methods are ineffable, intuitive, or irreproducible. Such implications would play into the biases of many reviewers against subjectivist methods. All investigators, objectivist and subjectivist, are guided significantly by intuition, and the entire scientific community tacitly acknowledges that fact.

Ethical, Legal, and Regulatory Considerations During Evaluation

Ethical Issues

Evaluation raises a number of ethical issues, some of which have been introduced earlier in this chapter or in earlier chapters of this volume. The recurring theme of confidentiality is of special concern when data must be processed off-site or includes items likely to be sensitive to patients (e.g., their HIV status or psychiatric history) or professionals (e.g., their performance or work load). One approach is to "anonymize" the data by removing obvious identifiers, although, especially in the case of rare diseases or professionals with unique skill sets, it may still be possible to identify the individuals concerned by a process of triangulation.[12] Physical security measures (locking up servers in a secure room) and shredding of discarded paper are underutilized but effective methods of restricting access to confidential data.[13] Software access controls on databases and encryption of data sent over the Internet are also useful safeguards.

Another ethical consideration for evaluation invokes the entire domain of human subjects research, introduced earlier in this chapter. Is it, for example, acceptable to make a clinical information resource available to care providers during a demonstration study without requesting the approval of the patients whose management it may indirectly influence or, conversely, to withhold advice of an information resource from the physicians caring for a control group? Within the scope of this volume, it is only possible to alert investigators to this broad category of concerns and to emphasize the necessity of requesting the approval of the appropriate IRB (or body with analogous authority) before undertaking a function or impact study. Studies of information technology applied to health care, research, and education invoke these human subjects' considerations in slightly different ways, but no application domain is exempt from them. The IRBs will offer investigators specific instructions regarding, for example, from whom informed consent must be obtained and how. These instructions make the life of the investigator easier in the long run by removing these difficult considerations from the sphere of the investigator's sole judgment, and allowing the evaluation study to proceed without concern that appropriate ethical procedures are not being followed.

The final ethical issue discussed here concerns the evaluator's integrity and professionalism.[14] Evaluators are in a strong position to bias the collection, interpretation, and reporting of study data in such a way as to favor—or disfavor—the information resource and its developers. One mechanism to address this concern would restrict the pool of potential evaluators to independent agents, commissioned by an independent organization with no strong predispositions toward or profit to be made from specific outcomes of the evaluation. While there is a role for evaluations conducted with this extreme level of detachment, it is impractical and perhaps suboptimal as a general strategy. The more removed the investigators are from the environment in which a resource is developed or deployed, the steeper their learning curve about the key issues relating to the resource that drive the generation of the evaluation questions. Some "incest" in evaluation is often inevitable, and, some would argue, desirable to enhance the relevance and the legitimacy of the study.

In the extreme case, where the developers of an information resource are the sole evaluators of their own work, the credibility of the study can be preserved through an external audit of decisions taken and data collected. Otherwise, no matter how careful the methods and clear the results, there may remain a suspicion that the reported study attesting to the statistically significant benefits of an information resource was the 20th study conducted, after 19 negative studies were conducted and their results suppressed. When the evaluation group for a project includes many of the same people as the development group, it is advisable to create an advisory committee for the evaluation that can perform an auditing, validation, and legitimating function. A recent systematic review of 100 randomized trials of clinical decision support systems emphasizes these concerns, as it showed that about three quarters of studies carried out by system developers showed improvements in clinical practice, contrasting with only one quarter of the studies carried out by independent evaluators.[15]

TABLE 12.4. Asymmetry in the reporting of studies according to their results.

Study produces positive result	Study produces negative result
Congratulations all round	Secrecy
Prompt publication	Delay/cancel publication
Conclude that the results can be widely applied	Conclude that the results should be applied with caution, if at all
No need to repeat study	Repeat study in other settings
Sweep any biases, confounders under the carpet	Search carefully for biases or confounders to explain the "anomalous" result

Increasingly, journals are requiring authors to sign a declaration describing their involvement, and that of other bodies such as study sponsors, in all key stages in the study process. These include the writing and approval of the study protocol; collection and analysis of data; decisions about when to stop the study and submit to a journal; and exactly who wrote, revised, and approved the final article. Table 12.4 depicts the temptations that might afflict individuals strongly interested in seeing an information resource cast in a highly positive light, as a function of whether the results of an evaluative study are favorable or not.

Legal and Regulatory Issues

The developers and users of biomedical information resources may be concerned about the possible legal implications if, for example, a patient takes legal action against a clinician who had access to an information resource during a demonstration study and who might have based the patient's care in part or in whole on the advice of the resource. This topic raises numerous and complex considerations,[16,17] but in summary both developers and clinician-users would probably be immune from negligence claims if they could demonstrate the following:

1. The information resource had been carefully evaluated in laboratory studies.
2. The information resource provided its user with explanations, well-calibrated probabilities, or the opportunity to participate in the decision-making process.
3. No misleading claims had been made for the information resource.
4. Any error was in the design or specification of the information resource rather than in its coding or hardware.
5. Users had been adequately trained and had not modified the information resource.

The intent of these measures is to persuade a court that system developers had acted responsibly and were providing clinicians with a service to enhance their professional skills, not a black-box product. This diminishes a developer's risk exposure because those who provide services are judged by whether they acted responsibly.* By contrast, those who provide products are deemed negligent once a fault is proved, no matter how much care they have taken to avoid faults.[17]

There is increasing interest in Europe, North America, and elsewhere, in the regulation of some forms of medical information resources. In the United Kingdom, for example, the National Institute for Clinical Excellence (NICE) (www.nice.org.uk) has announced a plan to accredit decision support systems intended for use in the National Health Service. To carry this out, NICE will form an advisory committee that will apply criteria relating to safety, usability, efficacy and cost effectiveness to the information resource, including the results of evaluation studies that decision support system (DSS) vendors provide about their products. With increasing concern about the safety and efficacy of decision support and similar systems it seems likely that other countries will follow suit, placing much greater emphasis on the need for carefully conducted evaluation studies of all kinds. It seems that, while having been an entirely unregulated market in the past, the efficacy and safety of clinical information systems are increasingly attracting attention, creating new challenges, opportunities, and requirements for evaluation.

Conclusion: Evaluation as the Core of Evidence-Based Informatics

Planning and running an evaluation study is a complex, time-consuming effort that requires both technical skills and the ability to compromise between often-conflicting constraints. Once the study is complete, it must be reported in such a way that the context, results, and implications are clear. Evaluation does raise a number of ethical and legal issues that must be carefully considered; for example, the separation of the information resource developer from the evaluators is now becoming an important consideration. Increasingly, it appears that careful and complete evaluation will become a component of the development and implementation of biomedical information resources, and in some cases will be necessary before these resources can be used in the field.

Complementing the tendency toward regulation of clinical information resources, the arrival of evidence-based policy and decision making is a further worldwide trend. This started in health care in the 1980s but in the last decade has moved into education, social policy, and broader fields, and is leading to more evaluation studies. We propose that our own field, bio-

---

* This criterion is known as the Bolam test within the United Kingdom and British Commonwealth legal traditions.

medical informatics, should also move toward an evidence-based model. This would require us to be clear about the question before we start a research or implementation project, and either to search for relevant results of evaluation studies already completed or to propose new studies, taking care to avoid threats to external and internal validity. In an evidence-based informatics model, we would also adopt an appropriately skeptical view toward the results of individual studies, and seek instead systematic reviews that combine the results of all rigorous studies—whether positive or negative, objectivist or subjectivist—to generate the best evidence to address a question of interest. Systematic review methods[7] can also be valuable in uncovering insights about which classes of information resources generate positive results. As an example, Table 12.5 depicts results from the systematic review by Garg et al.[15] of the impact of clinical decision support on health professional actions. In this review the investigators identified 100 randomized controlled trials (RCTs) covering the period 1974 to 2002. Performance improved in 62 (64%) of the 97 RCTs for which health care provider behavior was the focus, while patient outcomes improved in only 7 (13%) of the 52 RCTs in which outcomes were studied. The table shows the proportion of trials in which a statistically significant improvement in health professional behavior was observed by type of DSS. Absent this systematic review, it would have been hard or impossible to predict, for example, the results for diagnostic DSSs, which appear to be half as likely to be effective as preventive care systems.

Finally, certain systematic reviewing methods, specifically meta-regression,[7] can be used to improve our evaluation methods, by uncovering evidence about which methods lead to study bias. Table 12.6 shows an example from a related domain because relevant data for informatics are not yet available. The table summarizes the results of a systematic review by Lijmer et al.,[18] looking at the effect of various study faults on the results of 218 evaluations of laboratory tests. In the table, a high figure for relative diagnostic odds ratio suggests that the class of studies is overestimating the accuracy of the test in question. The table shows that, for example, case—control studies and those with verification bias (different reference standards for positive and negative test results) were biased, as they were

TABLE 12.5. The probability of a decision support system (DSS) leading to improved health professional behavior, by focus of the DSS.

Target behavior for the DSS	Percentage (number) of the randomized trials showing improvement in clinical practice
Diagnosis	40% (4/10)
Prescribing, drug dosing	66% (19/29)
Disease management	62% (23/37)
Preventive care	76% (16/21)

Source: Data redrawn from Garg et al.[15]

TABLE 12.6. Systematic review evidence of bias in studies of diagnostic tests.

Study fault (number of studies displaying this fault)	Relative diagnostic odds ratio (95% confidence interval)
Case-control (5) vs. clinical population (213)	3.0 (2–4.5)
Verification bias (48)	2.2 (1.5–3.3)
No criteria described for carrying out test (23)	1.7 (1.1–2.5)
No description of population studied (86)	1.4 (1.1–1.7)
Poor description of reference standard (80)	0.7 (0.6–0.9)
No blinding of test result when assigning reference standard (148)	1.3 (1.0–1.9)
Retrospective study (28)	1.0 (0.7–1.4)
Partial verification bias (54)	1.0 (0.8–1.3)
Not consecutive cases (121)	0.9 (0.7–1.1)

Source: Data redrawn from Lijmer et al.[18]

associated with much more optimistic results than retrospective studies or those in which there was no blinding.

The implications for biomedical informatics are clear. As experience with our own practice in evaluation accumulates, an analogous table will lead to assertions, backed by data as well as professional judgment, as to what kinds of study methods to adopt and avoid. In the future, we hope to offer readers these kinds of evidence to support assertions about evaluation methods that are preferred and those that should be avoided.

Biomedical informatics is a diverse domain in which to conduct evaluation studies, and as has been discussed many times in this volume, a wide array of evaluation approaches are employed across the life cycle of information resources to address a wide range of questions and inform a wide range of decisions. The methods that have been developed for aggregating study results so far apply only to the main kinds of objectivist study. Subjectivist studies clearly too provide evidence about what works and what does not, and why. The fact that the results of these studies are somewhat less straightforward to aggregate does not make them any less a part of an evidence-based approach to informatics.

References

1. Miller RA, Patil R, Mitchell JA, Friedman CP, Stead WW. Preparing a medical informatics research grant proposal: general principles. Comput Biomed Res 1989;22:92–101.
2. U.S. Department of Health and Human Services, Public Health Service. Grant Application (PHS 398). Form approved September 30, 2004, OMB No. 0925–0001.
3. Miller PL, Sittig DF. The evaluation of clinical decision support systems: what is necessary versus what is interesting. Med Inf (Lond) 1990;15:185–190.
4. Timpka T, Arborelius E. A method for study of dilemmas during health care consultations. Med Inf (Lond) 1991;16:55–64.

5. Sackett DL, Wennberg JE. Choosing the best research design for each question BMJ 1997;315:1636.
6. Moher D, Schulz KF, Altman D, the CONSORT Group (Consolidated Standards of Reporting Trials). The CONSORT statement: revised recommendations for improving the quality of reports of parallel-group randomized trials. JAMA 2001;285(15):1987–1991.
7. Chalmers I, Altman DG, Egger M, Smith GD, eds. Systematic Reviews in Health Care: Meta-Analysis in Context. London: BMJ Books, 2001.
8. Jones R. Why do qualitative research? BMJ 1995;311;2 [editorial].
9. Lindberg DA, Siegel ER, Rapp BA, Wallingford KT, Wilson SR. Use of MEDLINE by physicians for clinical problem solving. JAMA 1993;269:3124–3129.
10. Russell J, Greenhalgh T, Boynton P, Rigby M. Soft networks for bridging the gap between research and practice: illuminative evaluation of CHAIN. BMJ 2004;328(7449):1174.
11. Ziebland S, Chapple A, Dumelow C, Evans J, Prinjha S, Rozmovits L. How the internet affects patients' experience of cancer: a qualitative study. BMJ 2004;328(7439):564.
12. Anderson R. NHS-wide networking and patient confidentiality. BMJ 1995;311: 5–6.
13. Wyatt JC. Clinical data systems. II. Components and techniques. Lancet 1994;344:1609–1614.
14. Heathfield H, Wyatt JC. The road to professionalism in medical informatics: a proposal for debate. Methods Inf Med 1995;34:426–433.
15. Garg AX, Adhikari NK, McDonald H, et al. Effects of computerized clinical decision support systems on practitioner performance and patient outcomes: a systematic review. JAMA 2005;293(10):1223–1238.
16. Berner ES. Ethical and legal issues in the use of clinical decision support systems. J Healthcare Inf Manag 2002;16(4):34–37.
17. Brahams D, Wyatt J. Decision-aids and the law. Lancet 1989;2:632–634.
18. Lijmer JG, Mol BW, Heisterkamp S, et al. Empirical studies of design related bias in studies of diagnostic tests. JAMA 1999;282:1061–1066.

Suggested Reading

Popham WJ. Educational Evaluation. Englewood Cliffs, NJ: Prentice-Hall, 1988. (An amusing, widely applicable chapter on reporting evaluations.)
Smith NL, ed. Communication Strategies in Evaluation. Beverly Hills, CA: Sage, 1982. (A somewhat old but very interesting book that outlines many nontraditional modes of communicating evaluation results is.)

Appendix A: Proposal Quality Checklist for Authors and Referees

A. Specific aims
   1. Establishes a numbering system (Aim 1, Aim 2 . . .)
   2. Includes preamble followed by a list of numbered aims

B. Background and significance
   1. Establishes the need for this study/project (not a general need for studies of this type)
   2. States how we will be better off if we know the answers to these questions
   3. Uses the literature extensively (30+ references)
   4. Does not cite too much of the investigator's own work
C. Progress report/preliminary studies
   1. Describes relevant previous work of principal investigator or collaborators
   2. Emphasizes results of this work and how proposed study builds on these results
   3. Does not paraphrase investigator's curriculum vita
   4. Reports pilot data
D. Design and methods
   1. Does the proposal use the structure of the aims to organize the research plan? Are the following included?
      a. (Re)statement of aims and specific hypotheses or questions
      b. Overview of design
      c. Management plan
      d. Reporting plan
      e. Timeline in as much detail as possible
   2. For objectivist studies
      a. Participants and their selection/recruitment
      b. Experimental procedures/intervention
      c. Independent and dependent variables
      d. How variables will be measured (instruments and any reliability/validity data not previously reported)
      e. Data analysis plan (which statistical tests in what sequence)
      f. Power analysis and discussion of sample size
   3. For subjectivist studies
      a. Kinds of data that will be collected
      b. From whom data will be collected
      c. How study documents will be maintained
      d. Plan for consolidating and generating themes from data
E. In general
   1. Does the format/layout help the reader understand the project?
   2. If there is an unsolved problem, does principal investigator show awareness of the issues involved and how others have addressed them?
   3. Is the cascade problem (if any) adequately addressed?
   4. Are specimen data collection forms included in the appendix?

Glossary

The glossary in the first edition of this book was adapted from an earlier version produced by the authors for a conference on evaluation of knowledge-based information resources, sponsored by the National Library of Medicine and held in 1995. Some terms defined here are not explicitly used in this book but may be encountered elsewhere by readers as they read evaluation reports or the methodological literature. We thank Bruce Buchanan, Gregory Cooper, Brian Haynes, Harold Schoolman, Edward Shortliffe, Mark Roberts and Bonnie Webber for their suggestions for terms and definitions. This second edition glossary has been revised and expanded to reflect revisions in the text itself.

Accuracy: (1) Extent to which the measured value of some attribute of an information resource, or other object, agrees with the accepted value for that attribute or "gold standard" (qv.[†]); (2) extent to which a measurement in fact assesses what it is designed to measure (roughly equivalent to "validity").

Action research: A disciplined method for intentional learning from experience characterised by intervention in real world systems followed by close scrutiny of the effects. The aim of Action Research is to improve practice and it is typically conducted by a combined team of practitioners and researchers. Originally formulated by social psychologist Kurt Lewin. [Adapted from Wikipedia definition, www.wikipedia.org].

Alerting resource: Resource that monitors a continuous signal or stream of data and generates a message (an alert) in response to patterns or items that may require action on the part of the care provider.

Allocation concealment: Ensuring that those recruiting participants to a randomized trial have no knowledge of the group to which each participant will be allocated. Failure to conceal allocation has been shown (using meta regression techniques [qv]) to be a major cause of bias in such studies, and

---

[†] qv. = see also

is best avoided by recruiting participants only by communication with a central trials office.

Analysis of variance (ANOVA): General statistical method for determining the statistical significance of effects in experimental studies. The F test is the basic inferential test statistic for analysis of variance. (See Chapter 8).

Attribute: Specific property of an object that is measured, similar to "construct."

Baseline study: Study undertaken to establish the value of a variable of interest prior to an intervention such as the deployment of an information resource.

Before-after study: A comparative study (qv.) in which something is measured during a baseline period and then again after an intervention has occurred, eg., an information resource is installed. Because of confounding (qv.), no reliable inferences about cause and effect can be made in such a study without extra information such as that provided by internal or external controls (see Chapter 7). However, before-after studies are a reliable cause of the *post hoc ergo propter hoc* fallacy (after the event therefore because of the event).

Bias: (1) *Measurement bias:* Any systematic deviation of a set of measurements from the truth. (2) *Cognitive bias:* A set of consistent tendencies of all humans to make judgments or decisions in ways that are less than optimal. (3) Bias in demonstration studies—see confounding.

Blinding: In a comparative study, ensuring that participants in a study and those making measurements on them are unaware of the group to which the participant has been allocated. This is done to avoid the placebo effect and biased measurement, respectively. A study in which only the participant is blinded is called a single-blind study; if observers are also blinded, this is a double-blind study. It is also possible, but rarely necessary, to blind those processing and analyzing the study data to which group is the intervention and which the control; this is called triple-blinding.

Bug report: User's report of an error in a program. The rate of bug reports over time may provide a measure of improvement in an information resource.

Calibration: (1) Extent to which human participants' estimates of the probability of an event agree with the frequency with which the event actually occurs. (2) Extent to which appraisals by judges actually agree, as opposed to being correlated.

Case-control study: A retrospective correlational study which compares an outcome (e.g., prescribing error notes) between participants that varied in some way (e.g. who did or did not use an information resource). Usually impossible to intrepet so best avoided. (See Chapter 7).

Clinical trial: Prospective experimental study where a clinical intervention (e.g., an information resource) is put to use in the care of a selected sample of patients. Clinical trials almost always involve a control group, formed by random allocation, which receives either no intervention or a contrasting intervention.

Cohort study: Prospective study where two or more groups (not randomly selected) are selected for the presence or absence of a specific attribute, and are then followed forward over time, in order to explore associations between factors present at the outset and those developing later.

Comparative study: Experimental demonstration study where the values of one or more dependent variables are compared across discrete groups corresponding to values of one or more independent variables. The independent variables are typically manipulated by the investigator, but may also reflect naturally occurring groups in a study setting.

Confounding: Problem in experimental studies where the statistical effects attributable to two or more independent variables cannot be disaggregated. Also, the "hidden" effects of a bias or a variable not explicitly included in an analysis, that threatens internal validity.

Consultation system: Decision support system that offers task- and situation-specific advice when a decision-maker requests it.

Content analysis: Technique widely used with narrative data to assign elements of verbal data to specific categories (see Chapter 10). Usually, the categories are defined by examining all or a specific subset of the data.

Context of use: Setting in which an information resource is situated. It is generally considered important to study a resource in the context of use as well as in the laboratory. Synonym: "field."

Contingency table: Cross-classification of two or more nominal or ordinal variables. The relation between variables in a contingency table can be tested using the chi-square or many other statistics. When only two variables, each with two levels, are classified: it is called a "two by two table (2×2)." (See Chapter 8).

Control (control group): In experimental studies, the intervention(s) specifically engineered to contrast with the intervention of interest. It can be no treatment other than the normal treatment, an accepted alternative treatment, or no treatment disguised as a treatment (placebo). (See Chapter 7).

Controlled before-after study: A kind of before-after study (qv) in which either external or internal controls, or both, are used to reduce confounding. (See Chapter 7).

Correlational study: Non-experimental demonstration study, conducted in a setting in which manipulation is not possible, that establishes correlations or statistical associations among independent and dependent variables.

Cost Benefit Analysis: Economic analysis in which both costs and outcomes are measured in terms of money. It requires methods to value clinical benefit in terms of financial resources. The result is a statement of the type "running the reminder system cost $20,000 per annum but saves $15 per patient in laboratory tests."

Cost-Consequence analysis: Economic analysis that simply lists the costs in terms of money and the outcomes in whatever measure is appropriate for the particular condition. The number of outcomes may be single or multiple, and no attempt is made to analytically compare costs and outcomes.

Cost Effectiveness Analysis: Economic analysis that measures costs in dollars, and outcomes in a single health care outcome (such as life expectancy, number of infections averted) that is consistent across options. The result is a statement of the type "running the reminder system costs $20,000 per annum but saves one laboratory test per patient."

Cost Minimizing Analysis: Economic analysis that chooses the lowest cost strategy out of several options. A fundamental assumption is that the outcomes are equivalent.

Cost to charge ratio: The ratio of the overall costs a department or hospital spends related to the global measure of charges for the services it provides. It is used to develop individual cost measures for specific services or items by assuming that the same cost-charge ratio found for the organization as a whole applies to each component of the organization.

Critiquing system: Decision support system in which the decision maker describes the task (such as a patient) to the system then specifies his or her own plan to the system. The system then generates advice—a critique—which explores the logical implication of those plans in the context of the task data and the resource's stored knowledge.

Decision support system (decision-aid): Information resource that compares at least two task characteristics with knowledge held in computer-readable form and then guides a decision maker by offering task-specific or situation-specific advice. Such information resources, by definition, offer more than a summary of the task data. For example, a prescribing decision support system might offer a doctor advice based on the patient's diagnosis, age, allergies etc..

Demonstration study: Study that establishes a relation—which may be associational or causal—between a set of measured variables. (See Chapters 7 and 8).

Dependent variable: In a correlational or experimental study, the main variable of interest or outcome variable, which is thought to be affected by or associated with the independent variables (qv.). (See Chapter 7).

Descriptive study: A one-group demonstration study that seeks to measure the value of a variable in a sample of participants. A study with no independent variable.

Direct Costs: In health care analyses, direct costs represent the actual purchase of goods and services related to a particular chosen strategy. (See also Indirect costs).

Double-blind study: Clinical trial in which neither patients nor care providers are aware of the treatment groups to which participants have been assigned.

Emergent design: Study where the design or plan of research can and does change as the study progresses. Characteristic of subjectivist studies.

Errors of commission (analogous to type I error, false-positive error): Generically, when an action that is taken turns out to be unwarranted or an observed positive result is, in fact, incorrect. In statistical inference, a type I error occurs when an investigator incorrectly rejects the null hypothesis.

Errors of omission (analogous to type II error, false-negative error): Generically, when an action that should have been taken is not taken or a negative test result is incorrect. In statistical inference, a type II error occurs when an investigator incorrectly fails to reject the null hypothesis.

Ethnography: Set of research methodologies derived primarily from social anthropology. The basis of many of the subjectivist, qualitative evaluation approaches.

Evaluation (of an information resource): There are many definitions of evaluation, including (1) the process of determining the extent of merit or worth of an information resource; (2) a process leading to a deeper understanding of the structure, function, and/or impact of an information resource.

Experimental design: Plan for a study that includes the specification of the independent and dependent variables, the process through which participants will be assigned to groups corresponding to specific combinations of the independent variables, and how and when measurements of the dependent variables will be taken.

Experimental study: A comparative study purposefully designed by an investigator to explore cause-and-effect relations through such strategies as the use of control, randomization, and analytic methods of statistical inference.

Facet: A source of measurement error that is purposefully explored in measurement studies, analogous to independent variables in demonstration studies.

Feasibility study: Preliminary "proof-of-concept" evaluation demonstrating that an information resource's design can be implemented and will provide reasonable output for the input it is given. Similar to a pilot study.

Field study: Study of an information resource where the information resource is used in a real life context such as ongoing health care. Study of a deployed information resource (compare with Laboratory study).

Formative study: Study with the primary intent of improving the information resource under study by answering developer questions rapidly enough to allow the results to influence decisions they take. An example would be providing the developers with regular feedback or user comments during a pilot (compare with Summative study).

Gold standard: Expression of the state of the art in the application domain or the "truth" about the condition of a task (such as the diagnosis of a patient) against which performance of an information resource can be compared. In practice, gold standards are usually not knowable, so studies often employ the best approximation to the "truth" that is available to the investigator.

Human factors: Those aspects of the design of an information resource that relate to the way users interact with the information resource, primarily addressing the issues involved in a user interface design (related to ergonomics and human-computer interaction).

Impact: Effect of an information resource on an application area such as health care, usually expressed as changes in the actions or procedures undertaken by workers or as client outcomes such as patient morbidity and mortality.

Incremental Costs: In economic analysis in health care, these are the costs of implementing the next logical "option", irrespective of the magnitude of effect on costs and benefits. In general, the incremental costs are defined as the total costs that will be incurred by choosing one strategy over another.

Independent variable: In a correlational or experimental study, a variable thought to determine or be associated with the value of the dependent variable (qv.).

Indirect Costs: In economic analyses in health care, indirect costs are those that result from the choice of a strategy on the individuals who are treated, such as lost productivity, missed days of work, etc. This is quite different from the accounting definition of indirect costs. (See also Direct costs).

Information resource: Generic term for a computer-based system that seeks to enhance information management or communication in a biomedical domain by providing task-specific information directly to workers (often used equivalently with "system").

Instrument: Technology employed to make a measurement, such as a paper questionnaire. The instrument encodes and embodies the procedures used to determine the presence, absence, or extent of an attribute in an object.

Intention to treat analysis: In an experiment or clinical trial, analysis of the study results keeping all participants in the groups to which they were originally allocated, irrespective of whether a control participant gained access to the intervention or an intervention participant failed to use it. This reduces bias and makes the trial results more generalizable. (See Chapter 8).

Interrupted time series study: A comparative study design in which several measurements are made before and several after the intervention. The analysis attempts to show that a step change in the dependent variable (qv.) is statistically more likely to have occurred during the interval associated with the intervention than during any other interval. This makes attribution of a cause and effect relationship more reliable than in a simple before-after study [qv.]. However, the need for repeated measurements may make an interrupted time series study more expensive than the more rigorous randomized controlled trial.

Interval variable: A continuous variable in which meaning can be assigned to the differences between values, but there is no real zero point so it lacks ratio properties. Interval variables can support addition and subtraction but not division and multiplication (compare with Ratio variables).

Intervention: In an experimental study (qv.), the activity, information resource, treatment etc., that distinguishes the study groups.

Judge: Human, usually a domain expert, who, through a process of observation, makes an estimate of the value of an attribute for an object or set of objects.

Knowledge-based system: Class of information resource that provides advice by applying an encoded representation of knowledge within a biomedical domain to the state of a specific patient or other task.

Laboratory study: Study that explores important properties of an information resource in isolation from the application setting (compare with Field study).

Level: In measurement situations, one of the discrete values a facet can take on. In demonstration studies, one of the discrete values a nominal or ordinal variable can take on.

Marginal costs: In economic analyses, the marginal cost is defined as the cost of a single extra unit of output. Often in health care this measure has little meaning, as many activities are bundled: for example, many components of a clinical information resource are bundled, and there is no option of dividing either the inputs or expected outputs of their use, so true marginal costs cannot be calculated. (See also Direct costs, Indirect costs).

Measurement study: Study to determine the extent and nature of the errors with which a measurement is made using a specific instrument (cf. Demonstration study). (See Chapters 5 and 6).

Member checking: In subjectivist investigation, the process of reflecting preliminary findings back to individuals in the setting under study; one way of confirming that the findings are truthful.

Meta-analysis: a set of statistical techniques for combining quantitative study results across a set of completed studies of the same phenomenon to draw conclusions more powerful than those obtainable from any single study of that phenomenon. Used in many systematic reviews or overviews.

Meta regression: the use of systematic review (qv.), meta-analysis (qv.) and regression (qv.) techniques on a large body of primary studies to uncover significant associations between aspects of the study design, intervention etc., and a single outcome variable.

Nominal variable: Variable that can take a number of discrete values but with no natural ordering or interval properties.

Non-parametric tests: Class of statistical tests (such as the chi squared and Mann Whitney U tests) that requires few assumptions about the distributions of values of variables in a study (e.g., that the data follow a normal distribution).

Null hypothesis: In inferential statistics, the hypothesis that an intervention will have no effect: that there will be no differences between groups and no associations or correlations among variables.

Object (of measurement): Entity on which a measurement is made and to which a measured value of a variable is assigned.

Objective: (1) Noun: state of practice envisioned by the designers of an information resource, usually stated at the outset of the design process. Specific aims of an information resource. (2) Adjective: a property of an observation or measurement such that the outcome is independent of the observer (cf. Subjective).

Objectivist approaches: Class of evaluation approaches that makes use of descriptive, correlational or comparative designs and emphasizes statistical analyses of quantitative data.

Observational study (naturalistic study): Approach to study design that entails no experimental manipulation. Investigators typically draw conclusions by carefully observing users with or without an information resource.

Ordinal variable: Variable that can take a number of discrete values which have a natural order (compare with Nominal variable).

Outcome variable: Similar to "dependent variable," a variable that captures the end result of a health care, research or educational process; for example, long-term operative complication rate, citation rate of an article or mastery of a subject area.

Outcomes: See Impact.

Panel study: Study design in which a fixed sample of respondents provides information about a variable, often at different time periods.

Participant: In an evaluation study, the entities on which observations are made. Although persons are often the participants in informatics studies, information resources, groups, or organizations can also be the participants in studies.

Pilot study: Trial version of a study (often conducted with a small sample) to ensure that all study methods will work as intended or to explore if there is an effect worthy of further study. (See also Feasibility study).

Power: Statistical term describing the ability of a study to provide a credible negative result; if a study design has low power, usually because of small sample size, little credence can be placed in a "negative" result. The power of a study equals one minus beta, the probability of making a type II error.

Practical significance: Difference or effect due to an intervention that is large enough to affect professional practice. With large sample sizes, small differences can be statistically significant but may not be practically significant, usually because the costs or danger of the intervention do not justify such a small benefit. In health care, similar to "clinical significance."

Precision: In measurement studies, the extent of unsystematic or random error in the results. High precision implies low error. Similar to Reliability.

Process variable: Variable that measures what is done by staff in an evaluation study, such as accuracy of diagnosis or number of tests ordered by health care workers.

Product liability: When a developer or distributor of an information resource is held legally responsible for its effects on staff decisions, regardless of whether they have taken due care when developing and testing the information resource.

Prospective studies: Studies designed before any data are collected. A cohort study is a kind of prospective study, while most data mining activities are retrospective studies (qv.).

QALY (Quality adjusted Life Years): QALYs are a method for adjusting measures of the quantity of life / survival by the quality of being in a particular state. Utility weights (between 0 and 1) are assigned to health states, and the value of being in that health state is defined as the length of time in that state times the utility of being in that state. So, if a person lives for 10 years in a health state that has a utility of only 0.8, the person accrues only 8 QALYs.

Random sample: A sampling method used in any kind of study for picking participants to ensure that the study findings will be generalizable to the entire population. Entails obtaining a complete listing of all participants and randomly selecting a sample (eg., every 10th participant in a randomly ordered listing, or the first name on 100 pages selected at random using a random number generator).

Randomized allocation: A method used in comparative demonstration studies for reliably determining whether an intervention, such as a research information resource, causes a change in some dependent variable, such as research productivity. Entails the allocation of each eligible participant as soon as possible after recruitment to the intervention or control group using a random number generator. Randomized allocation ensures that at the end of the study, the study participant groups differ only in whether they had access to the intervention or not. (See Chapter 7 and www.jameslindlibrary.org).

Randomized studies: Experimental studies in which all factors that cannot be directly manipulated by the investigator are controlled through random allocation of participants to groups.

Ratio variable: Continuous variable in which meaning can be assigned to both the differences between values and the ratio of values (compare with Interval variable). Ratio variables support both division and multiplication, in addition to addition and subtraction.

Reference standard: See Gold standard.

Regression, linear: Statistical technique, fundamentally akin to analysis of variance, in which a continuous dependent variable is modeled as a linear combination of one or more continuous independent variables.

Regression, logistic: Statistical technique in which a dichotomous dependent variable is modeled as an exponential function of a linear combination of one or more continuous or categorical independent variables.

Reliability: Extent to which the results of measurement are reproducible or consistent (i.e., are free from unsystematic error).

Retrospective studies: Studies in which existing data, often generated for a different purpose, are reanalyzed to explore a question of interest to an investigator. A case-control study (qv.) is a kind of retrospective study.

ROC analysis: Receiver operating characteristic analysis. First used in studies of radar signal detection, it is typically used with a test that yields a continuous value but is interpreted dichotomously. ROC analysis documents the trade-off between false-positive and false-negative errors across a range of threshold values for taking the test result as positive.

Sampling strategy: Method for selecting a sample of participants used in a study. The sampling strategy determines the nature of the conclusions that can be drawn from the study.

Sensitivity: (1) Performance measure equal to the true positive rate. In an alerting information resource, for example, the sensitivity is the fraction of cases requiring an alert for which the information resource actually generated an alert. (2) In information resource design: the extent to which the output of the information resource varies in response to changes in the input variables.

Sensitivity analysis: in health economics, the extent to which the results of the economic modeling exercise vary as key input variables or assumptions are varied.

Single-blind study: Study in which the participants are unaware of the groups to which they have been assigned.

Specificity: Performance measure equal to the true negative rate. In a diagnostic information resource, for example, specificity is the fraction of cases in which a disease is absent and in which the information resource did not diagnose the disease.

Statistical significance: An observed difference or effect that, using methods of statistical inference, is unlikely to be due to chance alone.

Subject: See Participant.

Subjective: Property of observation or measurement such that the outcome depends on the observer (compare with Objective).

Subjective probability: Individual's personal assessment of the probability of the occurrence of an event of interest.

Subjectivist approaches: Class of approaches to evaluation that rely primarily on qualitative data derived from observation, interview, and analysis of documents or other artifacts. Studies under this rubric focus on description and explanation; they tend to evolve rather than being prescribed in advance.

Summative study: Study designed primarily to demonstrate the value of a mature information resource (compare with Formative study).

Systematic review: A secondary research method that attempts to answer a predefined question using an explicit approach consisting of: exhaustive searches for published and unpublished studies of the appropriate study design; critical appraisal of the internal and external validity of these studies; extraction of relevant data about their methods and results; assessment of study heterogeneity and, where appropriate, meta analysis (qv.) or other methods to synthesize their results.

Tasks: Test cases against which the performance of human participants or an information resource is studied.

Triangulation: Drawing a conclusion from multiple sources of data that address the same issue. A method used widely in subjectivist research.

Two by two (2 × 2) table: Contingency table (qv.) in which only two variables, each with two levels, are classified.

Type I error: In statistical inference, a type I error occurs when an investigator incorrectly rejects the null hypothesis, typically inferring that a study result is positive when it is in fact negative.

Type II error: In statistical inference, a type II error occurs when an investigator incorrectly fails to reject the null hypothesis, typically inferring that a study result is negative when it is in fact positive.

Usability testing: A type of pilot study (qv.) in which the focus is on evaluating the ease of use of the resource. (See www.useit.com).

Validation: (1) In software engineering: the process of determining whether software is having the intended effects (similar to evaluation). (2) In measurement: the process of determining whether an instrument is measuring what it is designed to measure. (See Validity).

Validity: (1) In demonstration studies or experimental designs: internal validity is the extent to which a study is free from design biases that threaten the interpretation of the results; external validity is the extent to which the results of the experiment generalize beyond the setting in which the study was conducted. (2) In measurement: the extent to which a instrument measures what it is intended to measure. Validity is of three basic kinds: content, criterion-related, and construct. (See Chapter 5).

Variable: Quantity measured in a study. Variables can be measured at the nominal, ordinal, interval, or ratio levels (qv.).

Verification: Process of determining whether software is performing as it was designed to perform (i.e., according to the specification).

Index

Health Informatics Series
(formerly Computers in Health Care)

(continued from page ii)

Consumer Informatics
Applications and Strategies in Cyber Health Care
R. Nelson and M.J. Ball

Public Health Informatics and Information Systems
P.W. O'Carroll, W.A. Yasnoff, M.E. Ward, L.H. Ripp,
and E.L. Martin

Advancing Federal Sector Health Care
A Model for Technology Transfer
P. Ramsaroop, M.J. Ball, D. Beaulieu, and J.V. Douglas

Medical Informatics
Computer Applications in Health Care and Biomedicine, Second Edition
E.H. Shortliffe and L.E. Perreault

Filmless Radiology
E.L. Siegel and R.M. Kolodner

Cancer Informatics
Essential Technologies for Clinical Trials
J.S. Silva, M.J. Ball, C.G. Chute, J.V. Douglas, C.P. Langlotz, J.C. Niland,
and W.L. Scherlis

Clinical Information Systems
A Component-Based Approach
R. Van de Velde and P. Degoulet

Knowledge Coupling
New Premises and New Tools for Medical Care and Education
L.L. Weed

Healthcare Information Management Systems
Cases, Strategies, and Solutions, Third Edition
M.J. Ball, C.A. Weaver, and J.M. Kiel

Organizational Aspects of Health Informatics, Second Edition
Managing Technological Change
N.M. Lorenzi and R.T. Riley

Information Technology Solutions for Healthcare
K. Zieliński, M. Duplaga, and D. Ingram